TEXTBOOK OF VOICE DISORDERS

Edited by

Albert L. Merati, MD, FACS
Steven A. Bielamowicz, MD, FACS

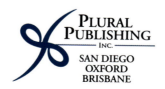

PLURAL PUBLISHING INC.

SAN DIEGO
OXFORD
BRISBANE

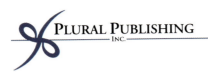

5521 Ruffin Road
San Diego, CA 92123

e-mail: info@pluralpublishing.com
Web site: http://www.pluralpublishing.com

49 Bath Street
Abingdon, Oxfordshire OX14 1EA
United Kingdom

Typeset in 11/13 Garamond by Flanagan's Publishing Services, Inc.
Printed in Hong Kong by Paramount Printing

For permission to use material from this text, contact us by
Telephone: (866) 758-7251
Fax: (888) 758-7255
e-mail: permissions@pluralpublishing.com

ISBN-13: 978-1-59756-137-2
ISBN-10: 1-59756-137-1

Library of Congress Cataloging-in-Publication Data

Textbook of voice disorders / [edited by] Albert L. Merati, Steven
   Bielamowicz.
       p. ; cm.
   Includes bibliographical references and index.
   ISBN-13: 978-1-59756-137-2 (hardcover)
   ISBN-10: 1-59756-137-1 (hardcover)
   1. Voice disorders.   I. Merati, Albert L. II. Bielamowicz, Steven
A.
   [DNLM: 1. Voice Disorders–diagnosis. 2. Voice Disorders
–therapy.   WV 500 T3558 2006]
   RF510.T49 2006
   616.85'5–dc22
                                        2006022882

Contents

Foreword

The patient with a voice disorder presents many challenges in diagnosis and management. Traditionally, voice disorders were managed by an otolaryngologist with either medication or surgery or the patient was sent off to a speech-language pathologist for voice therapy. Modern voice care relies on a different model, namely, combined interactive management of the patient by the otolaryngologist and speech-language pathologist who has acquired special training in voice disorders. The emphasis of *Textbook of Voice Disorders* fits the modern voice care model. This book brings together educators and clinicians from both specialties who have an understanding of the multifactorial etiology of voice disorders and who continually focus on the need for a team approach in the treatment of patients with voice disorders. The first chapter of this text immediately draws the reader into the study of voice with a cogent review of the anatomy and physiology of the larynx and phonation by a physician and speech-language pathologist, each of whom has an international reputation in the study of the larynx. The book follows with elegant details of state-of-the-art diagnostic and assessment protocols presented from the perspectives of otolaryngologists and speech-language pathologists in a team-like fashion.

A unique feature of this well-written text is the inclusion of study questions at the end of each chapter. This feature is especially useful to course instructors and to those who lead basic science lectures for residents and medical students.

Drs. Merati and Bielamowitz bring together a group of international otolaryngologists and speech pathologists who offer their special talents as teachers and clinicians to readers who have an interest in furthering their education in laryngology and voice. The references are current, the chapters are presented in an easy, readable format and the color photography is exceptional. This well-written text provides the necessary critical information for mature clinicians to update their knowledge of laryngology and for young clinicians to use as a reference of current clinical care of voice disorders.

I intend to make this text available to our residents and medical students in conjunction with our basic science lectures in laryngology and voice.

Thomas Murry, PhD
Professor
Department of Otolaryngology-Head and Neck
    Surgery
College of Physicians and Surgeons
Columbia University
New York, New York

Preface

"Love of learning is a pleasant and universal bond, for it deals with what one is and not what one has . . . "

Freya Stark, from *The Southern Gates of Arabia*, 1937

As we enter the 21st century, the re-emergence of Laryngology as a dynamic and vibrant sub-specialty has been a principal development in speech-language pathology. The *Textbook of Voice Disorders* deals with that most conspicuous of laryngeal functions, phonation.

As with the *Textbook of Laryngology*, it was our objective to provide a direct, cohesive, and instructional work that distills and collates the fundamentals of voice science and its direct clinical applications in one approachable volume. The major centers of clinical and research excellence are represented herein—this balance is crucial to ensure a credible and collaborative presentation.

Although there are many excellent references in laryngology, voice, and swallowing disorders, we believe that the *Textbook of Voice Disorders* is unique in its presentation of core information, key points, and review material. For every chapter, the authors were asked to present the central themes and knowledge in their main text, while material beyond these core concepts was placed in one of the three types of "Insert Boxes" located throughout a given chapter. These include the *Thought Box*, in which an author may present an interesting idea for the reader to consider; the *Controversy Box*, in which debatable or contentious matters in the field are noted; and finally, the *Emerging Concepts* boxes, in which cutting edge information is presented. The purpose of separating these boxes from the main text was to distinguish the areas of generally accepted and common knowledge from areas that are still controversial or in development. Of course the distinction of what belongs in an insert box and what is "established knowledge" is itself subject to debate.

We believe that the *Textbook of Voice Disorders* will serve well as a core textbook for graduate course work for speech language pathologists, as part of Otolaryngology residency reading, or as a resource for maintenance of certification review by established otolaryngologists.

The readers are welcome to contact the Editors or the authors directly for further questions. Each and every author was chosen for his or her commitment to education. We are all, first and foremost, teachers.

Al Merati
Steve Bielamowicz

Contributors

Mona M. Abaza, MD
Assistant Professor
Voice Program Director
Department of Otolaryngology
University of Colorado School of Medicine
Medical Director
National Center for Voice and Speech
Denver, Colorado
Chapter 12

Timothy D. Anderson, MD
Department of Otolaryngology-Head and Neck
  Surgery
Lahey Clinic Voice and Swallowing Center
Burlington, Massachusetts
Chapter 18

Gerald S. Berke, MD, FACS
Professor and Chief
Division of Head and Neck Surgery
UCLA Voice Center for Medicine and the Arts
UCLA David Geffen School of Medicine
Los Angeles, California
Chapter 14

Steven A. Bielamowicz, MD, FACS
Professor and Chief
  Division of Otolaryngology
Director, Voice Treatment Center
The George Washington University
Washington, District of Columbia
Editor

Diane M. Bless, PhD
Professor, Departments of Surgery and
  Communicative Disorders
University of Wisconsin-Madison
Madison, Wisconsin
Chapters 3 and 4

Andrew Blitzer MD, DDS
Professor of Clinical Otolaryngology
Columbia University

Director, New York Center for Voice and
  Swallowing Disorders
New York, New York
Chapter 11

Joel H. Blumin, MD, FACS
Assistant Professor
Department of Otolaryngology and
  Communication Sciences
Medical College of Wisconsin
Milwaukee, Wisconsin
Chapter 14

Nadine P. Connor, PhD
Assistant Professor
Departments of Surgery and Communicative
  Disorders
University of Wisconsin-Madison
Madison, Wisconsin
Chapter 3

Mark S. Courey, MD
Professor, Department of Otolaryngology-Head
  and Neck Surgery
Director, Division of Laryngology
The UCSF Voice and Swallowing Center
San Francisco, California
Chapter 10

Suzy Duflo, MD
Fédération d'Otorhinolaryngology, Head and
  Neck Surgery
265 rue St Pierre, Hôspital de la Timone
Marseille France
Chapter 1

Douglas M. Hicks, Ph.D., CCC-SP
Director, The Voice Center
Head, Speech-Language Pathology Section
Cleveland Clinic Foundation
Cleveland Ohio
Chapters 5 and 7

Felicia L. Johnson, MD
Director, Voice and Swallowing Clinic
Assistant Professor, Department of
  Otolaryngology-Head and Neck Surgery
University of Arkansas for Medical Sciences
Department of Otolaryngology, Head and Neck
  Surgery
Little Rock, Arkansas
Chapter 16

Elan Louis, MD, MS
Associate Professor of Neurology
Gertrude H. Sergievsky Center
Taub Institute for Research on Alzheimer's
  Disease and the Aging Brain
Department of Neurology
College of Physicians and Surgeons
Columbia University
New York, New York
Chapter 13

Christy L. Ludlow, PhD
Chief, Laryngeal and Speech Section
Clinical Neurosciences Program
National Institute of Neurological Disorders and
  Stroke
Bethesda, Maryland
Chapter 2

Nicole Maronian, MD
Assistant Professor
Department of Otolaryngology-Head and Neck
  Surgery
University of Washington Medical Center
Seattle, Washington
Chapter 6

Ted Mau, MD, PhD
Department of Otolaryngology-Head and Neck
  Surgery
University of California, San Francisco
San Francisco, California
Chapter 10

Albert L. Merati, MD FACS
Associate Professor and Chief

Division of Laryngology and Professional Voice
Staff Surgeon
Department of Otolaryngology and
  Communication Sciences
Zablocki VAMC
Medical College of Wisconsin
Milwaukee, Wisconsin
Editor

Tanya Meyer, MD
Assistant Professor, Department of
  Otorhinolaryngology-Head and Neck
  Surgery
University of Maryland Medical Center
Baltimore, Maryland
Chapter 11

Claudio F. Milstein, PhD, CCC-SP
Speech Scientist
The Voice Center
Cleveland Clinic Foundation
Cleveland Ohio
Chapters 5 and 7

Natasha Mirza, MD, FACS
Associate Professor, Otolaryngology, Head and
  Neck Surgery
Director Penn Center for Voice and Swallowing
  at Presbyterian Hospital
Philadelphia, Pennsylvania
Chapter 15

Rita Patel, MS
Research Assistant
Department of Surgery, Division of
  Otolaryngology
University of Wisconsin-Madison
Madison, Wisconsin
Chapter 4

James W. Ragland, MD
University of Arkansas for Medical Sciences
Department of Otolaryngology, Head and Neck
  Surgery
Little Rock, Arkansas
Chapter 16

Lawrence Robinson, MD
Professor and Chair
Department of Physical Medicine and Rehabilitation
University of Washington Medical Center
Seattle, Washington
Chapter 6

Adam D. Rubin, MD
Director, Lakeshore Professional Voice Center
Lakeshore ENT
St. Clair Shores, Michigan
Adjunct Assistant Professor, Department of
    Otolaryngology-Head and Neck Surgery
University of Michigan Medical Center
Chapter 9

Robert T. Sataloff, MD, DMA, FACS
Professor and Chairman, Department of
    Otolaryngology-HNS
Associate Dean for Clinical Management Specialties
Drexel College of Medicine
Professor of Otolaryngology-Head and Neck
    Surgery
Jefferson Medical College
Thomas Jefferson University
Chairman, The Voice Foundation
Chairman, American Institute for Voice and Ear
    Research
Chapters 8 and 9

Sarah Marx Schneider, MS, CCC-SLP
Speech-Language Pathologist

Robert T. Sataloff, MD and Associates
Philadelphia, Pennsylvania
Chapter 8

Jennifer Spielman, MA, CCC-SLP
Speech Pathologist and Research Associate
National Center for Voice and Speech
Denver, Colorado
Chapter 12

Lucian Sulica, MD
Director, Voice Disorders/Laryngology
Department of Otorhinolaryngology
Weill Medical School of Cornell University
New York, New York
Chapter 11 and 13

Susan L. Thibeault, PhD
Research Director
Department of Surgery,
Division of Otolaryngology-Head and Neck
    Surgery
School of Medicine, The University of Utah
Salt Lake City, Utah
Chapter 1

Riitta Ylitalo, MD, PhD
Karolinska Institute,
Department of Otolaryngology
Karolinska University Hospital Huddinge
Stockholm, Sweden
Chapter 17

For Dr. Javad Merati and Mrs. Adele Jalali Merati, for making me an American.
For Dr. Robert H. Ossoff and Dr. Robert J. Toohill, for making me a Laryngologist.

Al Merati

For my wife Anne, my boys Matthew and Nicholas, and my parents Albin and Patricia,
with great appreciation of your support and love.

Steve Bielamowicz

PART I

Anatomy and Physiology

1

Anatomy of the Larynx and Physiology of Phonation

Suzy Duflo, MD
Susan L. Thibeault, PhD

KEY POINTS

- Increases in length and tension of the vocal folds will result in an increase in pitch.

- During phonation, fundamental frequency is primarily determined by activity of the intrinsic muscles and to a lesser extent by subglottal pressure.

- The mean rate of vocal fold vibration per second represents the habitual pitch also known as fundamental frequency.

- Phonation threshold pressure (PTP) is the minimum subglottal pressure required for initiating and sustaining vocal fold oscillation and is an indication of vocal fold function.

- The high pitch exhibited by patients with vocal paralysis is a compensatory behavior, unconsciously developed to increase glottal contact during phonation. To achieve contact between the vocal folds, the cricothyroid muscle is activated, elongating the vocal folds and bringing them close together on adduction. This glottal position allows slightly louder and more consistent voice production in the patient with incomplete closure although it may be higher pitched.

ANATOMY OF THE LARYNX

Understanding the details of phonation requires knowledge of the anatomy of the larynx. The larynx is the principal structure for producing the vibrating airstream and the vocal folds, which are a part of the larynx, constitute the vibrating elements. The larynx is a musculocartilaginous structure located in the middle of the anterior neck region. It is suspended from the hyoid bone and sits on top of the trachea. Soft tissues and cartilage constitute the larynx. Cartilage forms a real skeleton for the larynx and the anatomy of the laryngeal muscles and ligaments can be defined in relation to this skeleton.

The Hyoid Bone

The hyoid bone is horseshoe-shaped, located immediately superior to the thyroid cartilage, and suspended in the neck by means of a sling of muscles and ligaments. It consists of a body with major and minor cornua projecting posterolaterally. Although not technically a part of the larynx, the hyoid bone plays an integral part in laryngeal motion and must be included in the laryngeal anatomy. Indeed, most of the "extrinsic" muscles of the larynx (see below) attach to the hyoid in some way.

The Laryngeal Cartilages (Figure 1–1)

Three unpaired and three paired cartilages are found in the larynx. The three unpaired are perhaps the most familiar to those outside of laryngology and speech-language pathology, the thyroid, cricoid, and epiglottic cartilages. The three smaller paired structures are the arytenoid, corniculate, and cuneiform cartilages. These cartilages articulate with each other in complex ways, including sliding and rotation in relation to one another, returning to their original positions after release of muscular forces, thus assuming different configurations to allow breathing, eating, and phonation.

The framework supports the specialized soft tissues of the larynx (ie, the vocal folds), and it is through motions of the cricothyroid and crico-arytenoid joints that the vocal folds are maneuvered into the positions for the different modes of phonation. Gross laryngeal motion can also be described in terms of degrees of freedom; it is a system with four degrees of freedom. The rotation and gliding of the cricoid and thyroid cartilages represent two degrees of freedom, and the rocking and rotation of the arytenoid cartilages represent the other two degrees of freedom.

The Thyroid Cartilage

The thyroid cartilage is made up of hyaline cartilage. This cartilage is the largest in the laryngeal skeleton, consisting of two flat plates called "laminae" that fuse together anteriorly to form an approximate 90° angle in the adult male and an approximate 120° angle in the adult female. Two pairs of horns, or cornua, extend upward (superior cornu) and downward (inferior cornu) from the posterior aspect of the thyroid cartilage. The superior horns attach to the hyoid bone via ligaments associated with the lateral aspect of the thyrohyoid membrane. On the lateral face of the laminae, there is an oblique line, which is an insert point for different laryngeal muscles. The thyroid cartilage articulates with the cricoid at the paired cricothyroid joints; this synovial joint permits the cricoid and thyroid cartilages to pitch forward around an imaginary horizontal axis drawn between the two joints.

The Cricoid Cartilage

The cricoid cartilage forms the lower part of the laryngeal framework and is located immediately above the uppermost tracheal ring. It is made of hyaline cartilage and consists of two parts: an anterior arch and a posterior quadrate lamina. It is a complete ring closed at the back where the massive lamina or plate extends vertically. Anteriorly, the cartilage becomes thinner to form the fine cricoid arch. It is connected to the thyroid cartilage by the cricothyroid membrane, the traditional site for immediate emergency surgical access to the airway. Another ligament, the *crico-tracheal* ligament, connects the cricoid cartilage to the trachea.

The Arytenoid Cartilages

The paired arytenoid (Latin for ladle or pitcher) cartilages are located on the sloping border of the cricoid cartilage. They have the shape of a pyramid with a base, an apex, and three surfaces. The anterior angle of these cartilages forms a pointed projection called the vocal process, which is the insertion point for the vocal ligament. The apices of the arytenoid are in contact with the *corniculate* cartilages. They may be fused with the arytenoid cartilages or be separated by an articulation containing synovial fluid. The corniculate cartilages are believed to be an embryonic vestige. The arytenoid cartilages are coupled to the cricoid cartilage via the cricoarytenoid joints. The movements of these cartilages on the cricoid are quite elegant; although they are thought of simplistically as opening and clos-

ing by sliding back and forth along the superior surface of the posterior cricoid, their motion is more complex. This is discussed further below.

The Epiglottis

The epiglottis is a broad fibrocartilaginous structure located just behind the hyoid bone and the base of the tongue. The space between the base of the tongue and the epiglottis forms the vallecula. The epiglottis is considered the superior edge of the larynx. Its upper edge is rounded and thin, the lower edge is narrow. It attaches to the thyroid cartilage by means of a thyroepiglottic ligament and to the arytenoid cartilages by means of the aryepiglottic folds. The aryepiglottic folds extend from the sides of the epiglottis to the arytenoids. They form a wall that separates the larynx from the lateral piriform fossae. The aryepiglottic folds extend inferiorly and medially in the larynx cavity to become the false vocal folds. The epiglottis closes over the glottal area during swallowing and prevents food from entering the larynx (Figure 1–1).

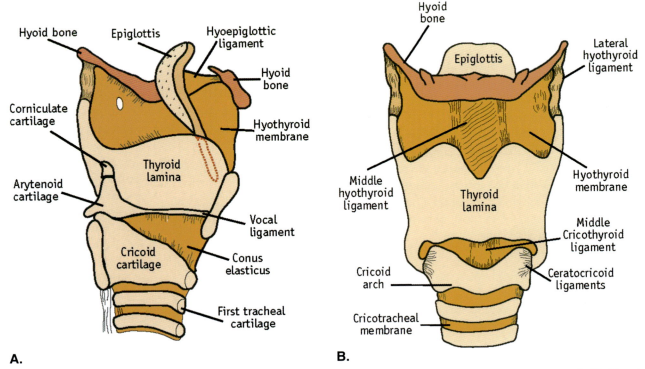

A.   **B.**

FIGURE 1–1. Laryngeal cartilages. **A.** Lateral view of the larynx (cuneiform cartilage not shown). **B.** Front view of the larynx.

Laryngeal Muscles

Two types of muscles are described in the larynx: *extrinsic* and *intrinsic* muscles. Extrinsic muscles are those that have one attachment to structures outside the larynx, intrinsic muscles have both attachments confined to the larynx. Both extrinsic and intrinsic muscles influence laryngeal function. The length and tension of the vocal folds are adjusted before and during phonation by means of rotation of the thyroid and/or cricoid cartilages as a result of the activation of laryngeal muscles.

Intrinsic Muscles (Figure 1–2)

The intrinsic muscles are attached at both ends to the cartilages of the larynx and are largely responsible for the control of sound production by moving those cartilages in relation to one another. They are abductor, adductor, tensor, and relaxer muscles and always act in pairs. Muscles on one side do not contract independently of the muscles on the opposite side. The abductor muscles, which separate the arytenoids and the vocal folds for respiratory activities, are opposed by the adductors, which approximate the arytenoid cartilages and the vocal folds for phonation and for protective purposes. The glottal tensors elongate and tighten the vocal folds. They are opposed by the relaxers, which shorten the vocal folds. They play an important role in the vibratory behavior of vocal folds. Each half of the larynx has a posterior and a lateral cricoarytenoid muscle, a cricothyroid muscle, and a thyroarytenoid muscle. There is also the interarytenoid muscle, a large, unpaired intrinsic muscle. The transverse and oblique portions extend between the two arytenoid cartilages.

Posterior Cricoarytenoid Muscle.
The posterior cricoarytenoid muscle originates from a shallow depression of the posterior surface of the cricoid lamina. It is divided into two parts: a lateral vertical muscle, which inserts on the upper surface of the muscular process of the arytenoid cartilage, and a medial part that inserts via a short tendon on the posterior surface of the muscular process. It abducts the vocal folds by pulling the arytenoids cartilage through its rocking motion. It is the primary abductor muscle of the larynx and is typically active during the inspiratory phase of the respiratory cycle when the abduction of the arytenoids opens the glottis widely. It is the only muscle that *actively* opens the glottis. Two muscles act as antagonists to the posterior cricoarytenoid muscle: the lateral cricoarytenoid and interarytenoid muscles.

Lateral Cricoarytenoid Muscle.
The lateral cricoarytenoid muscle originates along the upper border of the anterolateral arch of the cricoid cartilage and courses upward back to insert into the muscular process and anterior surface of the arytenoid cartilage. Some fibers blend with those of the thyroarytenoid muscle. The lateral cricoarytenoid muscle is an adductory muscle that permits rotation of the arytenoid cartilage and brings the vocal processes and vocal ligament toward midline. When the arytenoid cartilages are adducted for phonation, the lateral cricoarytenoid muscles may have the additional function of increasing the medial compression of the vocal folds.

Interarytenoid Muscle.
The interarytenoid muscle is a large muscle located on the posterior surface of the arytenoid cartilages. It consists of two parts, the oblique and transverse arytenoid. The oblique arytenoid muscle is the more superficial of the two parts. It originates from the posterior surface of the muscular process and adjacent posterolateral of one arytenoid cartilage and inserts close to the apex of the opposite cartilage. A few muscle fibers continue around the apex of the arytenoid cartilage laterally, upward, and forward to insert into the lateral border of the epiglottis forming the aryepiglottic muscle. The oblique arytenoid muscles regulate medial compression of the vocal folds and permit approximation of the arytenoid cartilages. The transverse arytenoid muscle originates from the lateral margin and posterior surface of one arytenoid cartilage, courses in a horizontal direction, and inserts into the lateral margin and posterior surface of the

opposite arytenoid cartilage. The deeper muscle fibers continue around the lateral margins of the arytenoid cartilages and blend with fibers of the thyroarytenoid muscle. Transverse arytenoid muscles permit approximation of the arytenoid cartilages toward the midline. The interarytenoid muscles rock the arytenoids during adduction. This action increases the medial compression of the vocal folds. Because it crosses the midline, the muscle's action on a given arytenoid is preserved even in the case of unilateral paralysis.

Cricothyroid Muscle.
The cricothyroid muscle originates from the upper rim of the cricoid arch and fibers diverge to insert into the lower rim of the thyroid as two distinct groups: pars recta and pars obliqua. The pars recta forms the upper or anterior fibers and courses nearly vertically upward to insert along the inner aspect of the lower rim of the thyroid lamina. The pars oblique forms the lower or oblique fibers and courses upward and back to insert into the anterior margin of the inferior horn of the thyroid cartilage. The cricothyroid muscle lengthens the vocal folds, decreasing fold thickness and increasing pitch. It is the primary antagonist of the thyroarytenoid muscle.

Thyroarytenoid Muscle.
The thyroarytenoid muscle comprises the main mass of the vocal fold. The thryomuscularis muscle (or *vocalis* muscle) inserts into the lateral and inferior aspect of the vocal process of the arytenoid cartilage and into the interior face of the thyroid angle cartilage. The contraction of the thyroarytenoid muscle permits a shortening and slackening of the vocal folds. It exerts an anterior traction on the vocal process, increasing vocal fold tension, thickness, and stiffness. Contraction of the thyroaryepiglottis muscle pulls the arytenoid cartilages forward, closing the glottis anteroposteriorly. The thyroarytenoid muscle also draws the arytenoid and thyroid cartilage toward one another, to shorten and relax the vocal folds. This action plays a role in pitch lowering. The thyroarytenoid muscle does not function as a single unit but in combination with the other laryngeal intrinsic muscles (Figure 1–2).

Extrinsic Muscles (Figure 1–3)

The extrinsic muscles are attached to structures outside the larynx. They are primarily responsible for the support of the larynx, for fixing it in position, and also for moving the larynx as a total unit, thereby changing its position in the neck. The elasticity of the trachea places a passive extrinsic force on the larynx. Three muscles are considered extrinsic: the sternothyroid, thyrohyoid muscle, and inferior pharyngeal constrictor. The suprahyoid and infrahyoid muscles play a role in deglutition and phonation.

Sternothyroid Muscle.
The sternothyroid muscle inserts into the posterior surface of the sternal manubrium and first rib; it then extends itself upward and slightly laterally in the anterior neck to insert on the oblique line of the thyroid cartilage. The sternothyroid muscle is a depressor muscle and its principal action is to draw the thyroid cartilage downward.

Thyrohyoid Muscle.
The thyrohyoid muscle is located in the anterior neck. This muscle originates from the oblique tendon or line of the thyroid cartilage and courses vertically upward to insert into the inferior edge of the greater horn of the hyoid bone. This muscle is an elevator as it decreases the distance between the hyoid bone and the thyroid cartilage. With the thyroid cartilage fixed, it depresses the hyoid bone and with the hyoid bone fixed, it elevates the thyroid cartilage.

Inferior Pharyngeal Constrictor.
The inferior pharyngeal constrictor consists of cricopharyngeus and thyropharyngeous muscles. These muscles influence the phonation by forming a principal resonating cavity of the vocal mechanism. They are also active during deglutition.

Suprahyoid and Infrahyoid Muscles.
Other extrinsic muscles, which for the most part have one attachment on the hyoid bone, may also influence the larynx. They are divided into suprahyoid and infrahyoid muscles. Functionally they are classified as laryngeal elevators and depressors.

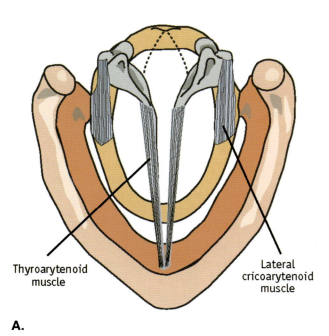

Thyroarytenoid muscle

Lateral cricoarytenoid muscle

A.

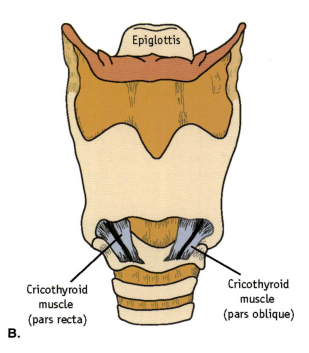

Epiglottis

Cricothyroid muscle (pars recta)

Cricothyroid muscle (pars oblique)

B.

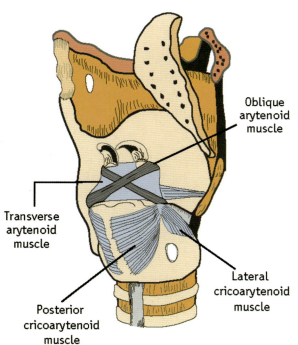

Oblique arytenoid muscle

Transverse arytenoid muscle

Posterior cricoarytenoid muscle

Lateral cricoarytenoid muscle

C.

FIGURE 1–2. Intrinsic laryngeal muscles. **A.** Thyroarytenoid muscle and lateral cricoarytenoid muscle. **B.** Cricothyroid muscle (pars recta and pars oblique). **C.** Posterior view of the larynx showing posterior cricoarytenoid muscle and lateral cricoarytenoid muscle.

The suprahyoid muscles are the laryngeal elevators (digastric, stylohyoid, mylohyoid, geniohyoid, hyoglossus, and genioglossus muscles), which play a role in deglutition. The infrahyoid muscles are laryngeal depressors (sternohyoid and omohyoid muscles). The sternohyoid muscle acts to draw the hyoid bone downward and the omohyoid muscle prevents the neck region from collapsing during deep inspiratory efforts and from compression of the vessels.

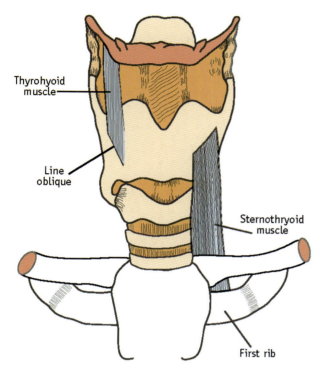

FIGURE 1–3. Extrinsic laryngeal muscles: Thyroid muscle and sternothyroid muscle (inferior pharyngeal constrictor, suprahyoid, and infrahyoid muscles not shown).

Larynx Cavity

The cavity of the larynx extends from the aditus laryngis to the inferior border of the cricoid cartilage. The aditus is a triangular opening including the epiglottis, aryepiglottic folds laterally, and apexes of the arytenoid cartilages. The vocal folds are oriented in the anterior/posterior direction and sit over the lower airway. The membranous vocal folds consist of mucosa and thyroarytenoid muscle, which is continuous with the conus elasticus. The cornus elasticus is represented by a membrane that arises in a full circle from the top of the cricoid cartilage.

The vocal folds are long, smoothly rounded bands of muscle tissue and can be lengthened, shortened, tensed, relaxed, abducted, or adducted. The medial borders of the vocal folds are free and they project like a shelf into the cavity of the larynx in a medio-lateral direction. In reference to the level of the vocal folds, the larynx can be divided into three areas: glottic, supraglottic, and subglottic areas. The space between the true vocal folds is designated the glottis or glottal area. Immediately superior to the vocal folds is a groove known as the laryngeal ventricle extending almost the entire length of the vocal folds. Superior to the ventricule is the paired ventricular or *false vocal folds*, which contain muscle fibers. The false vocal folds are not typically involved during normal phonation. The false vocal folds move with the arytenoid cartilages but they stand farther apart than the vocal folds. The space between the ventricular folds and the aditus is referred to as the vestibule of the larynx. The area superior to the true vocal folds, with the ventricle, the false vocal folds, and the vestibule, is called the supraglottis. The area immediately inferior to the true vocal folds down to the inferior aspect of the cricoid is called the subglottic region (Figure 1–4).

Laryngeal Motion[1,2]

When the glottis opens, each vocal fold changes shape by putting itself in abduction. The arytenoid cartilages rotate so that the vocal process moves outward, upward, and posteriorly. Abduction is accomplished by the posterior cricoarytenoid muscle pulling the muscular process posteriorly and inferiorly. Adduction is accomplished by the combined action of the lateral cricoarytenoid, interarytenoid, and thyroarytenoid muscles. The most powerful adductor is the lateral cricoarytenoid muscle which pulls the muscular process anteriorly and inferiorly. In addition to adduction and abduction, laryngeal muscle activity also changes vocal fold length, tension, and shape. The thyroarytenoid and cricothyroid muscles have opposing actions in this regard. Contraction of the thyroarytenoid muscle shortens and thickens the vocal fold whereas cricothyroid action stretches the vocal folds increasing length and tension and decreasing thickness. Simultaneous contraction to these two muscles can increase tension independent of length (Figure 1–5).

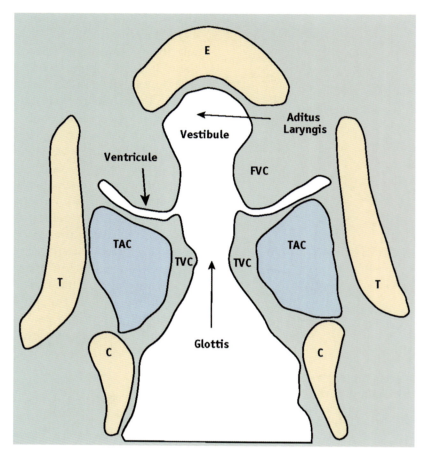

FIGURE 1–4. Larynx cavity: coronal view of the larynx. (E = epiglottis, FVC = false vocal fold, TAC = thyroarytenoid component, T = thyroid cartilage, C = cricoid cartilage, TVC = false vocal fold).

Criocoarytenoid (CA) Joint Motion

The CA joint is a diarthrodial joint that includes a synovial lining and a fluid-filled bursa. The joint capsule and the ligamentous attachments, including the CA ligament, vocal ligament, and false vocal folds, limit normal motion of the joint. The CA plays a crucial role in the adduction and abduction of the vocal folds. The rotation in which the anterior vocal process deviates medially causes adduction of the vocal folds, whereas a lateral rotation causes abduction. The vocalis ligament, CA ligament, and conus elasticus are most important in controlling abduction, whereas the posterior CA muscle and conus elasticus are crucial in limiting adduction. The vocalis ligament prevents posterior displacement of the vocal process, while the CA ligament and the posterior capsular ligament, restrict anterior vocal process migration. The anterior capsular ligament limits backward arytenoid cartilage tilting and lateral movement of the arytenoid cartilage on the cricoid cartilage facet.

VOCAL FOLD HISTOLOGY[3–5]

Most of the upper airway is lined by respiratory epithelium and contains mucous glands. The cover of the free edge of the vocal folds is adapted for vibration; subsequently the vibratory epithelium is squamous cell epithelium without mucous glands.

Hirano described five histologically distinct layers for the true vocal fold. The epithelium consists of stratified squamous cells. The superficial

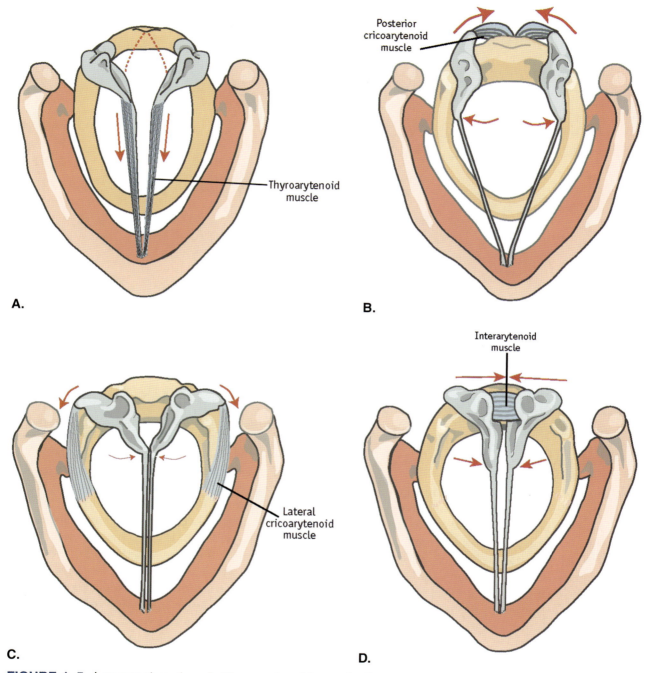

FIGURE 1–5. Laryngeal motion. **A.** Thyroarytenoid muscle. **B.** Posterior cricoarytenoid muscle. **C.** Lateral cricoarytenoid muscle. **D.** Interarytenoid muscle.

layer of the lamina propria (also known as *Reinke's space*), consists of loose fibrous components (elastin, collagen) and matrix. The intermediate layer of the lamina propria consists chiefly of elastic fibers, collagen, fibronectin, and hyaluronan.

The deep layer of the lamina propria consists of collagenous fibers. The intermediate and deep layers together comprise what is clinically referred to as the *vocal ligament.* The deeper layer of the vocal fold is the vocalis muscle (Figure 1-6).

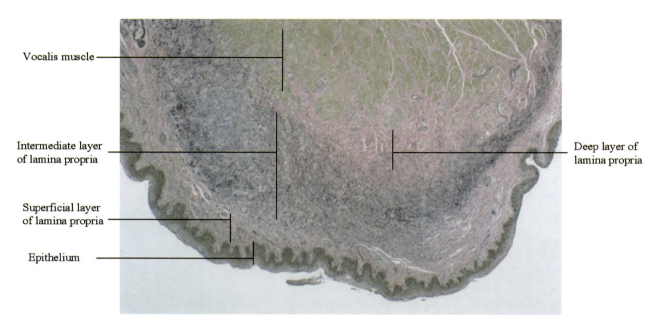

Vocalis muscle

Intermediate layer
of lamina propria

Superficial layer
of lamina propria

Epithelium

Deep layer of
lamina propria

FIGURE 1–6. Coronal histologic section through membranous portion of vocal folds.

LARYNGEAL VASCULAR SUPPLY AND LARYNGEAL INNERVATIONS[6]

Vascular Supply

The arterial vascularization of the larynx is provided by the inferior laryngeal artery, a small branch of the inferior thyroid artery and by the superior laryngeal artery, which comes from the superior thyroid artery. The superior laryngeal vein empties into the jugular vein and the inferior laryngeal vein joins the inferior thyroid vein. The lymphatic system of the larynx drains along the vessels both upward and downward into the deep cervical nodes.

Innervation

The vagus nerve (CN X) innerves the intrinsic laryngeal muscles and the trigeminal (CN V), facial (CN VII), and hypoglossal (CN XII) nerves are responsible for the innervation of the extrinsic muscles.

The vagus nerve comes from the *nucleus ambiguus* in the medulla and carries the motor and sensory supply of the larynx via two branches: the superior and recurrent laryngeal nerves. The superior laryngeal nerve exits the vagus just below the nodose ganglion and then branches into two divisions: the internal branch, which carries sensory fibers from the supraglottis and vocal folds, and the external branch, which carries motor fibers to the cricothyroid muscle. The recurrent laryngeal nerve follows a circuitous route, arising from the vagus nerve in the upper mediastinum and then ascending to the larynx in the tracheoesophageal groove. On the right side the nerve courses around the subclavian artery. On the left side the nerve curves around the aortic arch. The recurrent nerve carries motor fibers to the intrinsic muscle except for the cricothyroid muscle. The differences in intrinsic muscle innervation of the recurrent and superior laryngeal nerves are secondary to their embryonic etiology; branchial arches IV and VI form the superior laryngeal and the recurrent nerves, respectively.

Superior Laryngeal Nerve

The internal branch (ISLN) and external branch (ESLN) of the superior laryngeal nerve are supplied by their accompanying arteries in the upper pole of the thyroid gland. A topographic relationship between the ESLN, the superior thyroid artery, and the upper pole of the thyroid gland exposes the ESLN to high surgical risks during thyroidectomy[7-9] and anterior approach to the cervical spine.[10] The clinical evaluation of SLN lesions allows the diagnosis of vocal fold's hypomobility, with incomplete glottic closure and can result in detrimental voice changes, loss of airway protection, and effortful swallowing with aspiration in some cases. Injury of the ESLN produces no problem of respiration and deglutition but may result in changes in the quality of voice or even voicelessness. The consequences are important for patients like professional singers and speakers who depend on control of pitch and a clear and forceful voice. Several precautions when dissecting the superior pole of the thyroid gland seem to be necessary and sufficient to respect the ESLN. Moreover, neuromonitoring proved to be a reliable method to identify the nerve, prevent its injury,[11] and subsequently maintain optimal function of the larynx. During swallowing, the airway is protected from the aspiration of ingested material by brief closure of the larynx and cessation of breathing.

Mechanoreceptors innervated by the ISLN are activated by swallowing and connect to central neurons that generate swallowing, laryngeal closure, and respiratory rhythm. The injured ISLN causes effortful swallowing and an illusory globus sensation in the throat, sometimes with penetration of fluid into the larynx during swallowing. In contrast to the insufficient closure during swallowing after ISLN injury, laryngeal closure can be robust during voluntary challenges with the Valsalva, Muller, and cough maneuvers.[12] An afferent signal from the ILSN receptor field is necessary for normal deglutition by providing feedback that facilitates laryngeal closure during swallowing, but is not necessary for initiating and sequencing the swallow cycle, for coordinating swallowing with breathing, or for closing the larynx during voluntary maneuvers. A recent publication has also suggested that the ESLN supplies innervation to the cricopharyngeus muscle, which would further support SLN injury as a source of dysfunction in patients with dysphagia.[13]

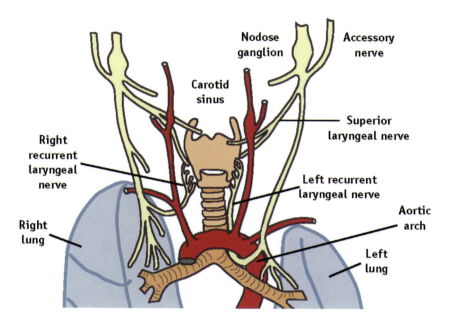

FIGURE 1–7. Nerve and blood supply of the larynx.

The trigeminal nerve supplies motor innervation to the mylohyoid muscle and the belly of the digastric. The facial nerve supplies motor innervation to the digastric and stylohyoid muscles. The hypoglossal nerve supplies motor innervation to geniohyoid, sternohyoid, omohyoid, thyrohyoid, and sternothyroid (Figure 1-7).

PHYSIOLOGY OF PHONATION

With the laryngeal anatomy detailed above, this chapter now reviews the physiology of phonation. Chapter 2 presents aspects of laryngeal physiology related to airway regulation.

Although phonation is not the most critical domain of the larynx, it continues to draw interest due to its elegance and close association with human communication. The phenomenon of phonation is defined by a rapid opening and closing of the vocal folds that periodically interrupt the airstream to produce a vocal or glottal tone within the pharyngeal, oral and nasal cavities.[14]

Galen (AD 130-200) was among the first to recognize the glottis as the source of vocal production. He suggested that vocal intensity was dependent upon the adjustment of the soft palate and uvula.[15] In 1543, the larynx was illustrated by Andreas Vesalius in *De Humani Corporis Fabrica*. Since then, others have contributed to our understanding of the physiology of phonation. Ferrein (1776) was the first to prove that vocal fold vibration was responsible for sound.[16]

Laryngeal Function

The larynx is used for speech but also to control and ensure the flow of air into and out of the lungs. Respiration is the primary function of the larynx. (This is reviewed in detail in the following chapter.) Effortful closure, also called the *Valsalva* maneuver, is another vital function of the larynx. This seals the larynx preventing air escaping from the lungs during physical effort such as coughing, throat clearing, vomiting, urination, and defecation. There is great contrast between the position of the vocal folds during phonation and effortful closing. During phonation, only the true vocal folds adduct, but during effortful closing, there is a massive undifferentiated adduction of the laryngeal walls, including both true and false vocal folds by means of the adductory muscles and the arytenoid cartilages. During effortful closing, the thyroid cartilage is elevated, approximating the hyoid bone, as subglottic pressure increases. Another function of the larynx is to prevent and avoid ingestion of solids and liquids in the trachea and consequently in the lungs, during swallow.

Physiology of Phonation[1,2,17,18]

Phonation must be coordinated with respiration. Phonation is a dynamic process. To drive vocal folds into vibration, a minimal subglottal pressure is required. This minimal subglottal pressure is referred to as phonation threshold pressure (PTP). The configuration of the glottal aperture and viscoelasticity of the vocal folds are both important factors that can alter PTP. Because vocal folds are shelflike elastic protuberances of muscles and mucosa, their tension and elasticity can be varied. They can be thinner, thicker, and shorter or longer, open wide, close together, or come together into an intermediate position. Additionally they can be elevated and depressed in their vertical relationship to the cavities above.

During normal breathing the vocal folds are spaced widely apart. During quiet inhalation, the vocal folds abduct moving away from the midline and widen the glottis. These movements are small and inconspicuous during quiet inhalation and they are extensive during forced inhalation. During exhalation they adduct slightly toward the midline. The entire larynx also moves during respiration. It moves downward during inhalation increasing the airway capacity allowing a larger volume of air to be inhaled. This movement is coupled with downward movement of the entire bronchial tree. During exhalation the larynx elevates readying for phonation.

During prephonation, the vocal folds are adducted slightly or completely but loosely, to restrict the flow of air from the lungs but always maintaining an open glottal airway. At the same time, the forces of exhalation produce an increasing amount of air pressure beneath the folds and when the pressure becomes sufficient, the vocal folds are literally blown apart, thus releasing a puff of air into the vocal tract. This release of air results in an immediate decrease of pressure beneath the vocal folds. The elasticity of the tissues and the reduction of air pressure simply allow the folds to snap back into their adducted position ready to be blown apart once again. At this moment, the air pressure has again built up, completing one cycle of vocal fold vibration. The vocal folds can then repeat the cycle. Lieberman (1975)[19] described this behavior as the *myoelastic-aerodynamic theory*. The muscle activity needed to adduct and tense the vocal folds simply readies them for vibration but *does not* cause the vibration itself. According to Lieberman, the two aerodynamic forces which produce vibration of the vocal folds are the positive subglottal air pressure applied to the lower part of the folds, forcing them open and the negative pressure which occurs as air passes between the folds increasing the velocity of airflow (Bernouilli effect). These positive and negative pressures set the vocal folds into vibration due to the elasticity of the folds.

To understand the negative air pressure, we need to refer to Bernouilli who formulated the following aerodynamic law:

$$d \times \tfrac{1}{2}(v^2p) = c$$

(d = density; p = pressure, v = velocity, c = a constant)

This means that if volume fluid flow is constant, velocity of flow must increase at an area of constriction, but with a corresponding decrease of pressure at the constriction. The Bernouilli effect applied to phonation assumes that the vocal folds are nearly approximated at the instant the airstream is released by the forces of exhalation. The airstream will have a constant velocity until it reaches the glottal constriction. Velocity will increase, as air passes through the glottis. The result of the Bernouilli force is a negative pressure between the medial edges of the vocal folds, producing a suction phenomenon. This suction and the static forces counterbalance the subglottic pressure from the lungs bringing the folds in a movement inward. The narrow channel causes an increase in suction snapping the vocal folds shut. Because the folds vibrate quickly, one puff of air follows another in an equally rapid succession. This repetition of air sets up a pressure wave at the glottis, which is audible. A necessary condition for voicing is that the air pressure below the folds must exceed the pressure above the folds. The vocal folds' elasticity permits them to be blown open for each cycle but the elastic recoil force works along with the Bernouilli principle to close the folds for each cycle of vibration (Figures 1–8 and 1–9).

Vertical Phase Difference in Vibration

Vocal folds begin to open posteriorly, and then anteriorly. Closure follows with the posterior, followed by anterior. Horizontally, typically the vocal folds close along the entire medial edge, with the posterior portion closing last. It is normal to have a gap in the posterior glottis that does not close. The posterior glottal gap (PGG) is more obvious and prominent in the female than the male. Young women demonstrate PGG and incomplete closure significantly more frequently than elderly women. This PGG is prominent in high phonation compared to normal phonation.

Voice Production, Frequencies and Harmonics, Loudness and Pitch, Voice Register, Quality of Voice

Frequencies and Harmonics

Phonation varies in intensity, frequency, and quality. As above, production of voice is the result of a steady flow of air from the lungs segmented at the laryngeal level into a series of air puffs at a fundamental frequency that generates harmonics in the cavities of the upper airway. The fundamental frequency is defined by the number of times the vocal folds open and close per second. The cavity resonation allows acoustic energy concentrations called "formant frequencies." Lieberman (1975)[19] has shown that a relationship between the fundamental frequency and the configuration of the supraglottic cavities does not exist. Increasing the subglottal pressure increases the intensity of the sound produced.

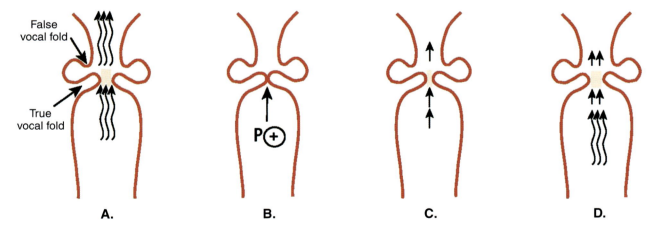

FIGURE 1–8. Vocal fold cycle vibration. **A.** Prephonation phase, the vocal folds are adducted slightly to restrict the flow of air from the lungs. An open glottal airway is maintained. **B.** The vocal folds are closed and the forces of exhalation produce an increasing amount of air pressure beneath the folds. **C.** The pressure is sufficient. Vocal folds are blown apart thus releasing a puff of air into the vocal tract. The velocity airflow is increasing and the pressure is decreasing (Bernouilli effect). **D.** The vocal folds are adducted again ready for another vocal fold cycle. The air pressure is again building up.

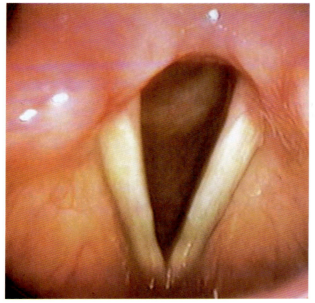

A.

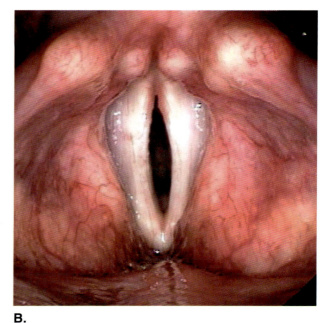

B.

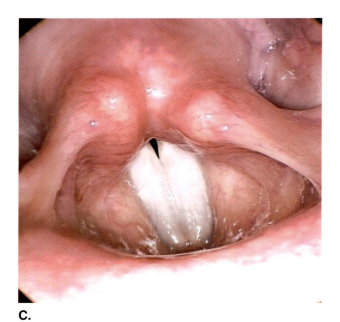

C.

FIGURE 1–9. Photographic sequence of the open and closed phases of one vibratory cycle. **A.** Vocal folds are abducted in rest position during normal breathing. **B.** Vocal folds adducted, open phase of vibration. **C.** Vocal folds adducted, closed phase of vibration.

In addition to subglottal pressure, the other major source of voice control is the larynx itself. Changes in the physical dimensions and characteristics of the vocal folds influence the sound that is produced. The fundamental frequency will change whenever the vocal folds are changed in some way that will allow them to move faster or slower. Increasing the subglottal pressure raises the fundamental frequency. According to the aerodynamic-myoelastic theory of voice production the tension of the vocal folds is considered to be one of the important forces of restoring the glottal closure. Longitudinal tension is a force that acts along the length of the vocal folds.

Physiology of Vocal Paralysis

Adequate diagnosis and treatment of unilateral paralysis of the vocal fold requires determining the cause of the immobility. The most common causes of unilateral vocal fold paralysis are surgical resection or injury of the recurrent laryngeal nerve (RLN). Examination of the larynx will show the affected vocal fold positioned in the paramedian position on the side of the paralysis. It is quite common for the aryepiglottic (AE) fold on the paralyzed side to collapse over into the glottis. Rarely, this causes symptoms of airway obstruction due to adequate abduction of the opposite vocal fold. However, in extreme cases, the AE fold on the paralyzed side may be pulled into the airway with vigorous respiratory exchange. The malposition of the arytenoid cartilage on the paralyzed side is caused by the lack of tension on the adductor muscles innervated by the RLN, which results in a rotation of the cartilage out of its normal physiologic position. The mobile vocal fold adjusts its length to match that of the paralyzed vocal fold on adduction. This is possible by reducing its length and descending inferiorly toward the midline such that the vocal processes are opposite one another during the glottal closure. However, this adaptation is insufficient to allow a normal phonation. The absence of muscle motion on one side involves a modification of pitch range and poor voice. Moreover, the larynx cannot prevent and avoid aspiration of solids and liquids because of insufficient glottal closure. Subsequently, there is a risk of increased morbidity (pneumonia) and mortality.

Many approaches have been proposed for the treatment of unilateral paralysis: speech therapy, expectant observation, intracordal injections, medialization laryngoplasty, arytenoid adduction, arytenopexy, and reinnervation of paralyzed muscle groups. None of the available methods are capable of restoring physiologic adduction and abduction to the paralyzed vocal fold. Medialization allows insertion of an implant deep to the thyroid cartilage displacing the vocal fold toward the midline. As the medialization has gained popularity, many different variations have been described.[20-22] Even in very experienced hands, some patients will obtain less than desired results or the initial good result may weaken over the follow-up period for many different reasons. Laryngeal reinnervation has been done using different nerves and methods with good results.[23,24] Studies have shown that reinnervation and medialization are both effective in the treatment of vocal fold unilateral paralysis, but the reinnervation also allows recovery of the thickness, elasticity, and tension of the vocal fold better than medialization.[25] Voice deterioration (6 months to 2 years postsurgery) is more common after medialization than reinnervation.[26] To avoid and prevent long-term deterioration of voice, combined surgical medialization and nerve-muscle pedicle reinnervation have been reported.[27] The results were significant, showing an improvement and a better quality of voice both short- and long-term. This is reviewed in detail in chapter 11.

The stretching of the vocal ligament will increase its longitudinal tension, which will accelerate the vocal fold movement and increase the rate of vocal fold vibration to raise the fundamental frequency.

Determinants of Loudness and Pitch

Vocal *loudness* increases as subglottic air pressure increases and as the duration of the closed phase of the vibratory cycle increases. Additionally, lateral excursion will increase with intensity. Glottal resistance is the resistance that the glottis places on airflow. When the vocal folds are closed longer, glottal resistance increases. Subsequently, increases in glottal resistance (with increased intensity) will be compensated with increased subglottal resistance.

For constant loudness during speech, subglottic pressure must be held constant. Frequency increases as (1) subglottic pressure increases; (2) the larynx rises in the neck, shortening the pharyngeal dimensions; and (3) vocal fold length and tension increase. In a study of excised human larynges, Kitajima et al (1979)[28] found that vocal pitch increased almost linearly with approximation of the cricoid and thyroid cartilages.

Photographic and x-ray studies have proved that fundamental frequency of phonation increases systematically with increased vocal fold length, which causes a decrease in cross-sectional area of the vocal fold. The decrease in mass causes an increase in frequency. The increase in length also creates an increase in tension that contributes to the increase in frequency. Vocal fold length

increases and thickness decreases with rising frequency in the modal registers. Pitch lowering is the result of a decrease in tension, and/or increase in mass per unit length (or the vocal folds shorten).

Vocal Registers. Although conceding that there are possibly more than three vocal registers, Hollien (1974)[29] recognizes the following:

1. *Pulse* register, the lowest range of phonation along the frequency continuum.
2. *Modal* register, the range of fundamental frequencies normally used in speaking and singing.
3. *Loft* register, the higher range of fundamental frequencies, including the *falsetto*.

In the untrained singer, transitions between registers are heard as changes in quality and even as a "break" in the voice.

Quality of Voice and Elastic and Viscoelastic Properties. The vocal tissues have two properties: elastic and viscoelastic. *Elastic* properties of vocal folds tissues are a key factor in the control of fundamental frequency in phonation,[30] but also a major determinant of the quality of voice. In 1974, Hirano[3] recognized that the morphological structure of the vocal folds is important for the control of tension in vibration; he called this the *cover-body* theory. The *cover* (epithelium and superficial layer of the lamina propria) is pliable, elastic, and noncontractile, whereas the body (muscle) is relatively stiff and has active contractile properties. The vocal ligament, composed of the intermediate and deep layers of the lamina propria, serves as a transitional layer between the two. The importance of the undulatory function of the mucosal covering of the vocal folds for normal phonation has been demonstrated in patients who have scarred vocal folds, where the mucosa has lost its mobility, resulting in breathiness and elevated pitch. Quality of voice depends on the quality of the cover and is also influenced by changes in the subglottal pressure. Normal vocal fold oscillations are an important precondition for a healthy voice.

Understanding normal laryngeal anatomy and physiology is imperative in the diagnosis and management of voice, airway, and swallowing disorders. This first chapter of the Anatomy and Physiology section presented the basic anatomy and physiology information for the chapter that follows.

Review Questions

1. The phenomenon of phonation:
   a. consists of a rapid opening and closing of the vocal folds which periodically interrupt the airsteam
   b. is independent and is not coordinated with respiration
   c. does not require air pressure to drive the vocal folds into vibration
   d. does not involve the Bernoulli effect
   e. requires the vocal folds to be in the abducted position

2. The range of fundamental frequencies normally used in speaking and singing is called:
   a. pulse register
   b. loft register
   c. vocal pitch
   d. modal register
   e. formant frequencies

3. The fundamental frequency of voice:
   a. depends on the configuration of the supraglottic cavities
   b. is always the same whatever the increase of the subglottal pressure
   c. will rise whenever the vocal folds move more slowly
   d. is the highest frequency which can be generate by the larynx
   e. is determined by the elasticity, tension, and mass of the vocal folds

4. The recurrent laryngeal nerve innervates:
   a. the thyrohyoid muscle
   b. the posterior belly of the digastric muscle
   c. the cricothyroid muscle
   d. the stylopharyngeus muscle
   e. the posterior cricoarytenoid muscle

5. The false vocal folds:
   a. allow the phenomenon of phonation
   b. move with the arytenoid cartilages
   c. are located in the subglottal area
   d. contain no muscle fibers
   e. move faster when the subglottal pressure increases

6. All the following occur during phonation except:
   a. the arytenoid cartilages rotate and the vocal process move outward, upward, and posteriorly
   b. adduction is accomplished by the posterior cricoarytenoid muscle
   c. the subglottal pressure increases and blows apart the vocal folds
   d. the release of air into the vocal tract entails a decrease of pressure beneath the vocal folds
   e. the Bernoulli effect results in an increase in airflow velocity

REFERENCES

1. Bless D, Abbs J. *Vocal Fold Physiology*. San Diego, Calif: College-Hill Press; 1983.
2. Titze I. *Vocal Fold Physiology*. San Diego, Calif: Singular Publishing Group; 1993.
3. Hirano M. Morphological structure of the vocal cord as a vibrator and its variations. *Folia Phoniatr.* 1974;26:89–94.
4. Hirano M. Structure of the vocal fold in normal and disease states: anatomical and physical studies. *ASHA Reports.* 1981;11:11–30.
5. Hirano M, Sato, K. *Histological Color Atlas of the Human Larynx*. San Diego, Calif: Singular Publishing Group; 1993.
6. Zemlin W. *Speech and Hearing Science Anatomy and Physiology*. Boston, Mass: Allyn and Bacon; 1998.
7. Furlan JC, Cordeiro AC, Brandao LG. Study of some "intrinsic risk factors" that can enhance an iatrogenic injury of the external branch of the superior laryngeal nerve. *Otolaryngol Head Neck Surg.* 2003;128(3):396–400.
8. Page C, Laude M, Legars D, Foulon P, Strunski Y. The external laryngeal nerve: surgical and anatomic considerations. Report of 50 total thyroidectomies. *Surg Radiol Anat.* 2004;26(3):182–185.
9. Friedman M, LoSavio P, Ibrahim H. Superior laryngeal nerve identification and preservation in thyroidectomy. *Arch Otolaryngol Head Neck Surg.* 2002;128(3):296–303.
10. Netterville JL, Koriwchak MJ, Winkle M, Courey MS, Ossoff RH. Vocal fold paralysis following the anterior approach to the cervical spine. *Ann Otol Rhinol Laryngol.* 1996;105(2):85–91.
11. Timmermann W, Hamelmann WH, Meyer T, et al. Identification and surgical anatomy of the external branch of the superior laryngeal nerve [in German]. *Zentralbl Chir.* 2002;127(5):425–428.
12. Jafari S, Prince RA, Kim DY, Paydarfar D. Sensory regulation of swallowing and airway protection: a role for the internal superior laryngeal nerve in humans. *J Physiol.* 2003;550(pt 1):287–304.
13. Halum S, Shemirani N, Merati AL, Jaradeh S, Toohill RJ. Electromyography findings of the cricopharyngeus in association with ipsilateral pharyngeal and laryngeal muscles. *Ann Otol Rhinol Laryngol.* In press.
14. Mimifie F, Hixon T, Williams F. *Normal Aspects of Speech, Hearing, and Language*. Englewood, NJ: Prentice-Hall; 1973.
15. Stroppiana L. Galen's treatise on section of the organs which produce sounds (translation and comment) [in Italian]. *Riv Stor Med.* 1970;14(2):131–148.
16. Joutsivuo T. Veraliu and De humani corporis fabrica: Galen's errors and the change of anatomy in the sixteenth century [in Finnish]. *Hippokrates.* 1997:98–112.
17. Borden G, Harris, K. *Speech Science Primer: Physuiology, Acoustics and Perception of Speech.* Baltimore, Md: Williams and Wilkins; 1980.
18. Van den Berg JW. Myoelastic-aerodynamic theory of voice production. *J Speech Lang Hear Res.* 1958;1:227–244.
19. Lieberman P. *On the Origin of Language*. New York, NY: Macmillan; 1975.
20. Odland RM, Wigley T, Rice R. Management of unilateral vocal fold paralysis. *Am Surg.* 1995;61(5):438–443.
21. Schneider B, Denk DM, Bigenzahn W. Functional results after external vocal fold medialization thyroplasty with the titanium vocal fold medialization implant. *Laryngoscope.* 2003;113(4):628–634.
22. Zheng H, Zhou S, Chen S, et al. Laryngeal reinnervation for unilateral recurrent laryngeal nerve injuries caused by thyroid surgery [in Chinese]. *Zhonghua Yi Xue Za Zhi.* 2002;82(15):1042–1045.
23. Zheng H, Li Z, Zhou S, Cuan Y, Wen W. Update: laryngeal reinnervation for unilateral vocal cord paralysis with the ansa cervicalis. *Laryngoscope.* 1996;106(12 pt 1):1522–1527.
24. Sercarz JA, Nguyen L, Nasri S, Graves MC, Wenokur R, Berke KS. Physiologic motion after laryngeal nerve reinnervation: a new method. *Otolaryngol Head Neck Surg,* 1997;116(4):466–474.
25. Wen W, Zhou S, Li Z. Treatment of the unilateral paralysis of vocal fold—comparison between laryngeal framework surgery and reinnervation [in Chinese]. *Zhonghua Er Bi Yan Hou Ke Za Zhi.* 1998;33(4):237–239.
26. Tucker HM. Long-term preservation of voice improvement following surgical medialization and reinnervation for unilateral vocal fold paralysis. *J Voice.* 1999; 13(2):251–256.
27. Tucker HM. Combined surgical medialization and nerve-muscle pedicle reinnervation for unilateral vocal fold paralysis: improved functional results and prevention of long-term deterioration of voice. *J Voice.* 1997;11(4):474–478.
28. Kitajima K, Tanabe M, Isshiki N. Cricothyroid distance and vocal pitch: experimental surgical

study to elevate the vocal pitch. *Ann Otol Rhinol Laryngol.* 1979;88(1 pt 1):52-55.

29. Hollien H. On vocal registers. *J Phonet.* 1974;. 2:125-143.

30. Titze IR, Talkin DT. A theoretical study of the effects of various laryngeal configurations on the acoustics of phonation. *J Acoust Soc Am.* 1979; 66(1):60-74.

Physiology of Airway Regulation

Christy L. Ludlow, PhD

KEY POINTS

- Each of these systems is controlled by overlapping neuronal circuits in the brainstem.

- These functions interact in awake humans. Dependent upon a certain state, one system may be dominant and modulate the function of other systems through suppression and/or excitation. Alterations in one system can alter the regulation of other upper airway systems.

- Sensory feedback from the larynx to the brainstem can trigger and/or enhance activity in several systems simultaneously.

- Abnormalities in sensory feedback from the larynx may cause both short- and long-term changes in each of the upper airway systems. Chronic abnormalities in laryngeal sensation due to inflammation, irritation, or injury may produce neuroplastic changes in brainstem function. Synaptic changes in brainstem circuits can produce long-term facilitation of some brainstem functions altering airway regulation.

- A better understanding of upper airway regulation both in normal human function and in disorders should lead to better diagnosis and treatment in patients with upper airway regulation abnormalities.

SYSTEMS INVOLVED IN UPPER AIRWAY REGULATION

The upper airway is composed of the larynx, hypopharynx, oropharynx, nasopharynx, and nasal and oral cavities. These regions are involved in respiration, swallowing, cough, voice, and speech. Each of these activities modulates the muscles of the upper airway to change the shape and function of this region. These functions are controlled by brainstem regulatory systems in addition to cortical volitional control. This chapter reviews each of the functions involved in upper airway regulation.

Respiration

During the two phases of respiration, inspiration and expiration, the airway is under control to enhance air exchange in the lungs. During inspiration, a traveling wave of muscle contractions develops to open the tract and reduce airflow resistance, starting at the nares, through the oral cavity, the hypopharynx, and finally the glottis. In this chain of muscle contractions from the alae nasi and genioglossus, to the posterior crico-arytenoid in the larynx all serve to maintain and enhance the opening of the upper airway on each inspiration. Inspiratory widening of the upper airway is often enhanced during sleep and exercise. If the levels of carbon dioxide in the blood are increased during hypercapnia, the drive to each of these airway-dilating muscles will increase.[1,2] On the other hand, if muscle tone decreases in the genioglossus, as occurs during some phases of sleep, tongue relaxation into the hypopharynx can interfere with airway opening producing an obstruction, which can be one cause of obstructive sleep apnea.[3]

During expiration, the vocal folds partially adduct[4] due to increased activity in the thyroary-tenoid muscles.[5,6] The respiratory control system in the brainstem includes a dorsal sensory input region involving the nucleus tractus solitarius and the ventral respiratory control centers. These include the pre-Bötzinger region, which provides rhythm generation, and the Bötzinger complex and rostral ventral respiratory groups, which contain premotor neurons with inputs to each of the motor neuron pools involved (Figure 2–1A).[7]

Swallowing

Swallowing also modifies the upper airway to prevent the entry of food or liquid through the vocal folds into the trachea during ingestion. After entry of food or liquid bolus into the oral cavity and mastication, the bolus is formed and moved to the posterior oral cavity where its presence triggers the initiation of the pharyngeal phase of swallowing. The pharyngeal phase involves elevation of the velum (preventing entry of the bolus into the nasal cavity), and anterior and superior movement of the hyoid bone and larynx to close the vestibule along with vocal fold closure. Cocontraction of the posterior tongue and the wall of the oropharynx push the bolus downward while reflexive and mechanical opening of the upper esophageal sphincter allows entry of the bolus into the esophagus and clearance from the hypopharynx. This coordinated pattern of multiple movements is rapid, smooth, and tightly coordinated, taking less than 1 second in healthy adults, and is under the control of central pattern generators in the brainstem. The medulla contains both a dorsal swallowing group, which receives sensory inputs and cortical control, and a ventral swallowing group, which provides input to the motor neurons for each of the upper airway muscles involved (see Figure 2–1B).[8]

Cough

Aspiration of a bolus through the glottis will produce tracheobronchial cough when contact is made with receptors in the trachea. Cough involves a chain of muscle actions to clear the bolus or a foreign body from the upper airway: first a quick inspiration to intake air, a rapid vocal fold closure to build up pressure in the subglottal region, and then a rapid expiratory expulsion of air involving the abdominal muscles with a

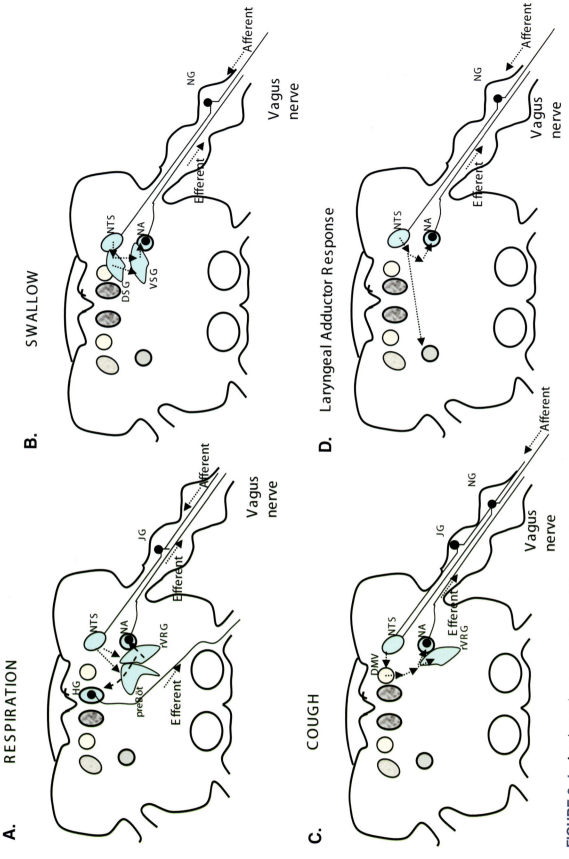

A. RESPIRATION

B. SWALLOW

C. COUGH

D. Laryngeal Adductor Response

FIGURE 2–1. A schematic representation of the neural pathways involved in respiration (**A.**), cough (**B.**), swallow (**C.**), and the laryngeal adductor response (**D.**). In each diagram the control pathway is only represented on the right side of the medulla oblongata at the level of entry of the vagus. (Abbreviations: DMV = dorsal motor nucleus of the vagus; DSG = dorsal swallowing group; HG = hypoglossal nucleus; JG = jugular ganglion; NA = nucleus ambiguus; NG = nodose ganglion; NTS = nucleus tractus solitarius; preBöt = pre-Bötzinger complex; rVRG = rostral ventral respiratory group; and VSG = ventral swallowing group.)

rapid abduction of the vocal folds. Laryngeal cough is elicited by stimulation of receptors in the mucosa overlying the arytenoid cartilages in the posterior glottis. There may be differences in the chemical and sensory regulation of tracheo-bronchial and laryngeal cough.[9] For laryngeal cough, the afferents are contained in the superior laryngeal nerve and have their cell bodies in the nodose ganglion.[10] Input to the brainstem from these afferent neurons terminates in the interstitial subnucleus of the nucleus tractus solitarius (see Figure 2–1C).[11,12] There is some interaction between the tracheobronchial and laryngeal cough systems; persistent stimulation of the trachea can increase the sensitivity of the larynx to stimulation lowering the threshold for laryngeal cough elicitation.[13] Chronic application of several stimuli such as smoke, sulfur dioxide and allergens will produce hypersensitivity of the trachea to stimulation, resulting in enhanced cough.[14] Although not as well studied, it is likely that chronic irritation in the larynx could similarly produce hypersensitivity and enhanced cough.

Laryngeal Adductor Response

The laryngeal adductor response is a spasmodic burst of thyroarytenoid muscle activity producing a rapid vocal fold closure of a short duration (less than 100 ms) following a single short stimulation of afferents in the superior laryngeal nerve.[15-17] In awake humans responses to a single electrical stimulation of the superior laryngeal nerve includes an ipsilateral early response around 17 ms referred to as an R1 and bilateral R2 responses around 60 ms (Figure 2–2), which produce bilateral vocal fold closure.[18] An air puff presented to the mucosa overlying an arytenoid cartilage will produce a short duration bilateral glottic closure due to bilateral thyroarytenoid muscle bursts similar to an R2 response in healthy adults.[19] In the event of strong or prolonged stimulation to the posterior glottis, this reflex can become prolonged producing a laryngospasm, which can be life threatening due to prolonged airway obstruction. Hypercapnia may reduce laryngospasm,[20] as well as depress thyroarytenoid

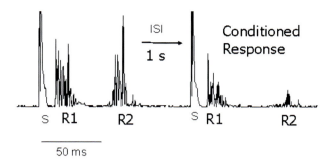

FIGURE 2–2. An example of a laryngeal adductor response to an initial electrical stimulus (*S*) to the superior laryngeal nerve and a response to a second pulse presented at an interstimulus interval (*ISI*) 1 second later.

muscle activity,[21] and was the basis for administering a carbon dioxide air mixture prior to extubation to prevent laryngospasm in pediatric anesthesia.[22] The laryngeal adductor response pathway in the brainstem involves inputs to the interstitial subnucleus in the nucleus tractus solitarius in the brainstem, the same sensory input region that is involved in cough and swallowing elicitation (see Figure 2–1D).[23]

Phonation

Vocalization can be elicited in mammals by electrical or chemical stimulation of neuronal pools in the central nervous system including the anterior cingulate and/or the periaqueductal gray, which projects to the brainstem, referred to as the indirect vocalization pathway (Figure 2–3).[24] Others have demonstrated that muscle patterning for vocalization may also be present in the nucleus retroambiguus[25] that projects to the nucleus ambiguus containing the motor neurons for the laryngeal muscles. The extent to which the indirect pathway that produces vocalization in animals (anterior cingulate, periaqueductal gray, nucleus retroambiguus) also controls voice production in humans during speech is not yet known and a matter of some controversy.[26] Jurgens proposed that voice during speech involves a direct corticobulbar pathway that may bypass the indirect system; whereas the indirect control

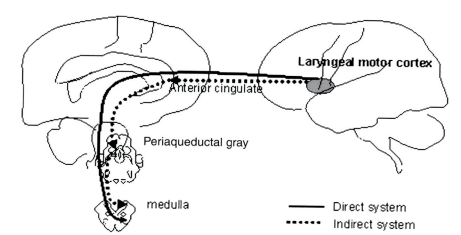

FIGURE 2–3. A schematic representation of the direct and indirect central pathways possibly involved in vocalization in humans.

system may be involved in emotional vocal expression in both humans and other mammals.[24] This may explain why patients with spasmodic dysphonia have symptoms during voice for speech while laughter and cry are symptom free. The disorder may affect the direct pathway but not the indirect pathway for voice production. Likely, both the direct and indirect systems are involved in speech while only the indirect system may be used during laughter and crying.

INTEGRATION OF UPPER AIRWAY SYSTEMS

Each of the upper airway systems involve several regions in the central nervous system from the cortex to the brainstem, where central pattern generators can produce these behaviors in an automatic fashion.[27–29] Studies in anesthetized or decerebrated animals have identified the location of neuronal pools in the brainstem, which can produce these behaviors in isolation. However, in awake humans, each of these systems must be regulated so that they do not interfere with each other. For example, every time a speaker is producing a word, he or she must maintain a controlled smooth flow of air on expiration and not swallow, cough, or inspire. In recent years, animal studies have begun to address how changes in neuronal firing within the same regions in the medulla are affected as

control is shifted between the different upper airway systems of cough, swallowing, respiration, and phonation.

Swallowing has a powerful influence on the other upper airway systems. The suppression of respiration occurs in the middle of expiration during the pharyngeal phase of swallowing. After the pharyngeal phase is complete, expiration resumes. Swallowing also has a suppressive influence on the laryngeal adductor response in humans. When electrical stimuli were presented to the superior laryngeal nerve prior to, during, and up to 5 seconds after a water swallow in healthy adults, the laryngeal adductor response was suppressed by swallowing. Both the frequency and amplitude of R1 and R2 responses were reduced when the subjects were swallowing and up to 3 seconds after they completed a swallow.[30] This demonstrates a suppression of neuronal activity in the laryngeal adductor response neural pathway during swallowing. The laryngeal adductor response is a subcomponent of the cough reflex pathway[23] (see Figure 2–1). The suppression of this pathway during swallowing may explain why coughing is reduced by taking a sip of water.

Cough also modifies respiratory control by producing a quick inspiration followed by forceful expiration. This demonstrates a modification of the neuronal firing in the ventral respiratory control system as the cough system modulates respiratory control within the medulla (see Figure 2–1B).[31]

The usual modulation of one airway system by another may be altered in certain states. If respiratory drive is increased by hypercapnia, for example, then swallowing can only occur at certain intervals within the respiratory cycles.[29] Such interactions between upper airway systems may play a role in patients with chronic obstructive pulmonary disease where patients' respiratory-swallowing coupling is altered so that more swallows occur during inspiration placing them at greater risk of aspiration.[32-35]

Effects of Sensory Inputs in Regulating Upper Airway Physiology

Each of the upper airway systems is triggered or modified by sensory feedback to the central nervous system. Stimulation of the laryngeal afferents plays a role in each of these systems. As mentioned earlier, mechanical stimulation of the mucosa overlying the arytenoid cartilages will elicit the laryngeal adductor response in the thyroarytenoid muscles.[19,36] Mechanoreceptors are contained in the superior laryngeal nerve, as are chemosensory and C fibers. Water applied to the larynx will produce both a laryngeal adductor response and a central apnea[37]; both being the result of stimulation of afferents contained in the superior laryngeal nerve.[38] Capsaicin has a powerful effect on the larynx causing vocal fold adduction and central apnea both when it is applied topically to the larynx or to the pulmonary C fibers by intravenous injection.[39-42] This may be one of the factors involved in heightened laryngeal reactivity when patients eat spicy foods.

Swallowing is highly dependent on the central effects of laryngeal sensation for the normal triggering of the pharyngeal phase. This was demonstrated in healthy adults following a bilateral block of the superior laryngeal nerve, which not only increased laryngeal penetration and aspiration[43] but also causes normal persons to feel incapable of initiating a swallow.

Although all the upper airway systems are affected by afferent input from the superior laryngeal nerve, the degree and effects of such stimulation on each system depend on the intensity and duration of stimulation. This has been carefully studied in animals where the rate of electrical stimulation to the superior laryngeal nerve may determine whether a swallow or a cough is produced.[44] A rapid rate of 30 stimuli per second can evoke repeated swallowing,[29] whereas slower rates of the same stimuli will produce coughing.[11,27,45] A central apnea due to a suppression of respiration rhythm generation will occur with high rates of electrical stimulation, between 10 and 50 stimuli per second, being presented to the superior laryngeal nerve.[46-49] Similarly the intensity of nerve stimulation will alter the effects on the central control of swallowing, cough, and respiration.[50] Inhibition of respiration occurs at a lower intensity of superior laryngeal nerve stimulation than elicitation of swallowing, indicating that some part of the same brainstem neural pathways may be involved in each.[29]

Laryngospasm, a prolonged laryngeal adductor response, is usually only elicited when a strong stimulus is applied to the larynx. This response is normally suppressed, most likely because of inhibitory mechanisms within the brainstem pathways. Conditioning studies are used to quantify inhibition of a response in central pathways. An initial stimulus excites a brainstem pathway producing a response while also activating inhibitory interneurons in the same pathway. If a second stimulus is then presented at a short interstimulus interval of 1 second or less, the responses to the second stimulus are reduced because of the active inhibition in the brainstem (see Figure 2–2). This was demonstrated in healthy adults by presenting paired air puff stimuli to the laryngeal mucosa. Each time, the response to the second puff was reduced in both occurrence (by about 50%) and amplitude.[51]

Besides brainstem inhibition of these responses, the responses are also modulated at higher levels in the central nervous system. With anesthesia, laryngospasm is less likely to occur, indicating that these responses are facilitated by brain mechanisms above the brainstem. Sasaki and his colleagues demonstrated that the bilateral laryngeal adductor response (the R2) producing a vocal fold closure is reduced with anesthesia both in an animal model as well as in humans.[52-54]

During phonation for speech, a speaker must use proprioceptive feedback in addition to audition for fine control of the laryngeal musculature. Activation levels must be controlled in all the laryngeal muscles simultaneously to control vocal fold length and tension and for accurate timing of vocal fold closing and opening to allow onset and offset of vowel production. The powerful role of hearing in the laryngeal muscle control was demonstrated by shifting the pitch of a speaker's own voice as it is fed back to him or her. This produces a rapid change in the speaker's pitch within about 100 ms.[55,56]

It has been postulated that speakers also use muscle and joint receptors to control muscles when initiating a target pitch for voice onset before they receive auditory feedback. A servo-motor was used to push the thyroid cartilage and stretch the cricothyroid muscle and then release it to stretch the thyroarytenoid muscle, which altered voice pitch by muscle stretch in healthy adults. However, this did not produce any reflex responses in the laryngeal muscles, indicating that muscle stretch receptors (spindles) do not contribute to phonatory control in humans.[57] The role of other sensory feedback mechanisms, such as mechanoreceptors in the vocal fold mucosa and subglottal tracheal pressure receptors, need to be evaluated for their contribution to phonatory control in humans.

Effects of Abnormalities in Sensory Modulation on Upper Airway Regulation

Given the powerful effects of sensory and chemical stimuli to the larynx on each of the upper airway systems, it is not surprising that abnormalities affecting laryngeal sensation may produce disorders in respiration, cough, swallow, and voice.

A loss of laryngeal sensation produces swallowing deficits in healthy controls,[43] and patients with laryngeal sensory deficits often have swallowing disorders. Aviv and colleagues have shown that, when a stroke interferes with the central perception of laryngeal sensation, patients are at a greater risk of having aspiration pneumonia.[58] This is not because of any injury to the superior laryngeal nerve or the vagus, but rather due to a brain lesion disrupting sensory input to the central pathways involved in swallowing generation at the brainstem and/or cortex.[59]

Laryngopharyngeal reflux will produce low pH stimulation of the posterior larynx that can increase thyroarytenoid muscle tone producing laryngospasm.[60] Laryngopharyngeal reflux may be responsible for paradoxical laryngospasm in some patients[61] and should be considered when patients present with a history of intermittent laryngospasm. Long-term exposure to irritants may cause a hyperreactivity in the brainstem pathways involved in the laryngeal adductor response and has been postulated to be the basis for the "irritable larynx" syndrome.[62]

There may be two different effects of chronic laryngopharyngeal reflux on laryngeal function. First, acute application of low pH to the laryngeal mucosa can produce a central potentiation of the brainstem pathways involved in the laryngeal adductor response.[60] In addition, there may be long-term chronic effects due to inflammation or injury. In respiration, as a result of heightened sensory stimulation of the brainstem respiratory system with heightened serotonin release, long-term facilitation of respiratory control has been demonstrated in animal models.[63] Similarly, animals models of prolonged exposure to smoke, sulfur dioxide, and allergens in the trachea produced increased neural reactivity in the brainstem pathways involved in cough.[14] Similar mechanisms may be involved in neuropathic pain when central abnormalities continue long after the initial injury has resolved.[64] Such effects may occur in the laryngeal brainstem pathways with chronic inflammation.

Aviv and his colleagues have shown that the chronic effects of low pH to the laryngeal mucosa due to laryngopharyngeal reflux result in reduced sensory function on air-puff testing. Presumably the mucosal inflammation and edema

> ### Peripheral or Central?
>
> Patients with chronic laryngophargeal reflux may also develop a central abnormality because of the prolonged mucosal injury due to either low pH and/or peptic injury. Patients with pharyngeal sensory complaints may have both a peripheral loss of sensory function and a centrally based hypersensivity in the brainstem pathways.

interferes with air pressure changes affecting the mechanoreceptors in the mucosa.[65]

Paradoxic breathing disorder, when the vocal folds approximate in the midline during inspiration rather than opening, is often associated with chronic cough. When such disorders are refractory to proton pump inhibitors, hyperreactivity may have resulted from chronic irritation.[14,66] Such patients may need behavioral training involving upper airway regulation to restore normal function, as was demonstrated in a small case series in which patients benefitted from respiratory patterning through retraining.[67] The central mechanisms for the hyperactivity of the laryngeal adductor muscles during inspiration are not yet known. One animal study demonstrated that chemically blocking glycine receptors, normally involved in inhibition in the brainstem, increased laryngeal thyroarytenoid activity during inspiration.[68]

CURRENT AND FUTURE DIRECTIONS

Most of our understanding of central nervous system control for the upper airway systems comes from research using anesthetized or decerebrate animals. We have limited knowledge about how these systems are regulated in awake humans. Many patients have complaints of sensory abnormalities in the larynx for which we need additional diagnostic testing methods and additional treatments. With the development of air-puff testing,[58] we can now determine whether patients can sense pressure changes to the laryngeal mucosa. However, as is known from animal models of chronic cough,[14] significant disturbances in airway physiology can also come from central changes producing increased drive to the neuronal pathways in the brainstem. At present, we have few resources for diagnosing exaggerated responses to sensory stimulation and treating central increases in sensitivity, except for withdrawal of the irritating stimulus. Patients who fail a trial of proton pump inhibitors may have also developed central abnormalities affecting their responses to sensory stimulation.

Little is known about the neural mechanisms involved in the regulation of upper airway functions above the brainstem. Recent noninvasive brain imaging methods such as functional magnetic resonance imaging and other methods of study of central neurophysiology such as magnetoencephalography can be used to probe the role of central cortical control mechanisms in upper airway abnormalities. Such knowledge is needed for improved treatment approaches to disorders affecting the upper airway.

Acknowledgments. Support for preparation of this manuscript was from the Intramural Program, National Institutes of Health, National Institute of Neurological Disorders and Stroke. Both Keith Saxon, MD, and Sandra Martin, MS, provided helpful comments on earlier versions of this manuscript.

Review Questions

1. Name two effects of prolonged stimulation of the sensory fibers in the laryngeal mucosa.

2. Which two upper airway functions activate the posterior cricoarytenoid muscle?

3. Name two disorders that are often associated with reduced responses to sensory stimulation at the larynx.

4. Name two functions that are suppressed during swallowing.

5. Names two types of cough.

REFERENCES

1. Haxhiu MA, van Lunteren E, Mitra J, Cherniack NS. Comparison of the response of diaphragm and upper airway dilating muscle activity in sleeping cats. *Respir Physiol.* 1987;70(2):183-193.

2. Strohl KP, Hensley MJ, Hallett M, Saunders NA, Ingram RH Jr. Activation of upper airway muscles before onset of inspiration in normal humans. *J Appl Physiol.* 1980;49:638-642.

3. Strohl KP, Saunders NA, Feldman NT, Hallett M. Obstructive sleep apnea in family members. *N Engl J Med.* 1978;299(18):969-973.

4. Bartlett DJ, Remmers JE, Gautier H. Laryngeal regulation of respiratory airflow. *Respir Physiol.* 1973;18:194-204.

5. Kuna ST, Insalaco G, Woodson GE. Thyroarytenoid muscle activity during wakefulness and sleep in normal adults. *J Appl Physiol.* 1988;65: 1332-1339.

6. Insalaco G, Kuna ST, Cibella F, Villeponteaux RD. Thyroarytenoid muscle activity during hypoxia, hypercapnia, and voluntary hyperventilation in humans. *J Appl Physiol.* 1990;69:268-273.

7. Rubin A, Mobley B, Hogikyan N, et al. Delivery of an adenoviral vector to the crushed recurrent laryngeal nerve. *Laryngoscope.* 2003;113(6): 985-989.

8. Jean A. Brainstem control of swallowing: neuronal network and cellular mechanisms. *Physiol Rev.* 2001;81(2):929-969.

9. Bolser DC, Davenport PW. Functional organization of the central cough generation mechanism. *Pulm Pharmacol Ther.* 2002;15(3):221-225.

10. Yoshida Y, Tanaka Y, Hirano M, Nakashima T. Sensory innervation of the pharynx and larynx. *Am J Med.* 2000;108(Suppl 4a):51S-61S.

11. Gestreau C, Bianchi AL, Grelot L. Differential brainstem fos-like immunoreactivity after laryngeal-induced coughing and its reduction by codeine. *J Neurosci.* 1997;17:9340-9352.

12. Ohi Y, Yamazaki H, Takeda R, Haji A. Functional and morphological organization of the nucleus tractus solitarius in the fictive cough reflex of guinea pigs. *Neurosci Res.* 2005;53(2):201-209.

13. Hanacek J, Porubanova M, Korec L, Beseda O. Cough reflex changes in local tracheitis. *Physiol Bohemoslov.* 1979;28(4):375-380.

14. Bolser DC. Experimental models and mechanisms of enhanced coughing. *Pulm Pharmacol Ther.* 2004;17(6):383-388.

15. Suzuki M, Sasaki CT. Laryngeal spasm: a neurophysiologic redefinition. *Ann Otol Rhinol Laryngol.* 1977;86:150-158.

16. Ikari T, Sasaki CT. Glottic closure reflex: control mechanisms. *Ann Otol.* 1980;89:220-224.

17. Sasaki CT, Suzuki M. Laryngeal reflexes in cat, dog and man. *Arch Otolaryngol.* 1976;102:400-402.

18. Ludlow CL, VanPelt F, Koda J. Characteristics of late responses to superior laryngeal nerve stimulation in humans. *Ann Otol Rhinol Laryngol.* 1992;101:127-134.

19. Bhabu P, Poletto C, Mann E, Bielamowicz S, Ludlow CL. Thyroarytenoid muscle responses to air pressure stimulation of the laryngeal mucosa in humans. *Ann Otol Rhinol Laryngol.* 2003; 112(10):834-840.

20. Nishino T, Yonezawa T, Honda Y. Modification of laryngospasm in response to changes in $PaCO_2$ and PaO_2 in the cat. *Anesthesiology.* 1981;55(3): 286-291.

21. Kuna ST, Vanoye CR, Griffin JR, Updegrove JD. Effect of hypercapnia on laryngeal airway resistance in normal adult humans. *J Appl Physiol.* 1994;77(6):2797-2803.

22. Ahmad I, Sellers WF. Prevention and management of laryngospasm. *Anaesthesia.* 2004;59(9):920.

23. Ambalavanar R, Tanaka Y, Selbie WS, Ludlow CL. Neuronal activation in the medulla oblongata during selective elicitation of the laryngeal adductor response. *J Neurophysiol.* 2004;92(5):2920-2932.

24. Jurgens U. Neural pathways underlying vocal control. *Neurosci Biobehav Rev.* 2002;26(2):235-258.

25. Zhang SP, Bandler R, Davis PJ. Brainstem integration of vocalization: role of the nucleus retroambigualis. *J Neurophysiol.* 1995;74(6):2500-2512.

26. Holstege G, Ehling T. Two motor systems involved in the production of speech. In: Davis PJ, Fletcher NH, eds. *Vocal Fold Physiology: Controlling Complexity and Chaos.* San Diego, Calif: Singular Publishing Group; 1996:153-169.

27. Bolser DC. Fictive cough in the cat. *J Appl Physiol.* 1991;71:2325-2331.

28. Nakazawa K, Umezaki T, Zheng Y, Miller AD. Behaviors of bulbar respiratory interneurons during fictive swallowing and vomiting. *Otolaryngol Head Neck Surg.* 1999;120:412-418.

29. Dick TE, Oku Y, Romaniuk JR, Cherniack NS. Interaction between central pattern generators for breathing and swallowing in the cat. *J Physiol.* 1993;465:715-730.

30. Barkmeier JM, Bielamowicz S, Takeda N, Ludlow CL. Modulation of laryngeal responses to superior laryngeal nerve stimulation by volitional swallowing in awake humans. *J Neurophysiol.* 2000; 83(3):1264-1272.

31. Shannon R, Baekey DM, Morris KF, Lindsey BG. Ventrolateral medullary respiratory network and a model of cough motor pattern generation. *J Appl Physiol.* 1998;84(6):2020-2035.

32. Martin-Harris B, Logemann JA, McMahon S, Schleicher M, Sandidge J. Clinical utility of the modified barium swallow. *Dysphagia.* 2000;15(3): 136-141.

33. Langmore SE. *Endoscopic Evaluation and Treatment of Swallowing Disorders.* New York, NY: Thieme; 2001.

34. Good-Fratturelli MD, Curlee RF, Holle JL. Prevalence and nature of dysphagia in VA patients with COPD referred for videofluoroscopic swallow examination. *J Commun Disord.* 2000;33(2): 93-110.

35. Shaker R, Li Q, Ren J, et al. Coordination of deglutition and phases of respiration: effect of aging, tachypnea, bolus volume, and chronic obstructive pulmonary disease. *Am J Physiol.* 1992;263(5 pt 1): G750-755.

36. Aviv JE, Spitzer J, Cohen M, Ma G, Belafsky P, Close LG. Laryngeal adductor reflex and pharyngeal squeeze as predictors of laryngeal penetration and aspiration. *Laryngoscope.* 2002;112(2):338-341.

37. Goding GS, Richardson MA, Trachy RE. Laryngeal chemoreflex: anatomic and physiologic study by use of the superior laryngeal nerve in the piglet. *Otolaryngol Head Neck Surg.* 1987;97:28-38.

38. Van Vliet BN, Uenishi M. Antagonistic interaction of laryngeal and central chemoreceptor respiratory reflexes. *J Appl Physiol.* 1992;72(2): 643-649.

39. Kaczynska K, Szereda-Przestaszewska M. Superior laryngeal nerve section abolishes capsaicin evoked chemoreflex in anaesthetized rats. *Acta Neurobiol Exp (Wars).* 2002;62(1):19-24.

40. Szereda-Przestaszewska M, Wypych B. Laryngeal constriction produced by capsaicin in the cat. *J Physiol Pharmacol.* 1996;47(2):351-360.

41. Diaz V, Dorion D, Renolleau S, Letourneau P, Kianicka I, Praud JP. Effects of capsaicin pretreatment on expiratory laryngeal closure during pulmonary edema in lambs. *J Appl Physiol.* 1999;86(5): 1570-1577.

42. Palecek F, Sant'Ambrogio G, Sant'Ambrogio FB, Mathew OP. Reflex responses to capsaicin: intravenous, aerosol, and intratracheal administration. *J Appl Physiol.* 1989;67(4):1428-1437.

43. Jafari S, Prince RA, Kim DY, Paydarfar D. Sensory regulation of swallowing and airway protection: a role for the internal superior laryngeal nerve in humans. *J Physiol.* 2003;550(pt 1):287-304.

44. Harada H, Sakamoto T, Kita S. *Role of GABAergic control of swallowing and coughing movements induced by the superior laryngeal stimulation in cats.* Paper presented at: Society for Neuroscience; 2002; Orlando, Fla.

45. Satoh I, Shiba K, Kobayashi N, Nakajima Y, Konno A. Upper airway motor outputs during sneezing and coughing in decerebrate cats. *Neurosci Res.* 1998;32(2):131-135.

46. Lawson EE. Prolonged central respiratory inhibition following reflex-induced apnea. *J Appl Physiol.* 1981;50(4):874-879.

47. Sutton D, Taylor EM, Lindeman RC. Prolonged apnea in infant monkeys resulting from stimulation of superior laryngeal nerve. *Pediatrics.* 1978; 61(4):519-527.

48. Bongianni F, Corda M, Fontana G, Pantaleo T. Influences of superior laryngeal afferent stimulation on expiratory activity in cats. *J Appl Physiol.* 1988;65(1):385-392.

49. Bongianni F, Mutolo D, Carfi M, Fontana GA, Pantaleo T. Respiratory neuronal activity during apnea and poststimulatory effects of laryngeal origin in the cat. *J Appl Physiol.* 2000;89(3): 917–925.

50. Miller AJ, Loizzi RF. Anatomical and functional differentiation of superior laryngeal nerve fibers affecting swallowing and respiration. *Exp Neurol.* 1974;42(2):369–387.

51. Kearney PR, Poletto CJ, Mann EA, Ludlow CL. Suppression of thyroarytenoid muscle responses during repeated air pressure stimulation of the laryngeal mucosa in awake humans. *Ann Otol Rhinol Laryngol.* 2005;114(4):264–270.

52. Kim YH, Sasaki CT. Glottic closing force in an anesthetized, awake pig model: biomechanical effects on the laryngeal closure reflex resulting from altered central facilitation. *Acta Otolaryngol.* 2001;121(2):310–314.

53. Sasaki CT, Ho S, Kim YH. Critical role of central facilitation in the glottic closure reflex. *Ann Otol Rhinol Laryngol.* 2001;110(5 pt 1):401–405.

54. Sasaki CT, Jassin B, Kim YH, Hundal J, Rosenblatt W, Ross DA. Central facilitation of the glottic closure reflex in humans. *Ann Otol Rhinol Laryngol.* 2003;112(4):293–297.

55. Larson CR, Burnett TA, Kiran S, Hain TC. Effects of pitch-shift velocity on voice Fo responses. *J Acoust Soc Am.* 2000;107(1):559–564.

56. Burnett TA, Freedland MB, Larson CR, Hain TC. Voice F_0 responses to manipulations in pitch feedback. *J Acoust Soc Am.* 1998;103(6):3153–3161.

57. Loucks TM, Poletto CJ, Saxon KG, Ludlow CL. Laryngeal muscle responses to mechanical displacement of the thyroid cartilage in humans. *J Appl Physiol.* 2005;99(3):922–930.

58. Aviv JE, Sacco RL, Mohr JP, et al. Laryngopharyngeal sensory testing with modified barium swallow as predictors of aspiration pneumonia after stroke. *Laryngoscope.* 1997;107:1254–1260.

59. Aydogdu I, Ertekin C, Tarlaci S, Turman B, Kiylioglu N, Secil Y. Dysphagia in lateral medullary infarction (Wallenberg's syndrome): an acute disconnection syndrome in premotor neurons related to swallowing activity? *Stroke.* 2001;32(9): 2081–2087.

60. Loughlin CJ, Koufman JA, Averill DB, et al. Acid-induced laryngospasm in a canine model. *Laryngoscope.* 1996;106:1506–1509.

61. Loughlin CJ, Koufman JA. Paroxysmal laryngospasm secondary to gastroesophageal reflux. *Laryngoscope.* 1996;106:1501–1505.

62. Morrison M, Rammage L, Emami AJ. The irritable larynx syndrome. *J Voice.* 1999;13(3):447–455.

63. Feldman JL, Mitchell GS, Nattie EE. Breathing: rhythmicity, plasticity, chemosensitivity. *Ann Rev Neurosci.* 2003;26:239–266.

64. Coderre TJ, Katz J, Vaccarino AL, Melzack R. Contribution of central neuroplasticity to pathological pain: review of clinical and experimental evidence. *Pain.* 1993;52:259–285.

65. Aviv JE, Liu H, Parides M, Kaplan ST, Close LG. Laryngopharyngeal sensory deficits in patients with laryngopharyngeal reflux and dysphagia. *Ann Otol Rhinol Laryngol.* 2000;109(11):1000–1006.

66. Altman KW, Simpson CB, Amin MR, Abaza M, Balkissoon R, Casiano RR. Cough and paradoxical vocal fold motion. *Otolaryngol Head Neck Surg.* 2002;127(6):501–511.

67. Murry T, Tabaee A, Aviv JE. Respiratory retraining of refractory cough and laryngopharyngeal reflux in patients with paradoxical vocal fold movement disorder. *Laryngoscope.* 2004;114(8):1341–1345.

68. Dutschmann M, Paton JF. Inhibitory synaptic mechanisms regulating upper airway patency. *Respir Physiol Neurobiol.* 2002;131(1–2):57–63.

PART II
Diagnostic Procedures in Laryngology

3

Videostroboscopy

Nadine P. Connor, PhD
Diane M. Bless, PhD

KEY POINTS

■ Video imaging of the larynx is a standard and critical part of a complete functional laryngeal and voice examination; Videostroboscopy is a video imaging method that is effective in most clinical situations.

■ Videostroboscopy provides information on both laryngeal structure and function, and also provides a permanent record that can be stored and referred to in the future to track changes in structure or function over time.

■ Videostroboscopy allows imaging and recording of apparent vocal fold motion, rather than actual cycle-to-cycle motion of the vocal folds.

■ Specialized, high-quality equipment is needed for videostroboscopy and is commercially available; training is necessary for performing and interpreting videostroboscopic examinations of the larynx.

■ Videostroboscopy scoring instruments are available in the literature and are recommended for ensuring that a complete examination protocol is followed, and that observations are recorded in a systematic manner. However, reliability of ratings is always a concern with any instrument.

Videostroboscopy is a technique that allows the clinician to image the larynx and the vocal folds, and also view the apparent motion of the vocal folds during a variety of phonatory tasks. In this manner, videostroboscopy offers a means of determining the etiology of the dysphonia.[1,2] For most clinical assessments of voice, videostroboscopic examination of the larynx is a critical and necessary part of obtaining an understanding of laryngeal structure and function. It is considered to be part of a basic, or minimal set, of procedures performed as part of a complete laryngeal and voice evaluation.[2]

A complete voice evaluation must include imaging of the vocal folds during phonation and videostroboscopy is an effective method for most clinical situations.[1] In a recent survey of speech-language pathologists specializing in voice disorders, 81% indicated they were likely to use videostroboscopy in voice assessments.[3] In addition, 94% of speech-language pathologists found videostroboscopy important in defining voice therapy goals, and 81% reported that videostroboscopy was an important tool to use in educating patients.[3] These are remarkable levels of utility, particularly in contrast to other voice

Does Videostroboscopic Examination Really Matter in Terms of Outcomes?

Videostroboscopic examination of the larynx assists the otolaryngologist and speech-language pathologist in forming a diagnosis and in planning treatment for individual patients. The presence of laryngeal pathology and the effect of that pathology upon vibratory function of the vocal folds can be directly discerned. In this vein, establishment of an accurate diagnosis is vital in formulating appropriate treatment decisions, and hence encouraging a positive treatment outcome. Studies completed by Woo et al[4] and Sataloff et al[13] demonstrated that videostroboscopy made a difference in diagnosis in approximately 30 to 47% of cases with voice disorders. Uncertain diagnoses were often confirmed with this procedure. To the extent that diagnosis is important in making correct management decisions and positive patient outcomes, the use of videostroboscopy appears critical.

Extensive use of videostroboscopy for determining voice therapy goals by the speech-language pathologist and for patient education has also been reported.[3] Specifically, Behrman reported that 94 and 81% of speech-language pathologists used videolaryngostroboscopy for these purposes, respectively. To the extent that definition of appropriate therapy goals and patient education are important to patient outcomes, the use of videostroboscopy appears to be a widely used and important assessment and educational method.

To summarize, it is the opinion of these authors that videostroboscopic imaging of the vocal folds is an essential part of a complete voice assessment and greatly influences patient outcomes due to its role in diagnosis, management, and patient education.

assessment modalities, such as aerodynamic assessments and electroglottography, where only 17% and 6% of speech-language pathologists, respectively, reported that these types of assessment methods were valuable.[3] As such, videostroboscopy is in common use, and has been found to be a valuable tool in diagnosing and treating patients with voice disorders. Videostroboscopic examination is completed by both speech pathologists and otolaryngologists, but only otolaryngologists use the images to make medical diagnoses.

By definition, a stroboscope is a device for studying the motion of a body in rapid vibration or revolution. In laryngeal examinations, the stroboscope causes vocal fold motion to appear to slow down or stop by periodically illuminating the larynx with pulses of light.[1] It is important to recognize that "apparent motion" is imaged with videostroboscopy, not actual cycle-to-cycle vibratory motion. Because humans cannot perceive more that 5 images per second, even 6 cycles per second is too rapid to observe. Thus, the vocal folds vibrating at a rate of 100 to 300/sec is clearly too rapid to allow vocal fold vibration to

be observed on a cycle-by-cycle basis. Furthermore, most available video recording equipment does not allow greater than 33 frames per second to be recorded, which is well below the habitual fundamental frequency of the human voice (see chapter 4, Laryngeal High-Speed Digital Imaging and Kymography). Videostroboscopy capitalizes on the limitations of human observation and recording frames. Depending on the mode selected, videostroboscopy allows the examiner to observe a composite vibratory cycle that appears to be the same point in time within a cycle to evaluate a particular phase of vibration or to examine vibration at different points of time within a cycle for appreciation of many points within the vibratory cycle.[1] In the former situation, a light is pulsed at a rate identical to the fundamental frequency of the voice. In the latter case, the light is pulsed at a frequency slightly faster than the actual fundamental frequency of vibration. This asynchronous light pulse allows the vocal folds to be observed at a different point in time within the vibratory cycle across many cycles of vibration. A schematic of this effect is shown in Figure 3–1. The net result is that the vocal fold vibration

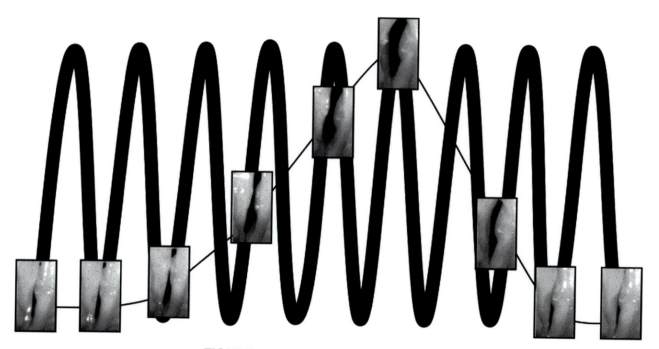

FIGURE 3–1. Apparent vocal fold motion.

appears to slow down. The eye is tricked into perceiving a continuous, slow-motion sequence of vocal fold vibration.[1,5]

EQUIPMENT

Specialized equipment is needed for videostroboscopy, as shown in Figure 3–2. This equipment includes a monitor, digital or video recording system, camera with microphone for recording an audio signal, a lens adaptor connected to either a flexible or rigid endoscope, a stroboscope that encompasses a pitch extractor and a light source, and a microphone or electroglottography (EGG) for pitch extraction. A speaker and printer are also necessary for complete functionality.[5]

The success of the technique is highly dependent on the quality of the equipment.[4] The light has to be bright enough, and pitch extraction must be accurate, have adequate range and speed, and must lock onto the patient's fundamental frequency quickly because many dyspho-

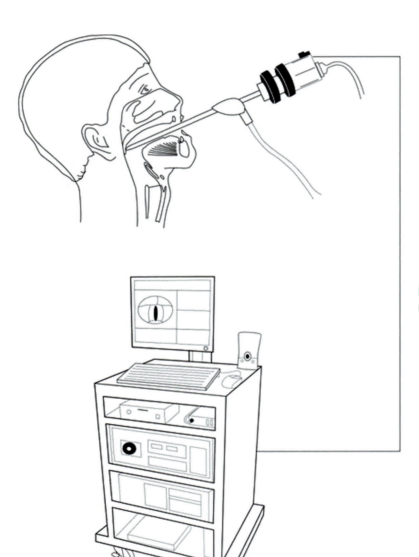

FIGURE 3–2. Diagram of equipment needed for videostroboscopy.

nic patients cannot sustain voice for long periods of time. In addition, the recording and camera equipment must be compatible and of high resolution. The resultant image will only be as good as the weakest link of the system.

Either flexible or rigid endoscopes can be used in videostroboscopy, with the goal of providing a bright image free of distortion. A flexible endoscope is passed through the nose, past the velum, and into the pharynx and has the advantage of imaging vocal fold vibration during connected speech, which is not possible with a rigid endoscope. The flexible endoscope is often better for individuals who tend to gag with something in their posterior oral cavity, those with a high tongue posture, or with young children (see further discussion below concerning children). A flexible endoscope can be used to examine a variety of exposure angles and also to examine velopharyngeal function.[6] However, its disadvantages include the need for anesthetic spray in the nose, lower magnification, and less light delivered to the vocal folds. As such, the resolution of the vocal fold images can be compromised. In rigid videostroboscopy, a 70-degree rigid endoscope is commonly used and generally obtains images of higher resolution than a flexible endoscope, and is less invasive. The high resolution chip-tip flexible endoscope with a built-in miniature chip video camera embedded in the end of the endoscope is an exception to resolution concerns expressed above for flexible endoscopy. The

Do Patients Need to Undergo Both Flexible and Rigid Endoscopic Examination with Videostroboscopy?

Ideally, most patients would benefit from receiving both rigid and flexible endoscopic exams with videolaryngostroboscopy due to the higher resolution images generally obtained via rigid endoscopy, and the greater variety of phonatory tasks that can be accommodated by flexible endoscopy. In this manner, rigid endoscopy could be used to document the presence of pathology and the vibratory correlates of the pathology on tissue mechanics during simple phonatory tasks, such as extended vowel production, whereas voicing during connected speech could be assessed via flexible endoscopy. However, time often prohibits this practice and the endoscopist must choose either a flexible or rigid endoscope for the videolaryngostroboscopic examination. For patients presenting with signs of spasmodic dysphonia and other neurologic disease without pathology, flexible endoscopy is indicated due to the need to evaluate vocal fold behavior during connected speech. While tip-chip endoscopes make it possible to obtain well-illuminated, high-resolution images of laryngeal tissue dynamics via flexible examination, not all clinics have access to this expensive equipment.

In summary, it is the authors' opinion that use of both flexible and rigid endoscopic examination with videostroboscopy is an ideal situation that is often not clinically realistic and likely not necessary for accurate observation of vocal fold behavior by the experienced clinician.

tip-chip endoscope provides good illumination and high resolution, but is significantly more expensive than a standard rigid or flexible endoscope.

Electroglottography (EGG) is often recorded in conjunction with videostroboscopy. There are two purposes for this simultaneous recording: (1) it can be used to trigger the strobe and (2) it provides a record of every cycle of vibration helping clinicians to interpret the apparent motion from the stroboscopic images. The EGG is strapped onto the neck and functions by recording the impedance to passage of a very low current across the glottis. The EGG activates the strobe, and triggers the device to turn on the light pulse, either at the fundamental frequency of the voice or slightly faster. As mentioned, when synchronous with the fundamental frequency, the resultant glottal image appears to stand still and the recorded image is very similar to that recorded with direct, rather than pulsed, light. In other words, when vibration is regular no motion is observed. However, if vibration is irregular the pulsed light appearing at slightly different places on the vibratory cycle will result in a slight shimmering of the image rather than the static image observed during regular vibration. When asynchronous, the light is pulsed at one or two cycles faster than the fundamental frequency, thus illuminating slightly different points along the vibratory cycle (albeit from different cycles of vibration). When these illuminated images are then presented in sequence at a rate of 33 frames per second, apparent vocal fold motion is created. The addition of the EGG signal to the recorded and displayed image provides a real time cycle-to-cycle signal of vocal fold vibration.[5]

EXAMINATION PROTOCOL AND TECHNIQUES

Direct imaging of the larynx during phonation, in a variety of tasks, is needed to ascertain the effect of a lesion, a particular laryngeal structure, or mode of vibration on phonatory function. Videostroboscopy is a very practical and widely used clinical technique for this purpose.[3] Although quantitative measures of acoustic and aerodynamic parameters of voice production provide valuable information about laryngeal function, clinicians can only infer, not directly observe, vocal fold vibratory information from these other quantitative measures.[5]

To perform videostroboscopy with rigid endoscopy, the patient should be seated and asked to lean forward with the chin extended at a 45-degree angle.[5] The EGG should be strapped gently on the neck. Patients should then be instructed to protrude the tongue and hold it out of the mouth with gauze. Then, the endoscope is inserted and a bright laryngeal image is obtained. A basic protocol can be followed during a videostroboscopic examination, with sufficient leeway for examining particular facets of a patient's case that are specific to the individual. At a minimum, a basic protocol should include the following tasks: inspiration, a gentle cough, a sustained vowel (usually the vowel /i/ is used), a sustained vowel with pitch and then loudness variations, a sniff immediately followed by a vowel, laryngeal diadochokinesis, and inspiratory phonation. For singers, it is useful to observe the singing of scales.[5] Flexible endoscopy does not necessitate an open mouth and permits adding connected speech tasks and whistling to the protocol. Connected speech tasks should be structured to include sentences loaded with vowels in contrast to sentences loaded with consonants.

The examiner should rate several parameters concurrently during the videostroboscopic examination. Recording the ratings and observations on a videostroboscopic protocol form can assist in data management, recall of the examination details at a later time, and also serve as a set of prompts to ensure that all examination tasks have been recorded. Several rating scales and forms have been proposed for use in videostroboscopic examination.[1,7-9] Use of these types of forms can allow observations of diagnostic importance to emerge during the examination. Intrajudge and interjudge reliability is always a concern in any type of perceptual rating instrument and has been shown to be variable for videostroboscopy evaluation forms, particularly when visual judgments need to be expressed as numerical entities or categories.[7,10] As mentioned throughout the literature on videostroboscopy, the training level of the rater is of primary importance to the validity and reliability of the use of an evaluation instrument. In developing the SERF, or Stroboscopy Evaluation Rating Form, Poburka[7] incorporated visual rating methods directly onto a drawing of a superior laryngeal view to remove the need to translate visual observations into numerical judgments.

Complete instructions and description of the examination to patients prior to starting is very important, so that patients know what to expect. Patients should be told at the onset that they can inform you if they experience discomfort. Instructions and a complete description will also assist in alleviating anxiety in patients and are particularly important when working with children.

VIDEOSTROBOSCOPIC EXAMINATIONS OF CHILDREN

Videostroboscopic examinations of children are generally undertaken via use of a flexible fiberoptic endoscope. Although cooperation can be limited, a rapid examination is generally sufficient to yield necessary information regarding vocal fold structure and function. Although higher resolution vocal fold images are generally obtained with a rigid endoscope, successful use of videostroboscopy can be negatively affected by gag reflexes in children, short phonation time, a highly oriented/posteriorly inclined epiglottis, increased pitch perturbation, and soft voice.[6] However, in a recent report, 74% of 42 children within the age range of 6 to 16 years old were successfully imaged via rigid videostroboscopy. Most of the failures in completing the rigid videostroboscopic examination were in children younger than 10 years old.[6] As such, flexible videostroboscopy is recommended for use in young children, whereas children over the age of 10 may benefit from a rigid videostroboscopic examination.

INTERPRETATION OF EXAMINATION RESULTS

Direct imaging of the larynx is critically important in obtaining a description of mass lesions or other pathophysiologic manifestations underlying the presence of a dysphonia. In most cases, videostroboscopy is a valuable addition to imaging with a straight light because it also provides information about laryngeal function.

Videostroboscopy must be performed, and resultant images interpreted, by an individual trained in the technique. The importance of training and experience cannot be overstated for obtaining excellent images and for correct interpretation of findings.[11]

Interpretation of videostroboscopic data involves a visual-perceptual task on the part of the examiner.[10] For this reason, experience in performing these types of interpretations is necessary. Knowledge of normal vocal fold anatomy and vibratory characteristics, and how anatomy and vibratory characteristics are altered by phonatory tasks or pathology is also critical for accurate interpretation.[10] Clinicians should recognize that a patient's history may introduce bias.[10] However, use of the patient's history to guide the examination is often necessary and certainly appropriate. Images should be recorded and saved for review after the examination has been completed.

When viewing the stroboscopic image, the examiner should evaluate all aspects of the appearance of the vocal folds, including the color (although this might be difficult to appreciate depending on the effectiveness of the light source, position of the velum, and characteristics of reflecting tissue), appearance of blood vessels, lesion location and size, mucus (amount, consistency), vocal fold free-edge characteristics, appearance of a microweb at the anterior commissure, symmetry of vocal fold motion during opening and closing phases, periodicity of vocal fold vibration, degree of vocal excursion for inspiration, glottic closure pattern such as presence of a glottal gap or other incomplete closure, closing phase, phase of motion, and vertical level differences between the left and right vocal folds.

Who Should Perform and Interpret Videostroboscopy?

Videolaryngostroboscopy should be performed by clinicians, whether otolaryngologists or speech-language pathologists, who have been trained to perform the examination and interpret the results. In clinical reality, local traditions and staff availability often dictate whether a speech-language pathologist or otolaryngologist performs and interprets the examinations. Performance of videolaryngostroboscopic examinations is within the scope of practice of speech-language pathologists, provided that they have appropriate training and experience.[12] A speech-language pathologist experienced in the role of performing videostroboscopic examination can increase efficiency in the clinic, allowing the physician's time to be dedicated to aspects of diagnosis and treatment not within the scope of practice of the speech-language pathologist. Interpretation of findings and treatment planning should involve a team approach.

To summarize, it is the opinion of these authors that speech-language pathologists, who are focused on acquiring an understanding of the physiologic mechanisms of vocal fold vibration, should perform recordings of laryngeal vibratory mechanics and also engage in the interpretation of findings, along with the otolaryngologist. The otolaryngologist, then, will have more time and better information to share with the patient when reviewing the medical diagnosis and surgical implications of the full voice assessment.

Most importantly, the presence and consistency of the mucosal wave and the stiffness of the vocal folds should be noted.[1,13]

During vocal fold vibration, symmetry is rated by observing the degree to which the vocal folds vibrate as mirror images of each other and reflects timing and extent of lateral excursions. Periodicity is observed during sustained phonation. Aperiodicity appears as vocal fold movement when the stroboscope is set to the patient's fundamental frequency. At this setting, the vocal folds appear to stand still when phonation is periodic, and aperiodicity is manifested as a noticeable quiver in the vocal folds. However, some caution should be used with this interpretation, as the apparent aperiodicity may also reflect difficulty with pitch tracking of the stroboscope. Vocal fold closure patterns refer to glottal shape when maximally closed for phonation and include entities such as glottal gaps and whether the closed phase is abnormally long or short indicating the pressence or absence of glottal hyper- or hypofunction. Vertical level differences between the right and left vocal fold are often best observed, or inferred, from out-of-phase motion. Mucosal wave is rated as absent if the normal traveling wave present on the superior surface of the vocal folds is not observed. Any particular areas of absent mucosal wave on the vocal folds should be noted as adynamic segments of the vocal fold. These adynamic segments likely have diagnostic significance and contribute to an overall rating of vocal fold stiffness. Similarly, limits in amplitude of vibration, or how much the vocal folds move laterally from the adducted position, also may reflect vocal fold stiffness. Limited amplitude of vibration may also result from high pitch, low effort, or poor respiratory support.

Particular attributes observed via videostroboscopy for various laryngeal pathologies are summarized in multiple volumes and cannot be discussed in proper detail here. The reader is directed to the interactive video textbook by Cornut and Bouchayer [13] and the interactive training CD by Bless and Poburka [5] for video samples of laryngeal pathologies recorded during videostroboscopic examination and the descriptions of laryngeal pathologies observed via videostroboscopy in the volume by Hirano and Bless. [1]

Because vocal fold vibration must be periodic or quasiperiodic for the stroboscope to track the fundamental frequency of vibration, videostroboscopy may not work well with severe voice disorders or aphonia. High-speed video imaging of the vocal folds is recommended in these cases, as discussed in detail in the following chapter.

In conclusion, it is critical to view the laryngeal structures, and record an image of the vocal folds in motion as part of a complete voice evaluation. Information gained during this type of procedure greatly enhances diagnosis, treatment, and patient education. Videostroboscopy is an imaging technique that is effective for this purpose for most patients with dysphonia. However, videostroboscopy requires that either a synchronized microphone or electroglottograph signal effectively tracks the fundamental frequency of the voice to trigger the light pulses in either a synchronous or asynchronous fashion. If fundamental frequency tracking cannot be done, for instance, in cases of very severe dysphonia or aphonia, then videostroboscopic examination is not the video imaging method of choice. Other methods, such as high-speed video imaging, should be used with severely aperiodic voices. In most clinical situations, however, videostroboscopy provides important information on both laryngeal structure and function, and also provides a permanent record that can be stored and referred to in the future to track changes in structure and/or function over time.

Review Questions

True or False?

1. Videostroboscopy does not track aphonic or highly dysphonic voices.

2. Videostroboscopy is a research, not a clinical, tool.

3. Videostroboscopic images are based on optical illusions.

4. Videostroboscopy does little more than straight light endoscopy recording.

5. Videostroboscopy takes too long to use in routine clinical practice.

6. Videostroboscopy need not be performed when an obvious lesion is present.

7. Videostroboscopy need not be performed over the entire range of voice.

8. Videostroboscopic interpretations do not take special training.

9. Videostroboscopy can be performed with pediatric patients.

Questions for Further Review

1. Describe the manner in which vocal fold motion is tracked by the stroboscope, and the way in which an optical illusion is generated that appears to result in slow motion.

2. What equipment and training is necessary for performing a videostroboscopic examination of the larynx?

3. What is included in a videostroboscopic examination protocol?

4. Describe aspects of laryngeal structure and function that should be observed, rated, and recorded during a videostroboscopic examination.

5. From further reading and observation, such as from the book by Hirano and Bless,[1] the training CD by Bless and Poburka,[4] and the video textbook by Cornut and Bouchayer,[11] appreciate and describe the aspects of laryngeal structure and function most commonly observed with different dysphonias and laryngeal pathologies.

REFERENCES

1. Hirano M, Bless DM. *Videostroboscopic Examination of the Larynx*. San Diego, Calif. Singular Publishing Group Inc; 1993.

2. Dejonckere PH, Bradley P, Clemente P, et al. A basic protocol for functional assessment of voice pathology, especially for investigating the efficacy of (phonological) treatments and evaluating new assessment techniques: guideline elaborated by the Committee on Phoniatrics of the European Laryngological Society (ELS). *Eur Arch Otorhinolaryngol.* 2001;258:77–82.

3. Behrman A. Common practices of voice therapists in the evaluation of patients. *J Voice.* 2005; 19:454–469.

4. Woo P, Casper J, Colton R, Brewer D. Diagnostic value of stroboscopic examination in hoarse patients. *J Voice.* 1991;5:231–238.

5. Bless DM, Poburka B. *Video Laryngeal Stroboscopy* [book on CD-ROM]. Clifton Park, NY: Thomson Delmar Learning; 2002.

6. Wolf W, Primov-Fever A, Amir O, Jedwab D. The feasibility of rigid stroboscopy in children. *Int J Pediatr Otorhinolaryngol.* 2005;69:1077–1079.

7. Poburka B. A new stroboscopy rating form. *J Voice.* 1999;13, 403–413.

8. Poburka BJ, Bless DM. A multi-media, computer-based method for stroboscopy rating training. *J Voice.* 1998;12:513–526.

9. Rosen CA. Stroboscopy as a research instrument: development of a perceptual evaluation tool. *Laryngoscope.* 2005;115(3):423-428.

10. Teitler N. Examiner bias: influence of patient history on perceptual ratings of videostroboscopy. *J Voice.* 1995;9:95–105.

11. American Speech–Language Hearing Association. Vocal tract visualization and imaging: technical report. *ASHA Suppl.* 2004;24:140–145.

12. American Speech-Language-Hearing Association. Vocal tract visualization and imaging: position statement. *ASHA Suppl.* 2004;24:140–145.

13. Cornut G, Bouchayer M. *Assessing Dysphonia. The Role of Videostroboscopy* [An Interactive Video Textbook]. Lincoln Park, NJ: KayPENTAX; 2004.

14. Sataloff RT, Spiegel JR, Hawkshaw MJ. Strobovideolaryngoscopy: results and clinical value. *Ann Otol Rhinol Laryngol.* 1991;100:725–727.

4

Laryngeal High-Speed Digital Imaging and Kymography

Rita Patel, MS
Diane M. Bless, PhD

KEY POINTS

- Video imaging of laryngeal motion is critical to understanding the structure and function of the larynx.

- High-speed digital imaging and kymography provide a permanent record of the actual cycle-to-cycle motion of the vocal folds.

- High-speed digital imaging and kymography can be used with all voice disorders regardless of the degree of dysphonia; the images can be used for both qualitative and quantitative descriptions of laryngeal behavior.

- Training is necessary for both recording and analyzing the images.

- Measures of vocal function can be obtained with high-speed digital and kymographic recordings that cannot be obtained with stroboscopy or acoustical analysis.

Fundamental to appropriate diagnoses and treatment of vocal fold pathology is direct visualization of vocal fold vibratory patterns. In the last several years, new concepts in the area of voice, voice diagnostics, image analysis, and modeling have been developed to shed light on mechanisms of irregular vocal fold vibrations.

Videostroboscopy, as detailed in the preceeding chapter, is routinely used in clinic for examination of vocal fold dynamics, but it is designed to examine periodic vocal fold vibrations, making it less valid for aperiodic voices. Moreover, videostroboscopy provides an *apparent motion* making it impossible to assess cycle-to-cycle vocal fold motions that are especially critical for comprehensive clinical appraisal of subjects with hoarseness. *High-speed digital imaging* (HSDI) and *kymography* appear to overcome these limitations because they are not limited to periodic voices, and initiate recording immediately regardless of vocal frequency or loudness,[1] or degree of dysphonia, a feat that cannot be said for stroboscopy. A comparison of advantages and disadvantages of videostroboscopy and clinical high-speed imaging are listed in Table 4–1.

TABLE 4–1. A Comparison of Advantages and Disadvantages of Stroboscopy and Clinical High-Speed Imaging Systems

No.	Stroboscopy	Clinical High Speed Imaging
1.	Sampling rate: 25 to 30 frames per second.	Sampling rate: 2000 to 4000 frames per second. Research systems with temporal resolution of up to 8000 fps available.
2.	Dependent on stable phonation. Fails in voiceless cases or very hoarse voice qualities.	Not dependent on stable phonation. Can analyze extremely aperiodic voice qualities.
3.	Requires phonation duration times of at least 2–3 seconds. Phonation of >1 second needed to observe one vibratory cycle as the frequency of strobe motion is about 1 to 2 Hz.[2]	No minimum requirements of phonation duration. Analysis of phonations >1 second possible. This permits observation of momentary breaks in phonation, vocal onset, and vocal offset.
4.	Maximum resolution of about 750 × 500 pixels.	Maximum resolution of about 256 × 256 pixels.
5.	Recording duration limited only by size of recording media (tape, computer memory, or disk).	Recording duration ranges limited from 2 to 8 seconds depending on selected resolution.
6.	Routinely used in clinic, but poor research tool for gaining insights into cycle-to-cycle variations of vocal fold motion.	Excellent for use in both clinic and research.
7.	Observing transient phenomena like voice breaks, extremely small aphonic segments, vocal tremor,[3] and onset of phonation impossible.	Detailed analysis of phenomena like voice breaks, extremely small aphonic segments, vocal tremor,[3] voice onset and voice offset possible.
8.	Yields an apparent vibratory motion.	Yields real time cycle-to-cycle vibratory motion.
9.	Quantification of "actual" glottal gap size, amplitude of vibrations, and size of vocal pathology[4] is difficult due to the resultant apparent vibratory motion.	Quantification for "actual" glottal gap size, amplitude of vibrations, and size of pathology possible.
10.	Availability of reliable and valid semi-automated software programs for easy extractions of glottal parameters limited.	Semi-automated software programs for easy extractions of glottal parameters readily available.
11.	Rigid and flexible endoscopy possible.	Color HSDI limited to 90° endoscope. Use of 70° endoscope possible for black and white HSDI. Flexible endoscopy not possible at this time.
12.	Simultaneous sampling of acoustic and electroglottographic signals possible.	Simultaneous sampling of acoustic and electroglottographic signals possible.

HISTORICAL REVIEW

High-speed imaging was first developed in 1942 by Bell Telephone Laboratories.[5] The early high-speed systems were bulky, difficult to use, recorded films required subsequent development that often revealed no usable data and usable recordings, and required laborious frame-by-frame analysis. Also the camera noise, limited recording duration, and problems with synchronizing additional signals for voice measurements prevented widespread clinical acceptance of high-speed imaging. Moore, von Leden, and Timcke in the late 1960s first used the above prototype high-speed system to study the vocal fold dynamics of normal and pathologic (unilateral vocal fold paralysis, edema, unilateral polyp, bilateral polyps, benign neoplasm, hematoma, vocal fold web) voices under various phonatory conditions (pitch and loudness variations).[6-9] Using high-speed recordings, these authors were also able to describe transient but complex vocal fold behavior for phenomena like cough, inspiratory phonation, laughter, and vocal fry. Nevertheless, the combination of difficulties encountered with equipment, recordings and analysis resulted in analysis of only a few seconds of phonation obtained from a few subjects. In fact, most of our current knowledge of normal dynamic vocal fold vibration is derived from a small number of subjects ranging from one subject[6,8] to a maximum of four subjects.[7] Even as late as the 1970s, attempts at quantification of vocal parameters and data reduction of high-speed images were technologically improved but still cumbersome and clinically impractical.[10-12]

Contemporary development of digital technology has led to much needed improvements in the camera, sensor systems, recording capabilities, and memory of the recording systems that were originally designed for nonmedical purposes, such as car crash tests,[9] thereby extending its application to clinical assessment of voice. As a result of technologic advancements, since the middle to late 1990s, there has been a surge of laboratory-based studies[13-17] investigating the research and clinical applications of high-speed digital imaging especially in the European literature. Efforts to develop semi-automated motion tracking and motion analysis software like the high-speed toolbox[18] and multidimensional voice analysis system (MVAS)[19] were initiated. More recently, Yan et al[20] proposed the glottal area waveform (GAW) method to analyze normal and abnormal vocal fold vibrations. These systems are fast, generally taking no more than a couple of minutes, and yield quantitative measurements of vocal fold vibratory patterns. One example of a commercially available program for extraction of quantitative glottal parameters is depicted in Figure 4–1.

Currently available high-speed systems reach a maximum speed of 8,000 frames per second but vary with duration and resolution. Commonly commercially available clinical systems record 2000 to 4000 frames per second with recording durations ranging from 2 to 8 seconds. Spatial resolution ranges from 160×140 pixels to 256×256 pixels for clinical high-speed systems. Simultaneous recording of both acoustic and electroglottographic signals are also possible. Measures identical to those obtained with stroboscopy are possible but represent *every cycle of vibration*. Interpretation of vocal fold amplitudes, glottal width, left-right asynchrony, temporal change of vibrations, mucosal waves, vertical plane difference between the vocal folds, and closure patterns can be judged using high-speed recordings. Characterizing the three-dimensional movement of the vocal fold vibrations in the lateral plane (adduction vs abduction), vertical phase shift (mucosal wave), and the inferior and superior margins, is also possible using high-speed imaging.

APPLICATIONS OF HSDI FOR LARYNGEAL IMAGING

Applications of HSDI for clinical imaging of the larynx are broad. However, because of recording limitations in its current form, it augments rather than replaces stroboscopy. Nevertheless, it is a valuable clinical tool that can be successfully used to evaluate various types of vocal fold vibrations, even extremely aperiodic voice qualities and phonations of less than 1 second.

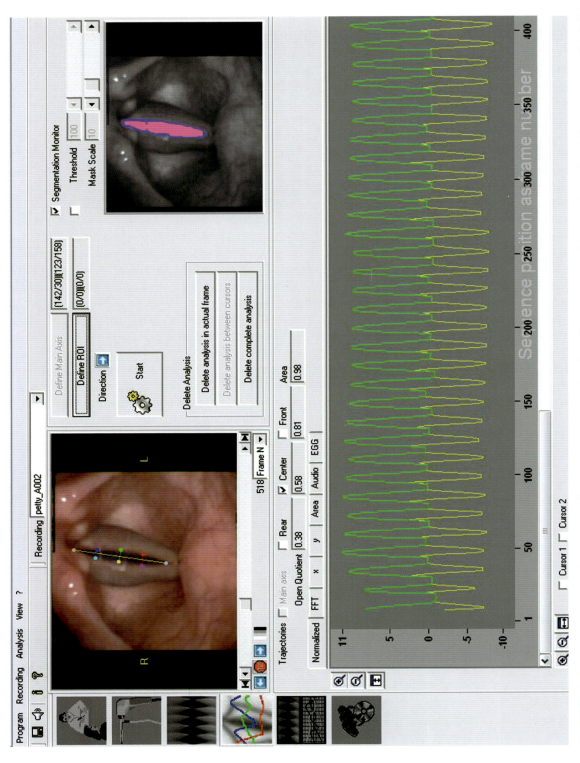

FIGURE 4–1. One example of commercially available automatic glottal feature extraction program. Vocal fold image on the left shows six points along the length of the vocal fold that tracts vocal fold amplitude across the anterior section, mid-membranous section, and posterior section of the right and left vocal fold. The graph below shows the extracted vocal fold amplitude of the mid-membranous section of the right (*green*) and left (*yellow*) vocal fold. (Courtesy of Richard Wolf Medical Instruments Corporation.)

Clinically, it is particularly useful in the setting of hoarseness that may not be explained or well characterized by stroboscopy; these abnormalities may include nonlinear dynamics such as subharmonics and bifurcations.

HSDI excels at the examination of phonatory onset and offset.[14] Traditional stroboscopy is not capable of delineating these subtleties. Furthermore, HSDI can simultaneously analyze vibratory motion with acoustic, electroglottographic, and inverse filtered signals.[21] The refined information from these imaging modalities may be able to detect even the minute return of function in cases of paresis and paralysis, as well as providing independent assessment of right and left vocal fold motions, glottal symmetry, and glottal area estimates. Specific transient vibratory phenomena, such as glissando, are better seen with these modalities as opposed to stroboscopy.[22]

In the area of basic research, high-speed imaging has been used for obtaining insights into glottal properties with use of the excised larynx setup,[23,24] as well as for the precise, noninvasive measurement of vocal fold length through the projection of two parallel laser beams onto the vocal fold.[25] In addition to the general vibratory dynamics and voice assessment applications, HSDI has been documented to be of particular

Do Clinical Impressions of Disorders Differ as a Function of Imaging Technique?

It is intriguing to contemplate how images of various voice disorders would differ between stroboscopy, high-speed imaging, and kymography. Would a malingering patient be more easily identified by one and not the other? The relatively long sample recorded from stroboscopy might make it more difficult for a speaker to maintain a false voice. On the other hand, the ability of kymography and HSDI to record initiation, whispering, and sudden but brief duration shifts in sustained vibratory modes (characteristics that may be present in malingerers) allows for subtle characterization not possible with stroboscopy. Even though HSDI is in its technological infancy, recordings of spastic dysphonic patients have already shown that laryngeal profiling of subgroups such as adductor, abductor, and mixed spastic dysphonia are possible with as little as 2 seconds of high-speed recording. The highly irregular patterns of severely dysphonic paralysis patients cannot be tracked longitudinally with stroboscopy because of high perturbation levels. Because this is not a limitation with HSDI or kymography, these findings may be used to predict return of function and aid in management decisions. Kymography makes interpretation of some of the images more objective consequently reducing observer bias. With kymography, it is straightforward to determine when there is no amplitude or a reduced mucosal wave, out-of-phase movement, or other aperiodicities of vibratory cycles. Software programs can be applied to both strobe and high-speed images to provide similar measures but one must question validity of measurements when the signal is highly irregular.

benefit to specific clinical cases. In some cases, it characterizes the disorder; in others it differentiates it from pathology with similar vocal characteristics; and in still others, it provides a means to document changes resulting from treatment.

The specific clinical indications reported for HSDI are numerous, and include the presence of diplophonia[26] and tremor,[4] as well as the detailed examination of benign vocal lesions and scar and stiffness of the vocal fold. HSDI is used for the assessment of moderate to severe voice disturbances[27] that cannot be reliably recorded with stroboscopy. Some authors have advocated its utility in distinguishing muscle tension dysphonia from spastic dysphonia.

At the extremes of vocal performance, HSDI has been investigated in determining the vibratory source of neoglottis and the pharyngoesophageal segment in laryngectomees.[28,29] Singers may be evaluated by these modalites, particularly for singing styles whose ranges may fall outside standard stroboscopy, such as rock singing[30] and Mongolian throat singing.[31] Finally, HSDI is useful in the investigation of low frequency or slow vibrations such as present in ventricular fold vibrations[32] and glottal fry. HSDI is relatively new; it is likely that future study will reveal additional clinical applications.

Although contemporary laryngology clinics would not function without stroboscopy, few have embraced high-speed imaging. This may be due, at least in part, to the cost of available high-speed systems and clinicians wishing to be responsible in helping control the rising costs of medical care. It also may be related to some of the current limitations of high-speed imaging. High-speed imaging requires greater skill from the examiner than does stroboscopy because: the recorded samples are shorter, flexible endoscopes cannot be used, some systems do not have color, it is difficult to use with pediatric cases, playback does not include simultaneous audio, and interpretations requires additional training. However, because technology is changing rapidly, some of the above limitations of high-speed imaging will likely be overcome in the near future.

KYMOGRAPHY

Recognition of the clinical importance of imaging every cycle of vibration in combination with the often prohibitive cost of these technologies motivated the development of video kymography, referred to as the "poor clinician's" HSDI because it has some of the advantages of high-speed imaging over stroboscopy but does so at one-fourth the cost. A kymogram or kymograph is a spatiotemporal image that shows a fixed horizontal line in the vocal fold image over time (see Figure 4–2). As the successive line images are presented in

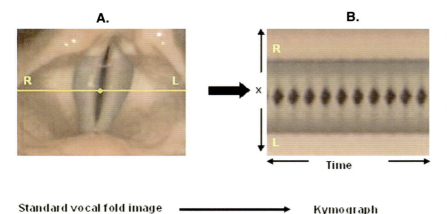

A.

B.

Standard vocal fold image ⟶ Kymograph

FIGURE 4–2. Generation of kymograph from high-speed digital imaging. **A.** A horizontal line along the mid-membranous portion of the vocal fold image obtained using high-speed digital imaging is used to generate a kymograph. **B.** When a kymograph is generated from high-speed imaging it is also called a digital kymograph.

real time, the system makes it possible to observe left-right asymmetries, open quotient, propagation of mucosal waves, and anterioposterior modes of vocal fold vibration.[33] Gall et al in 1970 first used a technique called "photokymography" to record vocal fold oscillations. Subsequent modifications of the above techniques in the 1970s were called larynx-photokymography, strip-kymography, and microphotokymography.[34] Modern kymographic techniques can be divided into two types: videokymography[35] and digital kymography.[34]

Videokymography

In 1994 videokymography (VKG) was developed by Švec and Schutte as a low-cost and better time resolution (8,000 frames per second) alternative to high-speed imaging.[35] VKG is obtained using a specialized CCD video camera that operates in two modes: standard and high-speed. In the standard mode, it records black and white images at 25 to 60 frames per second. In the high-speed mode, the system records black and white kymographic images at 8000 frames per second of an

Where We Have Come From: High-Speed Film

Paul Moore once said that there have been miles of high-speed film taken but only seconds of voice analyzed. This is not surprising when one takes a historical perspective. The development of HSDI is not unlike that of computer development. The early recordings required that a whole room be devoted to the large bulky recording apparatus. The systems needed to be table- or wall-mounted as they were far too heavy to be hand-held. They required a large water bath to cool the hot light so as not to burn the laryngeal tissue, camera housing to reduce the loud noise, and a rigid imaging apparatus that reflected light on a mirror used to illuminate the larynx. Subjects were positioned over the mirror with both neck and tongue extended. Once the larynx was visualized, they were asked to phonate /i/; when the camera was activated, a loud bang occurred followed by the buzz of the camera. The noise was sufficiently loud that it startled many patients so that they physically jumped and, in so doing, modified image placement. After the recording session was completed, the film was sent out to be developed and returned by the developers a week or so later. Often the recording started too early or late to record the phenomenon of interest. Sound synchronization was often not possible. The useful footage would be placed over a tracing, and later, a digitizing, plate, and laboriously traced frame-by-frame. *One second* (several thousand frames of film) would take hours and hours of measurement. New technology has made the current HSDI systems appear to be distant cousins. The ability to visualize the image while recording from a handheld instrument and subsequently use semiautomated software to analyze the waveform would have seemed impossible in the not too remote past.

examiner-selected single horizontal line section along the length of the vocal fold (Figure 4–3). It is critical to position this horizontal line perpendicular to the glottal axis for accurate interpretation of kymographs obtained from VKG. (Gross movements of the larynx could make the recording position inaccurate.) In VKG, positioning this horizontal line is achieved more readily with the use of a 90° rigid endoscope. To view oscillations across multiple horizontal sections along the length of the vocal fold separate endoscopic recordings are required for each horizontal section. The spatial resolution of the resultant kymographs is 768 pixels per line. Recording duration is virtually unlimited because fewer data have to be stored and processed when compared to HSDI. However, VKG lacks a full video image of the vocal folds.

Digital Kymography

Kymographs obtained from high-speed video recordings using software analysis methods of

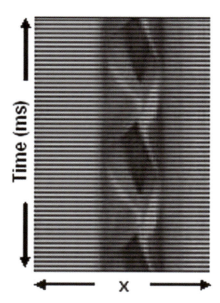

FIGURE 4–3. Videokymographic image obtained using a specialized CCD camera. Particularly note the black and white image and time along the ordinate compared to digital kymography where time is often depicted along the abscissa.

image processing are called digital kymographs (DK) or functional images.[34] In 1999, Wittenberg et al first reported extractions of multiplane kymographs from high-speed digital videos.[36] As the DK kymographs are obtained from high-speed digital video recordings the resultant DK are limited to the color, spatial, and temporal resolution of the original high-speed recordings. Presently the maximum possible spatial, and temporal resolution for clinical digital kymographs is 4,000 frames per second and 256 pixels per line, respectively. Both black and white and color DK can be obtained. Although more expensive than VKG, the DK are attractive because of the ease of examining vocal fold oscillations simultaneously from multiple horizontal sections along the vocal fold length from a single phonatory sample (Figure 4-4). This allows the examiner to easily study the tissue across a lesion and to compare anterior and posterior and lateral vibratory modes without making multiple recordings. Moreover, although general applications of VKG and DK are similar to those of HSDI, they can better define the extent of mucosal wave propagation, visibility of upper and lower margins of the vocal folds, glottal axis movement during closure, assess changes in opening and closing phases, and detect ventricular fold movements during phonation.[37]

In summary, HSDI and kymography allow for physiologically based interpretations of irregular vocal fold vibrations that can be based on the classic body cover theory[38] of vocal fold vibration. Interpretation involves the use of labels similar to those used in stroboscopy ratings (eg, mucosal wave, phase symmetry). Examiner retraining is required to make the finer qualitative vibratory pattern judgments made not from stroboscopic optical illusions of apparent motion obtained from frames of several segments of different cycles, but of thousands of frames reflecting individual vibratory cycles. Two sequential recordings, stroboscopy/endoscopy for structural examinations and simultaneous high-speed/kymographic, audio, and electroglottographic recordings may aid in complete analysis of vocal fold vibrations.

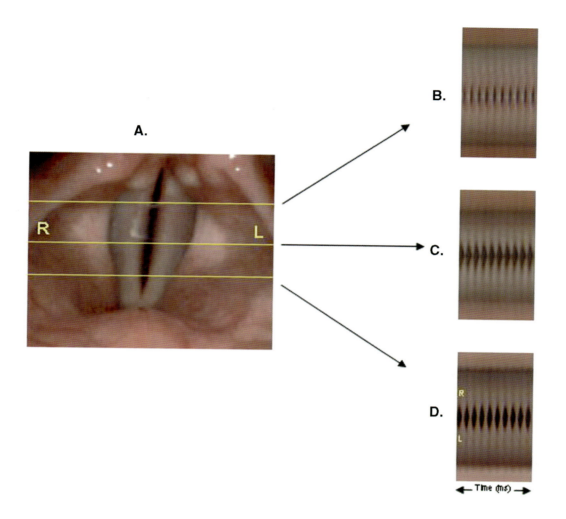

A.

B.

C.

D.

←—Time (ms)—→

Standard vocal fold image ——————————→ **Multi-plane Kymography**

FIGURE 4–4. Multiplane kymography from high-speed digital recording. **A.** Horizontal lines along the length of the vocal fold across to generate simultaneous multiplane kymography to compare vibratory characteristics across the anterior commissure, mid-membranous section, and posterior section of the vocal fold. **B.** Kymograph of the posterior section of the vocal fold **C.** Kymograph of the mid-membranous region. **D.** Kymograph of the anterior section of the vocal fold.

Review Questions

True or False:

1. High-speed imaging is not better than stroboscopy.

2. High-speed imaging is a research, not a clinical tool.

3. High-speed imaging and kymography give you the same information.

4. High-speed imaging depends on each and every cycle of vibration.

5. Kymographic imaging can be done with image processing software on high-speed images.

6. Kymographic imaging is unique in its ability to visualize the upper and lower lip of vibration.

REFERENCES

1. Eysholdt U, Mergell P, Tigges M, Wittenberg T, Proschel U. Direct evaluation of high-speed recordings of vocal fold vibrations. *Folia Phoniatr Logoped.* 1996;48:163–170.

2. Hertegård S. What have we learned about laryngeal physiology from high-speed digital videoendoscopy? *Curr Opin Otolaryngol Head Neck Surg.* 2005;13:152–156.

3. Colton R, Casper J. Understanding voice problems. 2nd ed. Baltimore, Md: Williams & Wilkins; 1996.

4. Hertegård S, Larsson H, Wittenberg T. High-speed imaging: applications and development. *Logoped Phoniatr Vocol.* 2003;28:133–139.

5. Fransworth DW. High-speed motion pictures of human vocal folds. *Bell Tel Rec.* 1940;18:203–208.

6. Moore P, von Leden H. Dynamic vibrations of the vibratory pattern in the normal larynx. *Folia Phonatr.* 1958;10:205–238.

7. Timcke R, von Leden H, Moore P. Laryngeal vibrations: measurements of the glottic wave. Part I. The normal vibratory cycle. *Arch Otolaryngol.* 1958;68:1–19.

8. Timcke R, von Leden H, Moore P. Laryngeal vibrations: measurements of the glottic wave. Part II Physiologic variations. *Arch Otolaryngol.* 1969; 69:438–444.

9. von Leden H, Moore P, Timcke R. Laryngeal vibrations: measurements of the glottic wave. Part III The pathologic larynx. *Arch Otolaryngol.* 1960; 71:16–35.

10. Booth JR, Childers DG. Automated analysis of ultra high-speed laryngeal films. *IEEE Transactions Biomed Eng.* 1979;26(4):185–192.

11. Tanabe M, Kitajima K, Gould W, Lambiase A. Analysis of high-speed motion pictures of the vocal folds. *Folia Phonatr.* 1975;27:77–87.

12. Koike Y, Hirano M. Glottal area time functiona and subglottal-pressure variations. *J Acoust Soc Am.* 1973;54(6):1618–1627.

13. Wittenberg T, Mergell P, Tigges M, Eysholdt U. Quantitative characterization of functional voice disorders using motion analysis of high-speed video and modeling. *IEEE Trans.* 1997;10:1663–1666.

14. Wittenberg T, Moser M, Tigges M, Eysholdt U. Recording, processing and analysis of digital highspeed sequences in glottography. *Mach Vis Applic.* 1995;20:100–112.

15. Tigges M, Wittenberg T, Mergell P, Eysholdt U. Imaging of vocal fold vibration by digital multiplane kymography. *Comp Med Imag Graphics.* 1999;23:323–330.

16. Eysholdt U, Mergell P, Tigges M, Wittenberg T, Proschel U. Direct evaluation of high-speed recordings of vocal fold vibrations. *Folia Phoniatr Logoped.* 1996;48:163–170.

17. Kiritani S, Hirose H, Imagawa H. High-speed digital image analysis of vocal cord vibration in diplophonia. *Speech Comm.* 1993;13:23–32.

18. Larsson H, Hertegård S, Lindestad P-A, Hammarberg B. Vocal fold vibrations: high-speed imaging, kymography, and acoustic analysis; a preliminary report. *Laryngoscope.* 2000;110:2117–2122.

19. Köster O, Marx B, Gemmar, Hess M, Künzel H. Qualitative and quantitative analysis of voice onset by means of a Multidimensional Voice Analysis System (MVAS) using high-speed imaging. *J Voice.* 1998;13(3):355–374.

20. Yan Y, Ahmad K, Kunduk M, Bless D. Analysis of vocal-fold vibrations from high-speed laryngeal images using a hilbert transform-based methodology. *J Voice.* 2005;19(2):161–175.

21. Granqvist S, Hertegård S, Larsson H, Sundberg J. Simultaneous analysis of vocal fold vibration and transglottal airflow; exploring a new experimental set-up. *Speech Music Hear.* 2003;45:33–46.

22. Hoppe U, Rosanowski F, Dollinger M, Lohscheller J, Schuster M, Eysholdt U. Glissando: laryngeal motorics and acoustics. *J Voice.* 2003;17(3):370–376.

23. Jiang JJ, Yumoto E, Lin SJ, Kadota Y, Kurokawa H, Hanson DG. Quantitative measurement of mucosal wave by high-speed photography in excised larynges. *Ann Oto Rhinol Laryngol.* 1998;107:98–103.

24. Berry DA, Montequin DW, Tayama N. High-speed digital imaging of the medial surface of the vocal folds. *J Acoust Soc Am.* 2001;110(5 pt. 1):2539–2547.

25. Schuberth S, Hoppe U, Döllinger M, Lohscheller J, Eysholdt U. High-precision measurement of the vocal fold length and vibratory amplitudes, *Laryngoscope.* 2002;112(6):1043–1049.

26. Kiritani S, Hirose H, Imagawa H. High-speed digital image analysis of vocal cord vibration in diplophonia. *Speech Comm.* 1993;13:23–32.

27. Titze I. R. (1995). *Workshop on Acoustic Voice Analysis, Summary Statement.* Iowa City: NCVS, Wendell Johnson Speech and Hearing Center, The University of Iowa; 1995.

28. Van As CJ, Op De Coul BM, Eysholdt U, Hilgers FJ. Value of digital high-speed endoscopy in addition to videofluroscopic imaging of the neoglottis in tracheoesophageal speech. *Acta Otolaryngol.* 2004;124:82–89.

29. Lundstrom E, Hammarberg B. High-speed imaging of the voicing source in laryngectomees during production of voiced-voiceless distinctions for stop consonants. *Logoped Phoniatr Vocol.* 2004;29(1):31–40.

30. Borch DZ, Sundberg J, Lindestad PA, Thalen M. Vocal fold vibration and voice source aperiodicity in 'dist' tones: a study of a timbral ornament in rock singing. *Logoped Phoniatr Vocol.* 2004;29(4):147–153.

31. Lindestad PA, Sodersten M, Merker B, Granqvist S. Voice source characteristics in Mongolian "throat singing" studied with high-speed imaging technique, acoustic spectra, and inverse filtering. *J Voice.* 2001;15(1):78–85.

32. Lindestad PA, Blixt V, Olsson JP, Hammarberg B. Ventricular fold vibration in voice production: a high-speed imaging study with kymographic, acoustic and perceptual analyses of a voice patient and a vocally healthy subject. *Logoped Phoniatr Vocol.* 2004;29(4):162–170.

33. Tigges M, Wittenberg T, Mergell P, Eysholdt U. Imaging of vocal fold vibration by digital multiplane kymography. *Comp Med Imag Graphics.* 1999;23:323–330.

34. Wittenberg T, Tigges M, Mergell P, Eysholdt U. Functional imaging of vocal fold vibration: digital multislice high-speed kymography. *J Voice.* 1997;14(3):422–442.

35. Švec JG, Shutte HK. Videokymography: high-speed line scanning of vocal fold vibration. *J Voice.* 1996;10:201–205.

36. Tigges M, Wittenberg T, Mergell P, Eysholdt U. Imaging of vocal fold vibration by digital multiplane kymography. *Comp Med Imag Graphics.* 1999;23:323–330.

37. Švec JG, Sram F. Kymographic imaging of the vocal fold oscillations. In: Hansen JHL, Pellom B, eds. *ICSLP-Conference proceedings.* Vol 2. 7th International Conference on Spoken Language Processing. September 16-19, 2002; Denver, Colo; Boulder, Colo: Center for Spoken Language.

38. Hirano M. *Clinical examination of voice.* 5th ed. Berlin: Springer-Verlag, 1981.

5

Clinical and Instrumental Evaluation of the Voice Patient

Claudio F. Milstein, PhD
Douglas M. Hicks, PhD

KEY POINTS

- An optimal voice evaluation is accomplished by teamwork between an otolaryngologist and an SLP with expertise in voice disorders.

- A mirror exam alone is not adequate for comprehensive evaluation of a voice patient. Videostroboscopy is the most useful instrumental tool for evaluation of voice disorders.

- The core voice evaluation is comprised of a thorough case history, perceptual assessment, and videoendoscopic examination, complemented by other objective diagnostic techniques.

Regardless of discipline or training, all practitioners routinely employ fundamental evaluation and management methods that are not unique to the laryngology patient, such as taking a case history, generating a clinical diagnosis, and offering treatment recommendations. The focus of this chapter, however, is to address more fully components unique to the voice disordered population to maximize patient outcome and clinical efficiency.

The chapter follows the format of the management tree outlined in the next section. Some of the points are self-explanatory and require no additional comment; whereas others will be the focus of more detailed discussion.

The gold standard of clinical care for laryngology patients involves a team approach between an otolaryngologist and a speech-language pathologist (SLP) with expertise in voice care. The assumption is that the combination of both disciplines renders better treatment than can be obtained by either discipline in isolation. This philosophy is implied in a joint statement between the American Academy of Otoloaryngology and the American Speech-Language-Hearing Association.[1]

OUTLINE OF EVALUATION— MANAGEMENT TREE

1. Training requirements
2. Review of information from referral sources and previous medical records
3. Case history
   a. Questionnaire
      i. Past and present symptoms
      ii. Onset and duration
      iii. Clinical course and variability
      iv. Previous treatments
      v. Vocal symptoms
      vi. Other related symptomatology
      vii. Medical history
      viii. Medications
      ix. Tobacco, alcohol, caffeine intake
      x. Family history
      xi. Voice use
      xii. Environmental issues
      xiii. Stress/anxiety
4. Patient's perception of the problem
   a. Voice quality of life measures (eg, V-RQOL, Voice Handicap Index, VHI-10)
5. Perceptual evaluation
   a. Listen to voice quality
      i. Physical appearance, age, weight, height, facial expression
      ii. Patient interaction with clinician and others
      iii. Posture
      iv. Breathing patterns
      v. Signs of musculoskeletal tension
   b. Administer standard perceptual evaluation scales (eg, GRBAS, CAPE-V)
6. Working hypothesis
7. Head and neck evaluation
8. Laryngeal and hypopharyngeal evaluation
   a. Endoscopic
   b. Videostroboscopic
9. Diagnostic probe therapy. Concept of stimulability.
10. Objective measures
    a. Acoustic
    b. Aerodynamic
    c. EMG, Sensory testing
11. Additional testing (eg, diagnostic imaging (CT, MRI, PET, blood tests, etc)
12. Diagnosis and recommendations

Training Requirements

Routine clinical interaction with voice-disordered patients confirms that their treatment requires special training and knowledge for both otolaryngologists and SLPs. It is not sufficient to simply have a grasp of normal and pathologic anatomy of the larynx and pharynx. Beyond sound fundamentals, the practitioner must keep abreast of new developments. As previewed in chapter 2, new research related to vocal fold histology, scar formation physiology, use of new biomaterials, nerve reinnervation, and implantable devices for nerve stimulation are continually advancing the field of laryngology/vocology.

Case History

The importance of a taking a complete and thorough case history cannot be stressed enough. Even in highly motivated and insightful voice patients, their inherent naiveté about laryngeal function may influence the revelation of critical information for proper diagnosis and treatment. Therefore, the burden of uncovering this information falls to the skilled clinician with a thorough case history.

Questionnaire

An invaluable tool for case history intake is a well-organized voice-related questionnaire, which serves several purposes: (a) it allows the patient to more accurately reflect on the nature and history of his or her problem before meeting with the clinician; (b) it helps the patient recall pertinent information, some of which may not seem intuitively relevant to their voice problem (eg, thyroid function, specific asthma medicines, late night eating habits); (c) it improves efficiency for the clinician by highlighting contributing factors unique to that patient. Several excellent examples of questionnaires can be found in published textbooks.[2,3]

Problem-specific questionnaires, such as the Reflux Symptom Index[4] (see chapter 17, Reflux and the Larynx) can be helpful. This tool conveniently addresses a number of symptoms or complaints that might suggest the presence of laryngopharyngeal reflux, which is now perceived as important to assess and treat in voice patients.

It may be helpful to have an additional questionnaire specifically designed for singers and professional voice users. Information related to the patient's level of vocal training, performance experience, as well as his or her current and upcoming professional schedule, can affect treatment, just as in the field of sports medicine with athletes.

Patient's Perception of Problem

The current trend in health care toward treatment efficacy and outcomes parallels the value in obtaining patient perception of their vocal problem. This can be accomplished effectively with several validated quality of life instruments, such as the Voice Handicap Index (VHI) and the Voice-Related Quality of Life Questionnaire (V-RQOL).[5,6]

An obvious benefit is to help patients clarify how the current vocal problem impacts their personal and professional life. This speaks to the "functional adequacy" of their voice, which directly relates to the clinician's insight for treatment recommendations. For example, a patient whose sole motivation is reassurance that they do not have a life-threatening condition may not be interested in pursuing treatment options to improve voice quality. In contrast, there are patients whose vocal demands and expectations are sufficient so even minor hoarseness cannot be tolerated, making them almost desperate for sophisticated treatment. Ultimately, with the aid of these tools, we can clarify individual patients' specific expectation for seeking help, as well as help them define their vocal problems. In this way, the clinician can provide prescriptive care, the essence of excellent clinical practice.

An extra value of these instruments is their ability to track progress as a function of treatment, as defined by patient's perception. As an example, changes in patient's ratings over time can be highly reassuring and motivate the patient for continued compliance with treatment strategies.

Perceptual Evaluation

Listening to the patient goes beyond the obvious hearing of their voice performance. It is essential that the clinician learns to attend to the message of concern, which is always expressed by the patient in some fashion. While taking the case history, the clinician informally begins a perceptual evaluation. This requires not only carefully listening to voice quality, but monitoring physical appearance, vocal behaviors, posture, breathing patterns, signs of musculoskeletal tension, and the patient's interaction with the clinician and others.

The formal perceptual evaluation represents a protocol of eliciting representative voice performance through the use of instructions, prompts, and demonstrations. This process is facilitated by categorizing the voice into various performance parameters (pitch, loudness, laryngeal quality, and resonance). Tasks specifically designed to elicit performance in these areas are standard among clinicians, although the exact protocol varies greatly from clinician to clincian. It should be strongly stated that this important step of clinical evaluation is not an objective evaluation of the voice, but rather a formal organization of one's subjective assessment of the voice.

Characterization of voice quality in terms of severity of dysphonia and specific voice parameters (such as hoarseness, breathiness, strain) can be addressed through several published classification systems such as GRBAS scale and CAPE-V (Figure 5–1).[7,8] These have evolved in an effort to establish standardization, thereby improving reproducibility of results within and across clinicians.

Working Hypothesis

The clinician should not lose sight of the fact that all information gathered to this point is a building process leading to a working hypothesis on the nature of the problem. This requires the clinician to actively evaluate this clinical information rather than simply collect it.

By the end of the case history intake and the perceptual evaluation, the clinician should be able to establish an initial working hypothesis on the nature of the problem. The remaining instrumental/objective evaluation phase allows either the confirmation or rejection of that hypothesis. Such an approach reduces the inefficiency of examining the patient out of context—avoiding diving into an exam with a blank slate.

Laryngeal and Hypopharyngeal Evaluation

A mirror examination alone is not sufficient for evaluating the complexities of phonatory function. Thankfully, the availability of sophisticated imaging tools allows any serious practitioner with voice patients to be well equipped. In particular, videostroboscopy is routinely perceived as the most valuable tool under objective voice assessment (see chapter 3, Videostroboscopy).

An important topic that transcends any endoscopic technique is garnering optimal patient cooperation. Patient participation is fostered by careful "prescoping" instructions so the patient is fully informed of the procedure (eg, briefly review the entire protocol including nose/mouth preparation, scope insertion, duration of procedure, and anticipated physical sensations). The benefits of taking a few extra moments to accomplish this cannot be underestimated. In essence, whatever the clinician can do to make the patient relax will benefit the accuracy and completeness of differential diagnosis based on the exam. Inherent in this philosophy is the additional requirement of obtaining a representative sample of voice and phonatory function, which is only possible by enlisting patient cooperation.

Is Confidence in Perceptual Evaluation Justified?

The time-honored tradition of our clinical practice is to make informed and expert judgments of a patient's voice and larynx. This requires reliance on the auditory and visual systems of the examiner. Even with intact systems and highly trained expertise, the evaluation process is still ultimately subjective. Furthermore, it is complicated by myriad factors related to anatomy, neurology, and psychology, in addition to variability introduced by technology. The practical reality of our clinical dilemma is highlighted with a

Consensus Auditory-Perceptual Evaluation of Voice (CAPE-V)

Name: _____   **Date:**_____

The following parameters of voice quality will be rated upon completion of the following tasks:
1. Sustained vowels, /a/ and /i/ for 3-5 seconds duration each.
2. Sentence production:
   - a. The blue spot is on the key again.
   - b. How hard did he hit him?
   - c. We were away a year ago.
   - d. We eat eggs every Easter.
   - e. My mama makes lemon muffins.
   - f. Peter will keep at the peak.
3. Spontaneous speech in response to: "Tell me about your voice problem." or "Tell me how your voice is functioning."

> **Legend:** C = Consistent   I = Intermittent
> MI = Mildly Deviant
> MO =Moderately Deviant
> SE = Severely Deviant

SCORE

Overall Severity _____   C   I   ____/100
MI   MO   SE

Roughness   _____   C   I   ____/100
MI   MO   SE

Breathiness _____   C   I   ____/100
MI   MO   SE

Strain   _____   C   I   ____/100
MI   MO   SE

Pitch   (Indicate the nature of the abnormality): _____
_____   C   I   ____/100
MI   MO   SE

Loudness   (Indicate the nature of the abnormality): _____
_____   C   I   ____/100
MI   MO   SE

_____ _____   C   I   ____/100
MI   MO   SE

_____ _____   C   I   ____/100
MI   MO   SE

COMMENTS ABOUT RESONANCE: NORMAL   OTHER (Provide description):_____

ADDITIONAL FEATURES (for example, diplophonia, fry, falsetto, asthenia, aphonia, pitch instability, tremor, wet/gurgly, or other relevant terms):

FIGURE 5–1. Consensus Auditory-Perceptual Evaluation of Voice (CAPE-V).

cursory review of research studies discussing intra- and interreliability outcomes, revealing low agreement. In other words, are observations reality or illusion?

Auditory perceptual evaluation of the voice is focused on characterizing both vocal quality and degree of dysphonia. This immediately relates to the field of psychoacoustics, which confirms that subjective human perception of sounds (from simple pure tones to very complex sounds such as human speech) is very complicated. While the air pressure waves of sound can be measured very accurately with sophisticated equipment, understanding how these waves are received and mapped in the brain is not easy. This process is further complicated by the filtering role of the examiner's psyche.

The problems are compounded for the field of visual perception, which is not as advanced as psychoacoustics, secondary to less research. Processing visual input not only requires the sophisticated imprinting of illumination patterns on the retina, but involves the influence of other sensory modalities, and past experiences as well. In the field of voice, routine clinical experience suggests that visual evaluation of the severity of laryngeal disease is influenced by the associated degree of perceived dysphonia—the rating is worse when we hear a poor voice. To complicate matters, one must take into account the high variability introduced by instrumentation. Factors that can potentially affect how one rates the status of laryngeal sites and signs (eg, edema, erythema, surface irregularity) include:

- Camera adjustments
- Color versus black and white
- Monitor camera adjustments
- Image focus
- Endoscope position (angle of vision and distance of the tip of the scope to structures of interest)
- Type of endoscope (flexible versus rigid).

All these factors (visual-perceptual and technologic) may account for the generally poor intra- and interreliability scores reported in studies related to visual-perceptual observation.

This points out that technology does not ultimately solve this inherently human subjective phenomenon called perception. Improved confidence in our assessment will only come with better understanding of the processes involved through careful study. Until that time, clinicians need to exercise caution by understanding their equipment, its optimal use, paired with developing rigorous evaluation protocols.

Videolaryngoscopy/Videostroboscopy

In addition to the detailed summary presented in the chapters on stroboscopy and laryngeal imaging, it should be noted that videotaped examinations can also be used as an effective biofeedback tool. A notable example of this would be in patients with vocal cord dysfunction, where they can observe laryngeal behavior and the effects of postural changes on airway management.

Therapeutic Probes

Even within the evaluation phase of clinical management, obtaining information about therapy potential is important. This can be accomplished through a variety of stimulability tasks known as therapeutic probes. These may be similar to exercises that are part of bona fide voice therapy, but are utilized here for their prognostic value. Examples of these include humming, throat clearing, digital laryngeal manipulation, pitch and loudness shifts, lips trills, laughing, and coughing. These tasks provide a quick and effective way to predict whether a patient may be stimulable for better voice production and, therefore, a candidate for voice therapy. They also may assist in determining whether there is a functional or malingering component to the problem.

Objective Measures of Vocal Function

The role of objective measures is important but complementary to the more crucial value of the evaluation components just discussed (see Table 5-1). Objective measures never provide a conclusive diagnosis but may confirm that which is suspected based on a thorough history, evaluation, and comprehensive endoscopic evaluation. This statement is not based on personal preference but rather the reality of the current instrumentation limitations: (1) both acoustic and aerodynamic measures represent indirect information about phonatory function as they capture the product at the mouth, thus requiring inference back to the voice source; (2) current technologies are restricted to sustained phonation samples of limited dura-

TABLE 5–1. Advantages and Limitations of Objective Voice Measures

Benefits of objective measures
Provide quantitative documentation of vocal function
Help understand underlying vocal mechanism
Useful in documenting treatment efficacy and outcomes
Assist with medicolegal issues
Efficacy issues regarding health insurance/managed care issues

Words of caution
The practitioner must know the equipment and its limitations
Understand the meaning of the measures, as well as normative data
Only use appropriate tasks and protocols for each technique
Limit interpretations to the scope of the information
Use the measures to complement, not dictate, clinical judgment

tion, which do not capture either representative or complex speech samples; (3) there is lack of consensus on the mathematical algorithms (eg, jitter) that generate the numerical values recorded; and (4) there is unevenness in the normative information against which a patient's profile can be compared—this is particularly true for aerodynamic measures. Although these current observations justify caution in the confidence of objective measures for everyday clinical practice, continued research may foster legitimate utility in the future. Nonetheless, it is important to be familiar with the terminology and the theoretical basis of each measure's utility in laryngology.

The following is a representative list of measures used in clinical practice and purported to be beneficial. Specific endorsement is difficult as particular selections are a function of patient population, clinician expertise, equipment availability, room acoustics, and personal preference.

Acoustic Measures (Christine M. Sapienza, personal communications, 2006)

- **Fundamental frequency (F_0)**—directly reflects the vibration rate of the vocal folds. It is the acoustic correlate of pitch.
  - unit of measure is hertz (Hz) or cycles per second
  - normative data = 100–150 Hz males; 180–250 Hz females
  - may be measured from sustained vowels, reading, or conversation
  - useful to estimate the appropriateness of F_0 for sex and age and for demonstrating pre- and post-treatment change

- **Frequency variability**—pitch sigma is the standard deviation of the fundamental frequency.
  - assesses and documents variation of F_0 during speech production

- **Phonation range**—range of frequencies from the highest to the lowest that a patient can produce.
  - may be expressed in Hz or semitones
  - normal young adults have about a 3-octave range; may vary with practice

- **Frequency perturbation**—the change of frequency from one successive period to the next.
  - unit of measurement is *jitter*; several algorithms are used to extract jitter; normative data for jitter percent is less than 1.00%
  - measures must be made from sustained vowels
  - may represent variation of vocal fold mass, tension, muscle activity, or neural activity, all of which may affect the periodicity of vocal fold vibration

- **Amplitude perturbation**—small cycle-to-cycle changes of the amplitude of the vocal fold signal.
  - unit of measurement is *shimmer*; several algorithms are used to extract shimmer; normative data for shimmer dB is less than 0.35 dB

  - measures must be made from sustained vowels
  - may represent variation of vocal fold mass, tension, muscle activity, or neural activity, all of which may affect the amplitude of vocal fold vibration

- **Intensity (I_0)**—directly reflects the sound pressure level (SPL) of voice. The direct correlate of loudness.
  - unit of measure is the logarithmic decibel (dB) scale
  - may be measured from sustained vowels, reading, or conversation
  - useful as pre- and post-treatment measure

- **Overall sound pressure level (SPL)**—average SPL in dB.
  - indication of the strength of vocal fold vibration (Norms: 75–80 dB conversation)

- **Amplitude variability**—standard deviation of the SPL during connected speech.
  - reflects loudness variability
  - Dynamic range—range of vocal intensities that a person can produce (Norms: 50–115 dB SPL).

- **Harmonics-to-noise ratio (H/N)**—a ratio measure of the energy in the voice signal over the noise energy; may be derived from different algorithms and expressed in various units.
  - greater signal or harmonic energy in the voice reflects better voice quality
  - large noise energy represents more abnormal function

- **Voice range profile (phonetogram)**—plots maximum and minimum intensities for entire frequency range.
  - resulting plot is ellipsoid-shaped frequency/intensity profile and the dimensions are expressed in semitones
  - most useful in pre- and post-treatment of professional voice users

- **Spectral analysis**—a sound spectrogram displays the glottal sound source and filtering characteristics across time.

- both formant frequency energy (vocal tract resonance) and noise components (aperiodicity) are presented in a three-dimensional scale
- horizontal axis = time
- vertical axis = frequency (lowest band = F_0; formants are above)
- gray scale (darkness) represents intensity change

Aerodynamic measures

- **Volume (vital capacity)**—available volume of air in the lungs.
  - measured in liters, will vary with age, sex, size, health
  - measured with a spirometer

- **Airflow rate**—rate at which air passes through the glottis during phonation.
  - measured in liters/sec, with normal rate = 50-200 ml/sec
  - Flow transducer

- **Maximum phonation time (MPT)**—maximum time that a vowel may be sustained while using maximum airflow volume.
  - will vary with lung capacity, age, sex, size, health

- **Subglottal air pressure (Psub)**—measure of air pressure beneath the vocal folds necessary to overcome the resistance of the approximated folds to initiate and maintain phonation.
  - measured in cm/H_2O with norm for conversational voice being 3-7 cm/H_2O
  - intraoral pressure measures reflective of Psub
  - vocal fold stiffness, hypo/hyperfunction, incomplete glottic closure will influence Psub

- **Laryngeal (glottal) resistance**—this is a calculated measure that utilizes measures of pressure and flow in a ratio. Laryngeal resistance is the quotient of peak intraoral air pressure (from unvoiced plosive) divided by the peak flow rate (measured from a vowel) as measured from a repeated consonant + vowel syllable such as /pi/pi/pi/.
  - estimates the overall resistance of the glottis and therefore the valving characteristics (ie, too tight, too loose, normal)

- **Phonation threshold pressure (PTP)**—a measure of the effort needed to initiate phonation.
  - measure is estimated indirectly using intraoral air pressure measured at the exact moment of voice onset for barely audible phonation
  - speakers with vocal pathologies often require greater effort to initiate phonation

- **Aerodynamic recording considerations:**
  - requires airtight seals around the lips or mask to face.
  - as natural speech as possible must be encouraged in this environment.
  - multiple trials are necessary to ensure a stable baseline.
  - instrument calibration is required prior to each examination session.

Diagnosis and Recommendations

The essential final component of a comprehensive voice evaluation involves counseling with the patient, providing conclusions, recommendations, and prognosis. Whether stated or not, the patient is assumed to be looking for answers to his or her problems in terms of "what's wrong, why is it wrong, and how do we fix it?" This places a burden of completeness on the clinician to satisfy this request through careful explanation using language appropriate for the patient's level. It is understood that success with this step requires an atmosphere of time and availability for patient comfort. In general, all voice disorders are treated through a combination of the four following options: behavioral (voice therapy, lifestyle changes, vocal hygiene, dietary modifications, as well as other complementary therapies like relaxation, biofeedback, or psychotherapy), medical therapy, and surgical intervention, or a combination of the three. This paradigm is repeated throughout this book for each of the specific laryngeal disorders presented. Finally, and frequently overlooked, is a definitive statement of prognosis. It is important to inform the patient as to the expected outcome both with and without treatment.

Review Questions

1. Can one get a representative sample of voice with sustained phonation tasks?

2. Is there value in utilizing therapeutic probes during the first evaluation contact with a voice disordered patient?

3. Can a diagnosis be reached based only on acoustic and aerodynamic measures?

4. Can a professional's original training suffice for adequate care of voice patients for an entire career?

REFERENCES

1. American Speech-Language-Hearing Association. (1998). Roles of otolaryngologists and speech-language pathologists in the performance and interpretation of strobovideolaryngoscopy. *ASHA.* 1998;40(suppl 18):32.
2. Loeh Koschkee D, Rammage L. *Voice Care in the Medical Setting.* San Diego, Calif: Singular Publishing Group; 1997.
3. Sataloff RT. *Vocal Health and Pedagogy.* San Diego, Calif: Singular Publishing Group; 1998.
4. Belafsky PC, Postma GN, Koufmann JA. Laryngopharyngeal reflux symptoms improve before changes in physical findings. *Laryngoscope.* 2001;111:979–981.
5. Hogikyan ND, Sethuraman G. Validation of an instrument to measure voice-related quality of life (V-RQOL). *J Voice.* 1999;13(4):557–567.
6. Jacobson BH, Johnson A, Grywalski C, et al. The Voice Handicap Index (VHI): development and validation. *Am J Speech Lang Pathol.* 1997;6:66–70.
7. Hirano M. *Clinical Examination of Voice.* New York, NY: Springer Verlag; 1981:83–84.
8. American Speech-Language-Hearing Association (ASHA). Consensus Auditory-Perceptual Evaluation of Voice (CAPE-V). 2003 document text available from: http://www.asha.org.

6

Laryngeal Electromyography

Nicole Maronian, MD
Lawrence Robinson, MD

KEY POINTS

- Laryngeal EMG can diagnose old versus new injuries to the laryngeal musculature and provide information about recovery.

- Prognosis for recovery of recurrent laryngeal lesions remains an area of intense research effort. Key factors in eventual recovery are likely the early presence of insertional activity and motor unit action potentials under voluntary control.

- Laryngeal dystonia is a disorder involving multiple laryngeal muscles. Fine-wire EMG provides a "roadmap" to document the most involved muscles and assist with treatment planning.

- Laryngeal dysmotility and immobility can be related to multiple factors. LEMG is the only method to definitively diagnose a neurologic cause for impaired vocal fold movement.

- The percentage of recruitment of the laryngeal muscles in a recovering injury is helpful in understanding the degree of nerve injury. The ability to reliably quantify recruitment by multiple practitioners may be challenging and should be actively evaluated.

This chapter focuses on the diagnostic capabilities of laryngeal electromyography (LEMG) as part of the workup and treatment of laryngeal disorders. Utilization of LEMG as well as techniques are discussed.

Electromyography provides the capability to detect electrical activity in muscles. In the case of the larynx, use of LEMG allows the practitioner to deduce information about the status of the efferent motor nerve or the recurrent laryngeal nerve (RLN), as well as the superior laryngeal nerve (SLN) and the laryngeal muscles they supply. Essentially, it can detect loss of neurons innervating a muscle. Utilizing muscle testing, information about prior injury, recovery from injury, or stability of RLN injury can be surmised. The testing provides reproducible patterns of muscle activity that can be combined with clinical information to provide a more robust understanding of the etiology of hoarseness or swallowing dysfunction.

Performing LEMG requires specialized equipment and ideally a combined effort between laryngologist and electromyographer. A standard EMG machine that can record muscle recordings either in digital or paper form is optimal. The team approach combines the expertise of the laryngologist in needle placement with the expertise of the electromyographer in interpretation of complex muscle activity patterns. Certification in electromyography requires 6 months full-time training and subspecialty boards. Thus, the team approach provides maximal information, interpretation, and reliability of the LEMG exam. Furthermore, physician expertise greatly increases with experience and time spent working as a team. Due to the complexity of interpretation, and because patient responses cannot be anticipated, the laryngologist needs to be present throughout the examination.

Laryngeal EMG was initially described in 1944 by Weddell in four patients in whom he attempted to characterize the cause of their laryngeal injury.[1] Just one year later, the first EMG machine made specifically for clinical use was introduced.[2,3] Electromyography of the limb muscles advanced steadily with eventual acceptance as the gold standard for muscle testing following injury, providing both vital diagnostic and prognostic information.

Laryngeal EMG was advanced in the 1950s by Faaborg-Andersen when he published a study detailing testing of multiple laryngeal muscles.[4] He documented muscle activity during voiced and unvoiced tasks, such as swallowing.[4] Hirano, in 1969, described the techniques currently utilized for localization of the laryngeal muscles during routine testing.[5] Concomitant with improved understanding of the electrodiagnostic findings in muscle injury, LEMG was utilized by investigators in research capacities to better understand speech production, effects of immobility, and swallow function.[6,7] In the late 1980s, LEMG became a clinical tool utilized for assessment of voice disorders and for localization of the laryngeal muscles for botulinum toxin injection in adductor laryngeal dystonia.[8,9]

EMG BASICS FOR LARYNGOLOGISTS

EMG Findings

The primary EMG responses evaluated for diagnostic and prognostic purpose include insertional activity, recruitment, denervation, reinnervation, and central response. Signs of peripheral injury are outlined with reference to central injury signs at the end of this section.

Insertional activity is the muscle activity initially identified upon advancement into a relaxed muscle. By advancing the EMG needle into the muscle, the individual muscle fibers are mechanically stimulated resulting in brief bursts of electrical activity exhibited as motor unit action potentials (MUAPs) (Figure 6–1). This pattern of response is present in normal and partially denervated muscle. In severely denervated muscle it is lacking and indicates a complete paralysis of the muscle, possibly with overlying fibrosis.

Testing then revolves around the appropriate voluntary **recruitment task** for the muscle. In the case of the adductor muscles, the thyroarytenoid, lateral cricoarytenoid, and interarytenoid, recruitment is tested by asking the patient to repeat /i/, /i/, /i/. The EMG recording shows brisk recruitment of multiple muscle fibers in response to each of the speech bursts (Figure 6–2).

Evidence of loss of neuron supply to a denervated muscle can be ascertained by specific muscle responses. **Denervation** results in spontaneous muscle fiber action potentials that occur without voluntary control while the muscle is at rest called fibrillations (Figure 6–3). They typically appear about 2 to 3 weeks following injury. Positive sharp waves are similar types of action potentials and typically precede fibrillations by several days (Figure 6–4). This pattern will remain until regeneration begins to occur or persist in the event of severe, irreparable injury. If a muscle becomes fibrotic, loss of these activity patterns, along with loss of insertional activity, may occur. In a densely denervated muscle, no electrical activity may be seen with attempts at voluntary activation with both voice and nonvoice tasks (eg, swallow, Valsalva) (Figure 6–5). If this response is elicited greater than 1 to 2 years from injury, a permanent paralysis is diagnosed without likely ongoing recovery.

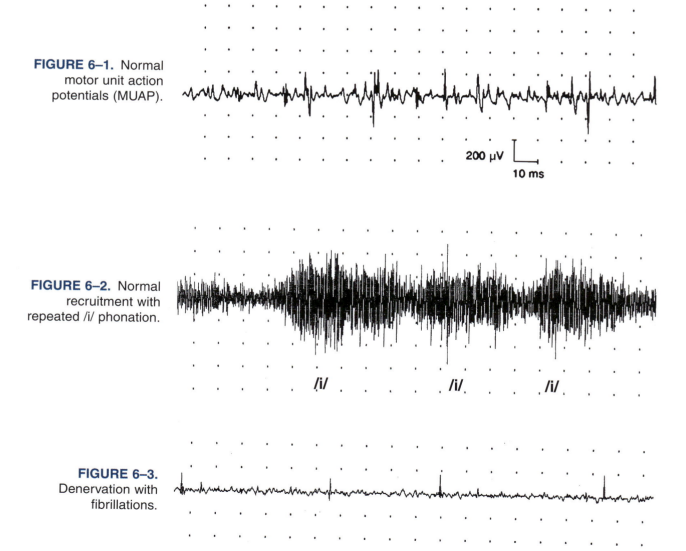

FIGURE 6–1. Normal motor unit action potentials (MUAP).

200 µV

10 ms

FIGURE 6–2. Normal recruitment with repeated /i/ phonation.

/i/   /i/   /i/

FIGURE 6–3. Denervation with fibrillations.

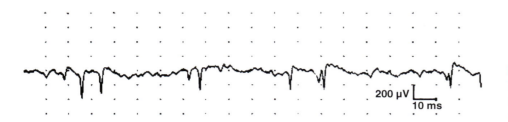

FIGURE 6–4.
Denervation pattern with positive sharp waves.

Note: By convention, the lower half of the EMG tracing is "positive," while the upper half is "negative."

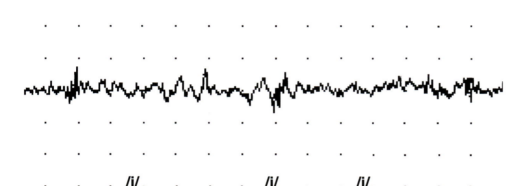

/i/ . . . /i/ . . /i/.

FIGURE 6–5.
Complete denervation without regeneration.

Reinnervation can occur by two different mechanisms, depending on severity of the lesion. In partial lesions, the remaining intact axons can sprout distally to reinnervate newly denervated muscle fibers, thus enlarging the existing motor unit territory. In complete lesions, axons may regrow from the point of injury to reinnervate the denervated muscle fibers. EMG evidence of reinnervation in partial lesions presents with muscle findings of polyphasic motor unit action potentials (MUAPs). These new sprouting fibers are not yet fully myelinated and thus conduct more slowly than mature nerve fibers. As the axons do not conduct at uniform speed, the motor unit becomes desynchronized and has multiple phases, characteristically more than five baseline crossings and a wider duration than a normal MUAP (Figure 6-6). Polyphasic MUAPs are signs of ongoing regeneration. They may recruit with voluntary contraction if an adequate amount of regeneration has occurred. In complete denervation, no motor units will initially recruit. Later, as axons reach the muscle, small polyphasic MUAPs, representing just a few muscle fibers, will be recruited. Over time, these will become larger and polyphasic.

Chronically, as the new nerve sprouts mature and myelinate, they begin to conduct at faster rates. The peaks, as well as the width of the MUAP, diminish as the muscle fibers begin to discharge more synchronously. The amplitude of the response (height) increases, however, as each motor unit now contains a larger number of active muscle fibers. This unit is now called a large-amplitude MUAP. These potentials indicate a stable, chronic injury that recruits with voluntary contraction tasks. The greater the number of motor units present, the greater the degree of reinnervation that has occurred. Even though fewer units may be present, they typically fire at appropriate or faster speeds in attempts to compensate for the peripheral injury. The term, "few firing fast" implies a stable peripheral process. Large MUAPs remain indefinitely as a sign of muscle injury (Figure 6-7).

Central injuries with intact peripheral recurrent laryngeal nerves can present with essentially normal MUAPs. The central nervous system, however, acts to coordinate the peripheral response.

Thus, rate and coordination of response at the laryngeal level can be affected. Typically, with poor central nervous system control, fewer MUAPs are able to be recruited and they fire at a slow rate (Figure 6-8). In normal recruitment the individual motor units cannot be identified due to their large number and varied appearance (see Figure 6-2) With a central pattern, the motor units are sparse and slow in response because of

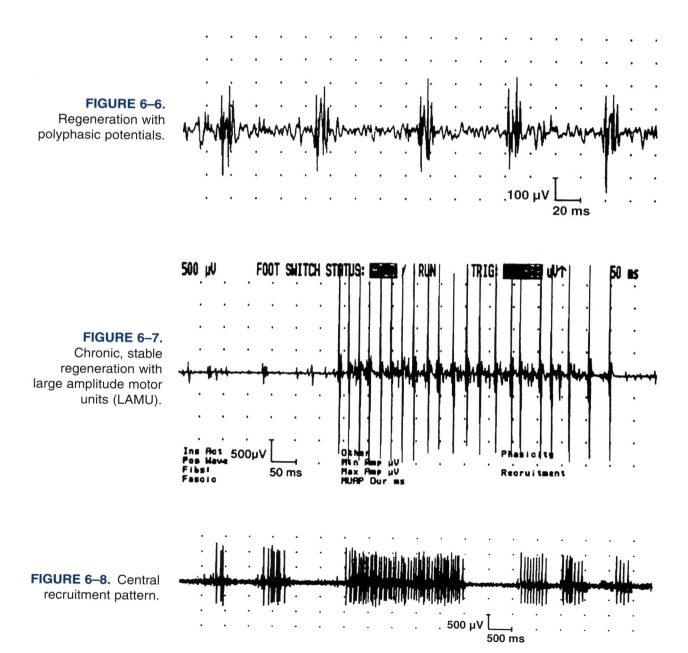

FIGURE 6–6. Regeneration with polyphasic potentials.

.100 µV
20 ms

FIGURE 6–7. Chronic, stable regeneration with large amplitude motor units (LAMU).

500 µV   FOOT SWITCH STATUS: / RUN   TRIG   uV   50 ms

Ins Act   500µV
Pos Wave
Fibs!   50 ms
Fascia

Other
Min Amp µV
Max Amp µV
MUAP Dur ms

Phasicity

Recruitment

FIGURE 6–8. Central recruitment pattern.

500 µV
500 ms

the reduction in upper motor neuron drive. Identifying the exact upper motor neuron process based on EMG response alone is challenging. Incorporation of clinical data and further neurologic testing is typically diagnostic.

Types of EMG

Two types of EMG, needle and fine-wire (FW-EMG), are currently utilized clinically to assist in diagnosis and treatment. Needle laryngeal EMG (LEMG) is performed primarily for evaluation of MUAPs in the setting of a vocal fold dysmotility or immobility. It allows for assessment of muscle recruitment and individual MUAP characteristics. LEMG recordings can be obtained from monopolar or concentric needle electrodes. The monopolar electrodes derive signals from all surrounding motor units providing information from approximately 10 motor units at one time. This is the most common method utilized to understand what is happening in the larger context of the laryngeal muscle being tested. Bipolar or single-fiber EMG recording details firing information from one to two motor fibers, thus giving more in-depth information about individual MUAPs. Controversy remains regarding the best method of testing using either monopolar or bipolar electrodes. Many laryngologists are familiar with using a monopolar botulinum toxin injection needle and thus utilize this same needle for their EMG procedures. Upcoming vector EMG techniques combine the ability to obtain both individual muscle fiber and composite information across the muscle simultaneously. Although currently it remains primarily a research tool, it holds promise as a more well-rounded method of characterizing injury to the intrinsic laryngeal musculature.[10]

FW-EMG utilizes fine 30-gauge hooked wire electrodes. This allows for placement within the muscle in a fixed position which combats the effects of needle dislodgement with swallowing, voicing, or coughing. The FW-EMG is optimally utilized when testing speech versus simple phonatory tasks. The FW-EMG can test multiple muscles simultaneously. It is typically utilized to define muscle involvement in spasmodic dysphonia and can be utilized when testing for laryngeal synkinesis to determine timing of muscle activation and overactive, inappropriate muscle involvement.[5,7]

TECHNIQUE

Needle LEMG is typically performed with the patient in the supine position with the neck in gentle extension. The laryngologist either sits at the side of the patient's neck or above the patient's head in the same position utilized for direct laryngoscopy in the operating room. A monopolar testing needle is typically a 27-gauge hollow bore Teflon-coated injection needle attached to a tuberculin (1-cc) slip-tip syringe. This needle is familiar to most laryngologists given that it is utilized with botulinum toxin injection. The addition of the syringe allows for increased length of the needle and improved angulation to access the laryngeal muscles under the thyroid cartilage.

The testing can stimulate coughing if the needle is introduced immediately below the subglottic mucosa. Coughing can be avoided by either placing the needle lateral to the mucosa or by performing a transtracheal block with 1 cc of 2% plain Xylocaine.

Muscle testing can then proceed based on techniques previously described by Hirano.[5] The thyroarytenoid (TA) muscle is approached via the cricothyroid (CT) space. It is important to stay strictly in the midline. The needle is advanced with steady light pressure through the CT membrane with EMG guidance. One feels a loss of resistance as the CT membrane is penetrated. Once the needle tip is past the CT membrane, inserting the needle at a 15- to 30-degree angle laterally and superiorly will result in strong TA muscle activity. In the female larynx, the vocal fold is typically lower and more lateral than in the male due to their small and broader laryngeal framework. Once the needle encounters muscle, the EMG signal will dampen and transmit muscle signal. The needle should be advanced until sharp recruitment is identified. Voluntary testing of this muscle is achieved by repetitive /i/ phonation, which should reveal sharp bursts of activity on the EMG monitor.

The interarytenoid (IA) muscle is approached by placing the needle through the CT membrane and then into airspace (with an open channel electrical finding). Staying in the midline, the needle is advanced posteriorly until it reaches the posterior cricoid. The EMG signal will again dampen as tissue is reached. The examiner then advances the needle slowly upward ("walking up the posterior cricoid") until the needle falls over the superior cricoid edge into the IA muscle. A burst of muscle activity will be identified. The patient will also note more sensitivity in this area perhaps due to the greater sensory innervation at the posterior glottis. Testing again occurs with repetitive /i/ phonation to activate the adductor muscle with repeated bursts visualized on the EMG. The IA is typically felt to have bilateral innervation; however, distinct differences may be apparent even in unilateral lesions.[11]

The posterior cricoarytenoid (PCA) muscle can be reached either via the CT membrane or from a lateral approach. It can be tested along with the TA and IA using the same needle insertion. Once the needle is in the airspace, the needle is directed laterally, maintaining the same level as the CT membrane. The EMG signal is dampened as the posterior cricoid is encountered. The needle can often be advanced through the cartilage into the PCA muscle with signs of MUAPs on the EMG. In some patients, the cricoid cannot be reached due to the limits of the EMG needle or advanced through the cricoid due to calcification. In that setting, the PCA is approached laterally. The larynx is grasped and rotated to one side. The lateral edge of the thyroid lamina is palpated. The EMG needle is inserted at the lower lateral border of the larynx and advanced inferiorly and medially toward the posterior cricoid until insertional activity is identified. Appropriate testing involves asking the patient to sniff three times and observing three bursts of activity on the EMG monitor.

The cricothyroid (CT) and lateral cricoarytenoid (LCA) muscles can be approached with one needle insertion. The CT membrane is identified and the needle advanced approximately one centimeter off midline. With insertion through the skin, the CT muscle is encountered. Testing for this muscle requires the patient to phonate with a low-pitched /i/, followed by a high-pitched /i/. The motor unit recruitment will increase significantly during high-pitched phonation. If no increase in recruitment is identified, then the needle may be in the strap muscle and the patient should be asked to elevate the head. If activity increases with this maneuver, then further redirection of the needle toward the CT membrane should occur.

The LCA muscle is localized after CT testing is complete. The needle is then advanced through the CT membrane, laterally and slightly upward. The muscle is encountered and demonstrates active recruitment with repetitive /i/ phonation only at the initiation of the phonation.

UTILIZATION OF EMG IN CLINICAL PRACTICE

LEMG plays a vital role in the laryngologist's diagnostic armamentarium. LEMG is a direct extension of the laryngologist's physical exam of laryngeal motion seen on an endoscopic examination. LEMG is the only modality that can discern between complete paralysis and denervation of the RLN, versus cricoarytenoid joint fixation/scar as the etiologies of an immobile vocal fold.[12,13] It can also diagnose synkinesis within the larynx. Synkinesis occurs after a peripheral nerve injury when a nerve carries muscle activity to multiple muscles. In the larynx, the RLN carries adducting fibers to the TA and LCA muscles and abducting fibers to the PCA. With synkinesis of the larynx, these fibers become crossed in a reinnervation state resulting in a hemilarynx with immobility and good muscle tone.[14]

EMG can be utilized to determine the timing of a permanent rehabilitative procedure to the vocal folds. In the acute setting of vocal fold immobility, limited information can be gleaned about eventual recovery based on the overall lack of muscle response during very early injury. After 4 to 6 weeks, some practitioners begin utilizing EMG for prognostication of eventual recovery with 44% specificity.[15] Overall, most investigators have reported variability in correct prediction of recovery utilizing early EMG.[11,16] However, the predictive nature of laryngeal EMG in patients 3 months out from injury has not been thoroughly studied.

Unfortunately, EMG can provide only one time point in the determination of neuromuscu-

lar regeneration. Thus, in injuries at a significant distance from the larynx, the regenerating axons may simply not have reached the intrinsic muscles which would result in a change in the type of motor units seen on EMG. Thus, findings on EMG may continue to show dense denervation, thereby overestimating the extent of injury if EMG is performed early. Multiple EMGs spaced out several weeks to months or an EMG at 4 to

---

Controversy: Laryngeal Reinnervation

The role of laryngeal reinnervation remains controversial in patients with vocal fold paralysis and is intimately associated with the debate over laryngeal synkinesis. As the RLN carries adductor and abductor fibers into the laryngeal muscles and branches immediately prior to the entrance into the larynx, significant injury to the RLN results in damage to both types of motor fibers. If the neural tubules remain intact, as occurs in a mild injury (eg, traction injury, mild thermal injury, compression), the proximal axons will find the appropriate target muscle and full recovery of muscle tone and appropriate function will occur. However, in patients with more profound RLN injury, nerve regeneration into the appropriate target muscle may be limited or absent. Those who argue for routine laryngeal reinnervation for patients with persistent immobility 9 to 12 months after an RLN injury assume that those patients have failed to develop a full neural recovery, have inadequate reinnervation, and would benefit from a reinnervation procedure. However, many believe that the majority of those patients have adequate muscle tone due to a synkinetic reinnervation pattern and would not benefit further by routine laryngeal reinnervation, therefore, a static medialization/augmentation is the procedure of choice. In a review of 75 patients with unilateral vocal folds paresis, only 19% of the patients demonstrated a severe level of denervation on preoperative LEMG.[30] In contrast, another study evaluated evoked EMG in patients prior to laryngeal reinnervation.[31] In this study, 15 patients with a clinical diagnosis of vocal cord "paralysis" (no preoperative diagnostic laryngeal electromyography), were tested intraoperatively for an evoked RLN response using either surface EMG via a custom endotracheal tube or bipolar concentric needles with direct stimulation of the RLN. In this study, only one patient demonstrated an evoked potential while a control group of eight patients undergoing thyroidectomy demonstrated a normal evoked potential. This clinical problem requires greater study.

6 months following initial injury will likely be more helpful in prognosticating recovery.[15] If early intervention is required for issues of aspiration or vocal requirements, then EMG can provide some guidance and reassurance particularly if early signs of recruitment are lacking. It does not, however, exclude that eventuality and ongoing recovery may occur over the next year. Clearly, the earlier that more favorable EMG signs are present (ie, preserved MUAPs with voluntary brisk recruitment), the more likely spontaneous recovery. However, lack of voluntary recruitment even at 6 months, does not preclude eventual recovery if the location of the lesion is near the skull base or the proximal aspect of the vagus nerve. The location of the lesion must be calculated into the therapeutic decision-making when applying EMG information to specific patients. In addition, the clinical interpretation of the EMG must be coordinated with the clinical findings and location of injury. For example, in patients with a vocal fold paresis after a left carotid endarterectomy, the length of time prior to reinnervation and return of motion will be much longer than in a patient who has suffered a right vocal fold paresis after thyroidectomy.

Final characterization of the neurophysiologic state of the vocal fold yields one of the following:

1. Dense denervation with no voluntary activity which can now be termed vocal fold paralysis.
2. Partial reinnervation with diminished motor units. This can range from very few units, indicating a severe peripheral nerve lesion, to many units with robust recruitment, indicating a mild injury.
3. Normal recruitment with complete recovery.

Varying degrees of reinnervation in vocal fold recovery is much more common than complete denervation.[17] The degree of reinnervation required to achieve paretic versus normal function remains unclear. A limb muscle that has sustained up to 45% MUAP loss may preserve the appearance of near-normal mobility or strength on clinical examination.[18] In the setting of a limb

paresis, partial to near normal reinnervation would be anticipated with a 50% neural injury.

It is helpful to judge the percentage of recruitment with voluntary activity. This has implications for eventual recovery and treatment planning. If near-normal recruitment is identified with standard testing but no movement is identified, then synkinesis should be suspected. If recruitment is zero or less than 10%, then reinnervation techniques should be considered.

Given that the RLN is a mixed nerve carrying abductor and adductor fibers, the consequences of a misdirected reinnervation can be significant.[19,20] This can result in a reinnervated but immobile vocal fold due to synkinesis. With simultaneous firing of the abductors and adductors, the vocal fold cannot move against these antagonistic muscle forces. The EMG definitions of synkinesis are divided into abductor and adductor types. Abductor synkinesis is commonly agreed upon to reflect PCA recruitment with phonation which is clearly abnormal.[14,19] Adductor synkinesis definitions are more challenging and variable in the literature due to the multiple glottic tasks that require TA activation.[14,19] The definition should reflect the normal function of the TA in comparison to its abnormal activation and remains an area of intense research interest.[14] Synkinesis does supply neuronal input to the vocal fold, thus resulting in improved bulk and tone and often more midline position with an upright arytenoid.[21]

Treatment decision-making will also change based on the presence of synkinesis and degree of reinnervation. In a planned therapeutic, laryngeal reinnervation procedure, the anticipated outcome is a synkinetic vocal fold that does not move but is improved in muscle tone and possibly improved position without need for a medialization implant. This approach utilizes a nonlaryngeal nerve to achieve new nerve supply to the intrinsic laryngeal muscles.[22-26] However, if a significant degree of reinnervation has occurred naturally, it is unlikely that new nerve ingrowth will be accepted by an already partially innervated muscle.[17] This has led some authors to propose that a vocal fold that is severely and permanently denervated would be the best reinnervation candidate. Other patients with partial denervation would best be served with a static repositioning procedure such as medialization with or without an arytenoid adduction suture.[21]

FW-EMG with fixed hooked-wire electrodes can also be utilized for patients with laryngeal dystonia to characterize muscle involvement and direct treatment with botulinum toxin.[27,28] In the setting of adductor laryngeal dystonia, routine testing of the TA, LCA, and IA muscles can provide a "roadmap" of predominant muscle involvement. This has been utilized to direct botulinum toxin therapy, particularly in patients less responsive to standard treatment protocols.[7,29]

EMG is a valuable adjunct to clinical decision-making in management of vocal fold movement disorders. Utilization, however, cannot occur in a vacuum. It requires amalgamation of clinical history, exam, patient needs, and EMG findings to determine the diagnosis and best treatment choice for each individual patient. It is limited by issues including patient tolerance, physician expertise, needle placement, and our present day understanding of neurolaryngeal reinnervation. Expertise in this area develops with repeated utilization and thus requires the investment of time by the laryngologist in combination with a skilled electromyographer. EMG used in context of other clinical information provides the crucial diagnosis, which cannot be gleaned from simple endoscopic observation of the vocal folds. As technical advances improve our understanding of neurophysiology, our ability to use EMG as a measurement of function will only improve our ability to care for patients with laryngeal disease.

Review Questions

1. The type of EMG utilized for diagnostic workup of vocal fold immobility or dysmotility is:
   a. needle EMG
   b. fine-wire EMG

2. In a stable, severe, longstanding paralysis of the recurrent laryngeal EMG, one may see the following EMG characteristics:
   a. fibrillations
   b. polyphasic potentials
   c. few, if any, motor unit action potentials
   d. poor insertional activity
   e. all of the above

3. EMG findings not consistent with vocal fold paresis include:
   a. polyphasic potentials
   b. reduced recruitment
   c. lack of insertional activity
   d. large motor unit action potentials

4. Adductor laryngeal dystonia involves which of the following muscles:
   a. TA
   b. LCA
   c. IA
   d. PCA

5. Laryngeal synkinesis of the abductor muscles is characterized by EMG as follows:
   a. PCA activation with phonation
   b. PCA activity with respiration
   c. TA and PCA activity with phonation
   d. cannot be characterized by EMG

REFERENCES

1. Weddell G, Feinstein B, Paattle R. The electrical activity of voluntary muscle in man under normal and pathological conditions. *Brain.* 1944;67: 178–242.
2. Golseth JG. Diagnostic contributions of the electromyogram. *Calif Med.* 1950;73:355–357.
3. Golseth JG. Electromyographic examination in the office. *Calif Med.* 1957;87:298–300.
4. Faaborg–Andersen K. Electromyographic investigation of intrinsic laryngeal muscles in humans. *Acta Physiol Scand.* 1957;41:1–150.

5. Hirano MJ. Use of hooked-wire electrodes for electromyography of the intrinsic laryngeal muscles. *J Speech Hear Res.* 1969;12:363–373.

6. Sataloff RT, Mandel S, Mann EA, Ludlow CL. Laryngeal electromyography: an evidence-based review. *Muscle Nerve.* 2003;28:767–772.

7. Hillel AD. The study of laryngeal muscle activity in normal human subjects and in patients with laryngeal dystonia using multiple fine-wire electromyography. *Laryngoscope.* 2001;111:1–47.

8. Ludlow CL, Naunton RF, Sedory SE, Schulz GM, Hallett M. Effects of botulinum toxin injections on speech in adductor spasmodic dysphonia. *Neurology.* 1988;38:1220–1225.

9. Blitzer A, Lovelace RE, Brin MF, Fahn S, Fink ME. Electromyographic findings in focal laryngeal dystonia (spastic dysphonia). *Ann Otol Rhinol Laryngol.* 1985;94:591–594.

10. Roark RM, Li JC, Schaefer SD, Adam A, De Luca CJ. Multiple motor unit recordings of laryngeal muscles: the technique of vector laryngeal electromyography. *Laryngoscope.* 2002;112:2196–2203.

11. Min YB, Finnegan EM, Hoffman HT, Luschei ES, McCulloch TM. A preliminary study of the prognostic role of electromyography in laryngeal paralysis. *Otolaryngol Head Neck Surg.* 1994;111:770–775.

12. Koufman JA, Postma GN, Whang CS, et al. Diagnostic laryngeal electromyography: The Wake Forest experience 1995–1999. *Otolaryngol Head Neck Surg.* 2001;124:603–606.

13. Rontal E, Rontal M, Silverman B, Kileny PR. The clinical differentiation between vocal cord paralysis and vocal cord fixation using electromyography. *Laryngoscope.* 1993;103:133–137.

14. Maronian NC, Robinson L, Waugh P, Hillel AD. A new electromyographic definition of laryngeal synkinesis. *Ann Otol Rhinol Laryngol.* 2004;113:877–886.

15. Munin MC, Rosen CA, Zullo T. Utility of laryngeal electromyography in predicting recovery after vocal fold paralysis. *Arch Phys Med. Rehabil.* 2003;84:1150–1153.

16. Gupta SR, Bastian RW. Use of laryngeal electromyography in prediction of recovery after vocal cord paralysis. *Muscle Nerve.* 1993;16:977–978.

17. Woodson GE. Configuration of the glottis in laryngeal paralysis. II: Animal experiments. *Laryngoscope.* 1993;103:1235–1241.

18. Beasley WC. Quantitative muscle testing. Principles and applications to research and clinic services. *Arch Phys Med.* 1961;42:398–425.

19. Crumley RL. Laryngeal synkinesis: its significance to the laryngologist. *Ann Otol Rhinol Laryngol.* 1989;98:87–92.

20. Blitzer A, Jahn AF, Keidar A. Semon's law revisited: an electromyographic analysis of laryngeal synkinesis. *Ann Otol Rhinol Laryngol.* 1996;105:764–769.

21. Maronian N, Waugh P, Robinson L, Hillel A. Electromyographic findings in recurrent laryngeal nerve reinnervation. *Ann Otol Rhinol Laryngol.* 2003;112:314–323.

22. Chhetri DK, Berke GS. Ansa cervicalis nerve: review of the topographic anatomy and morphology. *Laryngoscope.* 1997;107:1366–1372.

23. Crumley RL. Update: ansa cervicalis to recurrent laryngeal nerve anastomosis for unilateral laryngeal paralysis. *Laryngoscope.* 1991;101:384–387; discussion 388.

24. Paniello RC. Laryngeal reinnervation with the hypoglossal nerve: II. Clinical evaluation and early patient experience. *Laryngoscope.* 2000;110:739–748.

25. Tucker HM. Long-term results of nerve-muscle pedicle reinnervation for laryngeal paralysis. *Ann Otol Rhinol Laryngol.* 1989;98:674–676.

26. Zheng H, Li Z, Zhou S, Cuan Y, Wen W. Update: laryngeal reinnervation for unilateral vocal cord paralysis with the ansa cervicalis. *Laryngoscope.* 1996;106:1522–1527.

27. Maronian NC, Waugh PF, Robinson L, Hillel AD. Tremor laryngeal dystonia: treatment of the lateral cricoarytenoid muscle. *Ann Otol Rhinol Laryngol.* 2004;113:349–355.

28. Hillel AD, Maronian NC, Waugh PF, Robinson L, Klotz DA. Treatment of the interarytenoid muscle with botulinum toxin for laryngeal dystonia. *Ann Otol Rhinol Laryngol.* 2004;113:341–348.

29. Klotz DA, Maronian NC, Waugh PF, Shahinfar A, Robinson L, Hillel AD. Findings of multiple muscle involvement in a study of 214 patients with laryngeal dystonia using fine-wire electromyography. *Ann Otol Rhinol Laryngol.* 2004;113:602–612.

30. Bielamowicz S, Stager SV. Diagnosis of unilateral recurrent laryngeal nerve paralysis: laryngeal electromyography, subjective rating scales, acoustic and aerodynamic measures. *Laryngoscope.* In press.

31. Damrose EJ, Huang RY, Blumin JH, Blackwell KE, Sercarz JA, Berke GS. Lack of evoked laryngeal electromyography response in patients with a clinical diagnosis of vocal cord paralysis. *Ann Otol Rhinol Laryngol.* 2001;111:563–565.

PART III

Principles of Therapy

Laryngeal Hygiene

Douglas M. Hicks, PhD, CCC-SLP
Claudio F. Milstein, PhD, CCC-SLP

KEY POINTS

■ Laryngeal hygiene does not require, and usually does not involve, direct voice manipulation through the use of traditional exercises and drills.

■ Vocal wellness encourages prevention rather than treatment.

■ The principles of vocal care and nurturing are generally common sense but not intuitive; patients will benefit from education.

■ Insufficient or incorrect information about the larynx and about the voice in particular is a major cause of vocal career problems.

Hygiene is defined as the "establishment and maintenance of health" by facilitating "conditions or practices conducive to health."[1] Vocal hygiene, in particular, is focused on promoting laryngeal health, with appropriate phonatory function and normal voice production. Achieving health involves limiting trauma to laryngeal tissues by addressing diet, lifestyle choices, and vocal demands (Figure 7–1). Hygiene does not require, and usually does not involve, direct voice manipulation through the use of traditional exercises and drills. Therapeutic intervention instructs patients to care for their vocal folds rather than

teaching them voicing.[2] The impact of hygiene measures is well established in both amateur and professional voice users.[3,4] Just as importantly, the benefit of this education for teachers has been suggested,[5] although in a compelling prospective study,[6] instruction in vocal hygiene did not result in significant benefit when compared to vocal function exercises (see chapter 8, Speech-Language Intervention).

The principles of care and nurturing are often a result of common sense but not intuitive. As a result, naïveté about the larynx and vocal function becomes a major contributor to vocal

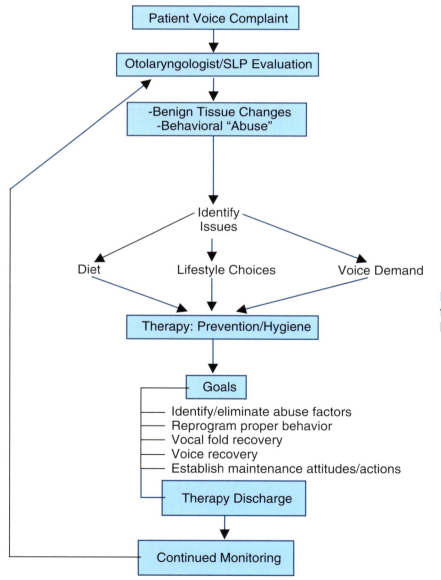

FIGURE 7–1. Management Tree for Treating Patients with Voice Disorders.

problems, sometimes chronic in nature. In all aspects of therapeutic intervention, patients are taught to be informed consumers of their problems by empowering them with knowledge that changes both their attitudes about voice and their actions. Therefore, the challenge for the patient is to increase the consistency of his or her behavior to provide a "larynx friendly" environment. This involves providing information about laryngeal function to the patient as well as reinforcing general health principles, such as the maintenance of adequate hydration.

Effective teaching of laryngeal hygiene by the speech therapist or phoniatrician, for example, is best served by initially providing several orientation concepts that explain the therapeutic process and provide a foundation for the patient's effective learning. The first concept is to clarify the nature of therapy as being cognitive—"information loading" rather than aimed at specific phonatory techniques. The "hard work" nature of therapy manifested in both consciousness and conscientiousness, is described below:

- **Consciousness:** a necessary part of any habit-changing process; requires patient to become temporarily preoccupied with a behavior previously produced unconsciously and automatically. Effective reprogramming of maladaptive behaviors demands this level of concentration.
- **Conscientiousness:** refers to an increased disciplined compliance in order to foster effective reprogramming of behavior. This process neither requires perfection nor paranoia about voice. Success should occur as long as the patient implements proper therapeutic changes "more often than not."

It is important to change as little as possible to produce the proper outcome; this reinforces the important principle that the cost of success through therapy is not for the patient to become uncomfortable with his or her new vocal profile. These principles are further discussed in chapter 10, Speech-Language Intervention. The practi-

tioner must make it clear that ultimate success is the patient's responsibility. Patients need to take personal ownership for both creating the problem through bad choices and achieving successful recovery. That process is not easy or guaranteed as recent research implies different stages of mental readiness to behavioral changes that may complicate patient compliance.[7] The majority of laryngeal hygiene intervention does not focus directly on actual voice performance. In contrast, most activity is focused on changing enough behavior (vocal choices) to promote recovery of laryngeal structure and function, which translates into voice restoration. The essence of vocal hygiene is an indirect focus on actual voice performance rather than a direct manipulation of specific performance parameters (pitch, loudness, laryngeal quality) through traditional exercises or drills. This is in addition to dietary and general health measures that should be emphasized in all patients, such as the avoidance of irritants (tobacco, alcohol, caffeine) and the maintenance of excellent hydration. This is discussed further in upcoming sections.

Two important therapy goals in patients suffering from vocal abuse are educating them on several key hygiene concepts and identifying/eliminating specific abusive factors. This information facilitates both proper attitudes about voice and recovery action plans.

There are several general concepts to keep in mind. Many therapists find it beneficial to emphasize the association between *structure*, *function*, and *performance*. The voice outcome represents a tangible behavioral indicator of vocal fold status. It is always available to be monitored contingent on the patient going beyond simple "hearing" of voice to the next step of analysis, implied in "listening." The patient may indeed become a self-sufficient monitor of both proper and poor vocal performances. They may learn to react properly to what they hear (and feel) by implementing appropriate therapy strategies, with each day constituting a series of decision points either for or against the larynx.

Vocal abuse must be defined in the instruction of laryngeal hygiene. Misuse can be defined as using the larynx beyond its physical limits (ie, screaming). Overuse, on the other hand, involves using the larynx within its physical limits but for too long or too often. Vocal abusers typically have evidence of both components; it is rare for an individual to manifest strictly one. The "abuse threshold" is variable even within a given individual as it may be a function of fatigue,

The Role of Complete Voice Rest in Vocal Hygiene Intervention

The traditional reliance on complete voice rest to resolve vocal fold nodules or other benign tissue changes has been replaced by a philosophy of conservation or caution. This is based on the realization that abusive behaviors underlying the tissue changes are ultimately maladaptive habit—chronically perpetuated as automatic, unconscious, and natural behaviors. Although complete cessation of voicing accomplishes the necessary reduction in tissue contact/collision forces, it does nothing to reprogram the patient's bad habits. Vocal conservation, in contrast, produces enough positive change to promote tissue recovery that will lead to voice improvement. Furthermore, these changes are accomplished in real-life circumstances rather than in an unrealistic world of silence. Long-term establishment and maintenance of new, vocally healthy habits are best formed in the very activities or settings that previously fostered abuse. By its nature, this process takes longer than what can be accomplished through complete voice rest. However, the strength and permanence of behavior reprogramming through a conservation approach is superior to the more aggressive silence approach. Cultivating patience in the patient is a necessary step for eventual success but acceptance is usually easy, given the benefit of generally maintained life routines possible with conservation.

This more contemporary practice pattern does not eliminate, however, a continued, valuable role for complete voice rest. Although more limited, its use in certain voice and larynx circumstances can be essential for positive outcomes with certain voice and larynx circumstances. These typically involve more acute or significant tissue impact as represented by acute laryngitis, laryngeal trauma, vocal fold hemorrhaging, or postphonosurgical care. The duration of complete rest for the first three conditions is usually dictated by recovery, through medical management, and/or natural healing time. Voice rest postsurgery is a far more variable time frame as a function of several factors including the specific surgical procedure; the extent, location, and nature of tissue insult; surgeon preference; healing response; and the nature of expected voice demands on recovery. In general, however, the weaning process back to normal promotes the shortest duration of complete voice rest that the tissue integrity and future positive vocal outcomes can allow.

In summary, complete voice rest has evolved in current practice to a limited but well-defined role that usually is not a part of routine vocal hygiene instructions.[11]

concurrent inflammation, and other medical and environmental issues. The important practical issue is for the patient to learn limits and operate within them.

A useful tool for managing vocal use and hygiene is the concept of "vocal finances." The patient may consider vocalization to be a tangible commodity that can be spent or saved. Although informal, the money analogy in which each use of the voice is considered a withdrawal from one's laryngeal "bank account" is highly effective with patients. It requires patient to assess the vocal expense of activities, scenarios, and life choices. The patient may ask him- or herself the following questions at each daily decision point: (1) Is there a vocal cost? (2) How much is that cost? and (3) Can I afford it?

The next major objective is to identify and eliminate specific abuse factors. The rationale is simple—focus on the major contributing factors that will increase both efficiency and effectiveness of treatment strategies. To accomplish that identification step, a simple but effective exercise can be used (Table 7–1).

The final step of hygiene intervention involves a review of numerous possible practical issues related to diet, lifestyle choices, and vocal demands. Perhaps the best studied of these factors is hydration. Several important studies have demonstrated the impact of systemic hydration on phonation threshold pressure and fatigue.[8] In a double-blinded, placebo-controlled study, Verdolini and colleagues demonstrated an inverse relation between phonatory effort and hydration level, although primarily for high-pitched phonation tasks.[9] Water should be each patient's primary beverage, with rare exception in the case of cardiac or renal disease. Even nasal obstruction and resultant oral breathing has been shown to negatively affect vocal effort.[10] In particularly harsh climates, consideration of whole house or room humidifiers is helpful.

In addition to drinking plenty of water, the patient should avoid known irritants such as caffeine, alcohol, and tobacco. See chapter 17, Reflux and the Larynx, for more information. Practitioners patients should be aware that decaffeinated products have their own potential liability as the chemicals used for decaffeination are

TABLE 7–1. Exercise to Identify and Eliminate Specific Voice Abuse Factors

1. Have the patient generate a generic detailed activity schedule for a full week from wake-up to bedtime, Monday through Sunday—using 30-minute intervals. Preferably this is done as a home assignment with patient returning for the next session with a written schedule printout.

2. Together, patient and therapist review *all* activities and overlay them with voice use/demand. To generate an accurate and comprehensive voice profile, it is important to be detailed.

3. In parallel with establishing voice use, identify the activities or scenarios that represent vocal abuse—previously defined and understood as either misuse or overuse. Compile a full list of abuse factors.

4. Rank-order the worst abuse factors (limit to maximum of five—requiring the patient to address additional factors reduces their effectiveness in strategy implementation and compliance).

5. Require the patient to generate at least two strategies to address and counteract the top-ranked factors. To stimulate his or her creativity, stress that effective action plans typically involve either elimination, reduction, or change-of-form thinking. Requiring patients to generate a strategy proposal markedly increases their ownership of the plan, usually improving subsequent implementation and compliance. The therapist role is strictly as a reactant—to confirm the patient's plan and offer edits when needed (usually because patient's suggestions are overly aggressive).

6. The final strategy decision step is ideally one of negotiation rather than unilateral dictation by the therapist. Re-emphasize the prior promise of changing as little as necessary to accomplish change. The ultimate litmus test for strategies is confirming the changes are specifically matched to a particular abuse factor, are easy to implement, and will be natural for the patient's use—in other words, "doable."

purported to also pro-mote reflux. Beyond that, the general well-being related to adequate rest and physical fitness provides the ideal environment for vocal and laryngeal health. Important tips for general laryngeal health and hygiene are noted in Table 7–2.

TABLE 7–2. Vocal Wellness and Laryngeal Health

Take personal ownership of your vocal health— be accountable

1. Practice proper vocal hygiene—be guided by common sense
2. Common sense—respond to how the voice sounds/feels
3. Count the vocal "costliness" of your lifestyle choices
4. Managing your voice requires discipline plus flexibility
5. Avoid physical/emotional exhaustion (eat/sleep wisely)
6. Hydration/humidification are key
7. Reduce caffeine intake
8. No smoking—active or second-hand
9. Alcohol in moderation
10. Avoid late night eating/drinking
11. No substitute for vocal training
12. Respond promptly to upper respiratory tract infections.

It is clear from clinical experience that maintenance of laryngeal hygiene is important in preventing and treating vocal dysfunction. Hydration is a key issue but the fundamentals of patient education and daily decision-making will provide for ideal long-term maintenance of laryngeal health. Factors that predispose the patient to vocal abuse should be identified and eliminated within the framework of the patient's wishes for vocal and laryngeal health.

Review Questions

1. Can the speaking voice harm the singing voice?
2. Do caffeinated beverages provide adequate vocal fold hydration?

3. Is the temperature of beverages irrelevant for my voice?
4. Is whispering a good "voice" alternative during laryngitis?

REFERENCES

1. Hygiene Definition; *Webster's Medical Desk Dictionary*. Springfield, Mass: Merriam-Webster, Inc; 1986.
2. Verdolini, K. *Guide to Vocology*. Iowa City, Ia: National Center for Voice and Speech; 1998:27.
3. Timmermans B, Vanderwegen J, DeBodt MS. Outome of vocal hygiene in singers. *Curr Opin Otolaryngol Head Neck Surg*. 2005;13(3):138–142.
4. Yiu EM, Chan RM. Effect of hydration and vocal rest on the vocal fatigue in amateur karaoke singers. *J Voice*. 2003;17(2):216–227.
5. Chan RW. Does the voice improve with vocal hygiene education? A study of some instrumental voice measures in a group of kindergarten teachers. *J Voice*. 1994;8(3):279–291.
6. Roy N, Gray SD, Simon M, Dove H, Corbin-Lewis K, Stemple JC. Evaluation of the effects of two treatment approaches for teachers with voice disorders: a prospective randomized clinical trial. *J Speech Lang Hear Res*. 2001;44(2):286–296.
7. Van Leer E, Hepner E. Toward a theoretical framework for patient adherence to voice therapy. *J Voice*. In press.
8. Solomon NP, DiMattia MS. Effects of a vocally fatiguing task and systemic hydration on phonation threshold pressure. *J Voice*. 2000;14(3):341–362.
9. Verdolini K, Titze IR, Fennell A. Dependence of phonatory effort on hydration level. *J Speech Hear Res*. 1994;37(5):1001–1007.
10. Sivasankar M, Fisher KV. Oral breathing increases PTH and vocal effort by superficial drying of vocal fold mucosa. *J Voice*. 2002;16(2):172–181.
11. Sataloff RT. Voice rest. In: Sataloff RT. *Professional Voice: The Science and Art of Clinical Care*. (2nd ed.) San Diego, Calif: Singular Publishing Group; 1997:453–456.

8

Speech-Language Intervention–Voice Therapy

Sarah Marx Schneider, MS, CCC-SLP
Robert T. Sataloff, MD, DMA

KEY POINTS

- Diagnostic and medical treatment of voice disorders are the responsibility of physicians, ideally otolaryngologists with expertise in this area. Behavioral evaluation and treatment of dysphonia in the professional voice user are the responsibility of speech-language pathologists.

- Interdisciplinary team relationships are crucial to improve patient care.

- Special information should be included when gathering the history of the professional voice user compared to the nonprofessional because of differences in vocal demand and expectations.

- The initial voice evaluation provides the clinician with valuable baseline information about vocal function, patient stimulability, possible therapy techniques, expectations of the voice user, and information regarding likely success and outcomes of therapy.

- Voice therapy is patient specific. A common diagnosis among patients does not indicate that the same facilitators will be appropriate for each. Multiple approaches must be available.

The practice of speech-language pathology includes prevention, habilitation, and rehabilitation of communication, swallowing, or other upper aerodigestive disorders; elective modification of communication behaviors, and enhancement of communication.[1] The American Speech-Language-Hearing Association (ASHA) states that the speech-language pathologist should provide prevention, screening, consultation, assessment, treatment, intervention, management, counseling, and follow-up services for speech, voice, language, swallowing, cognition, and sensory awareness for communication, swallowing, and upper aero-digestive functions. In the area of treating voice disorders, the speech-language pathologist is concerned not with diagnosis and treatment of laryngeal diseases or other physiologic disorders, but rather with understanding, analyzing, and modifying vocal function.

If, perceptually, the voice is within normal limits for the patient and is being produced in a reasonably efficient, nonabusive manner, then intervention by a speech-language pathologist need not be conducted. It is not within the speech-language pathologist's scope of practice to provide special training that will develop range, power, control, stamina, and the esthetic quality required for artistic expression. The speech-language pathologist is concerned with the voice that presents with a current or potential problem, identifying and analyzing the problem, then helping the voice user modify vocal behaviors to use the vocal mechanism with optimal efficiency. Responsibilities in ameliorating the voice problem include: analyzing vocal behaviors perceptually and objectively; analyzing vocational, educational, and psychological factors that may interact with vocal behaviors to precipitate, maintain, or exacerbate vocal difficulty; and then designing and implementing an individual program for modifying vocal behaviors.[2]

Just as do physicians, speech-language pathologists vary in their backgrounds and experience in the treatment of voice disorders. Furthermore, the curricula that speech-language pathologists complete during education and training varies widely and typically addresses normal and disordered voice production only at a general level. Curricula rarely provide extended education or knowledge about the professional voice. Therefore, prior to making a referral to a speech-language pathologist for voice therapy, his or her background and training should be considered.

This chapter focuses on the speech-language pathologist's treatment of voice disorders with special emphasis on the treatment of professional voice users. There are many factors to consider when working with professional voice users. The following is not meant to be an inclusive list but is intended merely to provide a framework of key considerations. Evaluation and treatment of a professional voice user requires increased sensitivity from the clinician. At first, when listening to the patient's voice, it may sound "normal. However, sounding "normal" is relative. The professional voice user, typically, has increased awareness of minute changes in the voice. Therefore, a speech-language pathologist must be "supersensitive to superspeaking." The goals of the professional voice user/performer are typically different from those of a nonperformer and must be considered as such. With that in mind, it is important to learn the patient's expectations and provide a realistic perspective on the possible outcome of therapy based on the diagnosis and response to trial therapy techniques during the initial assessment.

Further consideration must be given to body and self-awareness issues in performers versus nonperformers. Body- and self-awareness, in this sense, refers to the patient's awareness of his or her own behaviors and the ability to make changes as instructed. Depending on their previous depth of training, professional voice users may have increased awareness of vocal behaviors. Body- and self-awareness are important skills to develop or maximize in the voice user. They will aid the patient in developing, recognizing, and maintaining techniques for efficient voice use.

Environmental contributions also should be noted. As a professional voice user, the patient may be in situations that may not be obvious to a treating clinician. These may include poor acoustics while performing, interference of costumes and clothing, positional factors, and so forth, which can be significant contributing factors to suboptimal voice performance. Therefore, the clinician must ask specific questions or even attend a rehearsal or performance to make a complete assessment of conditions.

Psychological factors also commonly contribute to voice problems. The voice can be described as an emotional part of each person. Studies by Fonagy, described by Sundberg, have indicated that articulatory and laryngeal structures in addition to respiratory muscle activity patterns change in relation to 10 different emotions.[3] This is indicative of the emotional/psychological connection to the voice. Psychological factors may be related to the patient's response to the voice disorder and its effect on his or her life, or the voice disorder may be the manifestation of a larger psychological issue that is causing a voice disorder, as in psychogenic voice disorders. In either case, treatment should be tailored to the needs of each patient with careful history taking and thorough examination. The speech-language pathologist may act as a patient advocate speaking with the physician and acting as a catalyst for a referral to the appropriate psychological professional as deemed by the physician.

Emotional factors also can affect the patient's overall response to the voice disorder. Is the patient able to cope with the voice disorder?

How will it affect his or her current life, voice demand and expectations, and career? Are past vocal experiences, the diagnosis, or other people's responses affecting therapy sessions or outcomes?[4] These basic questions should be addressed with the patient.

Treating voice patients requires the interaction of many disciplines. Patients and clinicians alike will benefit from a team approach to the voice patient's care. In some centers, the interdisciplinary team may be in one facility, but not always. It is important to build relationships within the community to maximize patient care. Treatment by an interdisciplinary team is important when treating anyone with a voice disorder and crucial when treating the professional voice user. The members of the team may include a laryngologist, speech-language pathologist, singing voice specialist/singing teacher, acting-voice specialist, voice researcher/scientist, singing coach, and/or psychologist. Relationships with other medical specialists are also important, including neurologists, pulmonologists, gastroenterologists, endocrinologists, physiatrists, psychiatrists, and others (Table 8–1).

Additionally, in specific cases, other specialists may be included in the interdisciplinary

TABLE 8–1. Composition of a Typical Interdisciplinary Team

Member	Role
Laryngologist	Primary medical member of the team—responsible for diagnosis and medical/surgical intervention
Speech-Language Pathologist	Conducts evaluation and treatment of the voice problem by promoting efficient use of the vocal mechanism
Acting Voice Specialist	Develops singing technique and singing voice production—may be beneficial to a nonsinger in teaching more efficient breathing and coordination with voicing that can be carried over into speaking
	Focuses on honing vocal skills such as projected speech and communication skills as they relate to vocally demanding professions—typically utilized once a patient has become efficient in speaking voice production with a speech-language pathologist
The Patient	The most important member of the team—the patient must be motivated to participate in therapy, be knowledgeable about the voice disorder and techniques for treatment as instructed by the clinician, and be involved in therapy decision-making and planning

team. The *voice researcher/scientist* can provide valuable insight and perspective with regard to the care of a voice patient because of his or her specific knowledge and skill-set in acoustic measurement and voice production. Referral to a *singing voice coach* may also be useful following rehabilitation work with the speech-language pathologist and singing voice specialist. The singing voice coach will be a valuable aide in the development of artistic style and repertoire for the voice user. A *psychologist or psychiatrist* may prove valuable in a team setting, providing the patient with counseling for the management of emotional reactions to the voice disorder, as well as psychological issues that may have contributed to its occurrence. In addition, a *physiatrist* may offer contributions in the way of addressing areas of tension or other injury throughout the body.

Of note regarding the interdisciplinary team, both singing and acting-voice specialists, in addition to the singing coach, have no formal licensing or certification board. Therefore, it is important to understand that resources can vary widely from community to community, as can the backgrounds and knowledge of various voice professionals. For example, singing and acting-voice teachers/coaches are not trained to work with the injured voice and, therefore, may not have experience in this area. Singing voice specialists and acting-voice specialists are experienced teachers who have acquired such training, usually through apprenticeships.

EVALUATION

The initial voice evaluation should include a thorough review of case history, performance of objective and subjective evaluation, trial therapy,

Interdisciplinary Treatment of Voice Disorders

The interdisciplinary approach to the treatment of voice disorders is increasing and professional organizations are recognizing the development of these specialized relationships. The American Speech-Language-Hearing Association (ASHA) is working in conjunction with the National Association of Teachers of Singing (NATS), and the Voice and Speech Trainers Association (VASTA) to revise the joint statement, *Role of the Speech-Language Pathologists, the Teacher of Singing, and the Speaking Voice Trainer in Voice Habilitation.* This statement is intended to encourage interdisciplinary treatment of voice disorders and to encourage professionals working with voice patients to work within the scope of practice and laws regarding treatment. In addition, ASHA is working with the Speech, Voice, and Swallowing Committee of the American Academy of Otolaryngology-Head and Neck Surgery to generate a new joint statement, *The Use of Voice Therapy in the Treatment of Dysphonia,* which is currently under consideration for approval. This statement recognizes the importance of voice therapy in conjunction with medical and surgical management in treating voice disorders as supported by clinical research and expert experience.

and assembling initial impressions and recommendations. This will provide the clinician with baseline information about vocal function, patient stimulability and possible therapy techniques, expectations of the voice user, and information from which to draw conclusions regarding success of therapy and possible outcomes.

Case History

A thorough case history should be elicited from the patient beginning with the onset and development of the voice problem and the circumstances under which it ensued. The patient's previous and/or current medical diagnoses and treatments should be reviewed. The duration of the voice disorder and its constancy are also important factors. In some cases, voice problems can be intermittent over many years with the patient not having pursued treatment until the problem worsened significantly. Knowing this information can give the clinician perspective on the patient's overall voice disorder. Whether or not the patient had received voice therapy previously should be documented. If so, when the treatment took placed, its duration, techniques employed, and whether previous treatment was effective should be noted. These factors can be indicative of how receptive the patient will be to further intervention and how he or she will likely respond to different voice therapy techniques.

A complete inventory should be taken regarding vocal hygiene, abuse, and misuse including hydration, caffeine intake, yelling, shouting, loud talking, coughing, throat clearing, smoking, exposure to second-hand smoke, sleep patterns, overall rest, and other environmental factors. In addition, vocal demands should be reviewed and the patient should provide examples of voice use during a typical day. Throughout this inventory, the patient should explain the primary vocal complaints so as to provide the clinician with a possible starting point for intervention. The patient's initial concerns are addressed immediately and may increase his or her motivation to continue therapeutic intervention.

Special factors must be considered when eliciting a history from a professional voice user. Learning vocal complaints as they are related to their "performance voice" can be very helpful. The clinician should inquire about the history of professional voice use, whether it be singing, acting, public speaking, or a combination thereof. The clinician should also ask about the genre of music the patient is singing, voice classification, performance venues, and the size of his or her typical audience, if any. Knowing the extent of the professional voice user's vocal training is also valuable, particularly when and how long he or she has studied, the specific school of training and whether he or she is studying currently. This process provides information about the types of vocal techniques the patient may already employ or be aware of, or those that may need to be developed or reworked.

The clinician should request that the patient share his or her professional goals and expectations for voice. Ideally, voice therapy should be tailored to accommodate the patient's professional and career goals concurrently with satisfying the clinician's therapeutic objectives. Even though the singing voice specialist typically will perform a more thorough evaluation of the complaints of a singer, the speech-language pathologist can play an important role in singing voice rehabilitation and development. The clinician can use knowledge of a patient's background, education, and experience to assist in development of an efficient daily speaking voice and in articulating the relationship between daily speaking routines and singing or stage voice.

Objective Evaluation

Gathering and analyzing objective voice data is a crucial part of the complete voice evaluation. Completing pre- and post-therapy voice measures can supply objective data to assist in predicting therapy outcomes, for use in research, and to provide tangible voice statistics for use by insurance companies. The objective voice evaluation is discussed further in chapter 5.

Subjective Voice Evaluation

Respiration

The respiratory system is the source of power for voice production. Many voice problems can be related to uncoordinated breathing. The clinician should pay special attention to the manner in which the voice user inhales and then exhales air to produce voice during the evaluation. Observation of the patient's breathing pattern should be completed during reading and conversational speech. Breathing patterns that may be inefficient for voice production include clavicular breathing, upper thoracic breathing, or a combination of the two. So called "diaphragmatic breathing" can be the most efficient breathing pattern as it tends to provide optimal balance of inspiratory and expiratory muscle use. Speaking on residual air, shortness of breath while speaking, gasping for air during inhalation, forced exhalation, or decreased airflow during phonation are also common indicators of vocal misuse.

Phonation

Phonation is defined as the production of sound at the level of the vocal folds. A perceptual evaluation of phonation (vocal quality, loudness, and pitch) during reading and conversation should be completed. Vocal quality characteristics may include: hoarseness, breathiness, roughness, raspiness, vocal fry, diplophonia, voice breaks, pitch breaks, and others. Vocal intensity or loudness should be judged as appropriate, increased, or decreased for the particular setting. The pitch of the patient's voice should be judged as appropriate, high, or low for the age and gender. In addition, the frequency of hard glottal attacks should be assessed.

Resonance

Vocal resonance refers to the way sound is shaped acoustically as it travels through the vocal tract. Phonation begins at the level of the vocal folds and moves up through the pharynx, oral cavity, and nasal cavity. Frontal resonance or forward focus of sound is ideal for most efficient voice production. It optimizes acoustics of the vocal tract while balancing oral-nasal resonance. The use of resonant voice therapy, which places emphasis on frontal tone focus, can increase perceived vocal loudness levels which then may allow the voice to be heard better in noisy situations without excessive strain. A variety of resonance patterns may be observed while making a perceptual judgment of the voice including oral, oral pharyngeal, nasal, nasopharyngeal, and hypopharyngeal.

Articulation

A global assessment of articulation should be completed judging clarity and accuracy of articulatory movement for intelligible speech production.

Prosody

Prosody may have a subtle effect on voice production and should be assessed generally paying attention to the rhythm, fluency, rate, pauses, and intonation or inflection patterns used.

Locating Muscle Tension

Muscle tension can have an adverse affect on voice production causing vocal fatigue, pain, and/or changes in the ease and quality of voice production. Locating these areas of tension is vital in breaking patterns of tension and retraining efficient muscle patterns. Possible places of tension are outlined in Table 8–2.

Laryngeal palpation provides valuable information regarding specific areas of tension, which may include the thyroarytenoid muscle, suprahyoid area, strap muscles, and other related structures. The base of tongue should also be palpated to assess the presence and degree of tension. Digital manipulation and laryngeal massage of the extrinsic laryngeal musculature during evaluation can provide the clinician with valuable information regarding tension and may yield immediate improvement in vocal quality or an identifiable

TABLE 8–2. Possible Places of Muscle Tension

Tongue	Anterior/posterior neck
• Anterior	• Strap muscles
• Base of tongue	• Occipital area
Jaw	**Shoulders**
• Masseter	• High shoulder posture
• TMJ	• Tightness/stiffness
Laryngeal Tension	**Upper chest**
• Intrinsic laryngeal muscles	• Anterior/posterior chest muscles
	• Clavicular area

release in laryngeal tension. These changes are useful to provide the patient with an identifiable vocal change or release of tension and may be indicative of the patient's responsiveness to therapeutic intervention.

Oral Mechanism Exam

A general assessment of oral and facial structure and function should be completed to rule out abnormalities or asymmetries in strength, range of motion, and coordination that may affect functional communication. Structures include the face, mouth, dentition, tongue, and hard and soft palate. Abnormalities may be indicative of neurologic problems that warrant further evaluation.

Trial Therapy

During the initial evaluation, a period of trial therapy should be completed using facilitators to improve ease and quality of voice production. The facilitators are used to assess the patient's stimulability for improvement in voice production. Throughout the trial therapy period, the clinician attempts to provide the patient with a demonstration of possible improvement in voice production, which should in turn increase motivation and feelings of therapeutic success. While completing facilitating techniques, the clinician should gain information on the patient's self-awareness of existing habits and changes in voice production that may occur. Judgments can also

be made by the clinician on the patient's ability to learn new techniques, willingness to comply with voice therapy, and overall appropriateness for therapy. A statement of prognosis for outcomes through voice therapy should also be made.

Impressions/Recommendations

A complete voice evaluation provides the clinician with baseline data regarding voice production and the patient's view of his or her voice disorder, in addition to allowing the speech-language pathologist to develop an impression of the cause and/or contributing factors to the voice disorder. The review of vocal hygiene, vocal demand, and overall voice use provides the clinician with a place to begin educating the patient about his or her voice. Although the trial therapy portion identifies facilitators for improved ease and/or quality of voice production, it also provides an appropriate starting point for therapeutic intervention.

When a general impression has been formulated by the clinician, it should be discussed with the patient. The clinician should indicate to the patient if a course of voice therapy is recommended and identify expectations for follow-up sessions. The goals of therapy should then be discussed with the patient and consideration should be given, at that time, to the patient's personal goals. Once the goals are delineated, other referrals may be made including singing intervention, physical therapy, and so forth. Expectations for therapeutic intervention should be clear to the patient, including the approximate length of the therapy in months, weeks, or sessions, and how often the sessions should be scheduled (weekly, biweekly, monthly). The patient also should be aware that home practice is a crucial part to success in therapy. The clinician will teach the patient tools and provide support to improve vocal efficiency and carryover of efficient voice use. It is the patient's responsibility to attend sessions, complete home practice, and work to carry over efficient voice use in everyday life with the clinician's guidance so that therapy goals can be met and independence in efficient voice use can be achieved.

THERAPY

Initially, goals for therapy must be set forth. When treating the professional voice user the ultimate long-term goal is to produce an excellent speaking voice. The means to reaching this goal is to increase vocal efficiency during speaking. The therapy techniques presented in this chapter can be used to address behavioral voice problems that may or may not include organic or structural changes that have taken place in the vocal folds.

Therapy begins with educating the patient. A brief overview of the anatomy and physiology of voice production should be introduced and discussed with the patient; including coordinating breathing, phonation, and balancing oral-nasal resonance. This explanation should provide the patient with a foundation for understanding voice production and the primary focus of voice therapy. Vocal hygiene should be addressed and improved to eliminate vocal stressors and promote an optimal environment for improving vocal ease and quality. Furthermore, the voice user must be made aware of vocal habits that promote abuse and/or misuse of the vocal mechanism and should be provided with alternatives to abusive vocal behavior.

Voice conservation strategies should be taught to the patient in an attempt to manage voice use on a daily basis. Vocal exercises should then be introduced and practiced to begin retraining muscle patterns for voice production. The vocal exercises work to maximize efficiency of the vocal mechanism and promote carryover of targeted voice use into daily activities. Body- and self-awareness should be targeted from the onset of therapy to promote carryover of the efficient voice learned during therapy.

Areas of tension can have an adverse effect on efficient voice production. Areas of muscle tension that were identified during the initial evaluation should be addressed throughout therapy. The patient should be taught a daily routine for stretches and massage that may include those listed in Table 8–3. Laryngeal massage may also be taught to the patient and completed independently outside the therapy setting.

TABLE 8–3. Exercises to Reduce Muscle Tension

Sites of Tension	Sample Exercises (Partial List)
Tongue	
• Anterior	• Tongue stretches
• Base of tongue	• Base of tongue massage
Jaw	
• Masseter	• Massage
• TMJ	• Jaw stretch
	• Tension/relaxation awareness exercises
Laryngeal Tension	
• Intrinsic laryngeal muscles	• Digital manipulation of the suprahyoid area and thyrohyoid muscle
• Intrinsic laryngeal muscles	• Breathy, sighing
	• Gentle scales and glides
Anterior/Posterior Neck	
• Strap muscles	• Neck stretch
• Occipital area	
Shoulders	
• High shoulder posture	• Shoulder shrugs
• Tightness/stiffness	• Shoulder rolls

Postural alignment should also be addressed with special attention given to hip angle and shoulder and head placement. Slight misalignments in posture can cause increased muscle tension. For example, elevated chin placement will tighten laryngeal and neck muscles or an arched lower back will make relaxing the abdomen for lower abdominal breathing difficult.

Facilitators for Breath Control and Support

As respiration is the power source for phonation, the patient must be taught to balance inspiratory and expiratory muscles for efficient breathing. Exercises for breath management may start with a simple explanation of the respiratory system. This may include a description of the expansion of the lungs and diaphragm with subsequent expansion of the rib cage and abdominal area during inhalation. As exhalation takes place these areas begin to slowly deflate. Expiratory muscles may be engaged but should not be hyperfunctioning. The patient must understand that it is possible to coordinate breathing and vocalization without hyperfunctional muscle use.

Appropriate terminology should be used when teaching a new breathing pattern secondary to learned responses that many adults have to phrases such as "take a deep breath." When a patient is asked to do this, the stomach pulls in, the shoulders and chest rise, and the patient holds his or her breath. Phrases such as "expand for inhalation" versus "take a deep breath" and release/deflate for exhalation or engage the abdomen during exhalation rather than pushing/pulling in may be employed. In addition, the image of a newborn baby during quiet breathing with the belly rising on inhalation and falling on exhalation may elicit understanding of the target breathing pattern.

While establishing a more efficient breathing pattern, the patient may be placed in multiple positions to experience the targeted feeling of expansion during inhalation and active deflation during exhalation. Positions may include lying on the floor in the supine or prone position and concentrating on expansion of the lower rib cage and abdomen during inhalation and then slowly releasing air during exhalation. These two positions with the help of gravity provide tactile feedback during expansion and deflation. They also aide in decreasing shoulder and upper thoracic movement while breathing. However, these strategies alter respiratory function and should be used cautiously and with knowledge of their purposes and limitations. Another useful technique is instructing the patient to bend over at the waist with arms extended to a chair or table so that his or her back is parallel with the floor. The patient is instructed to expand the abdomen during inhalation and feel the abdomen actively deflate during exhalation. These breathing techniques/positions are not meant to be sustained but to increase body awareness of an efficient pattern of breathing that can be applied during daily activities. As the patient and clinician work through the therapeutic hierarchy and gradually introduce simple to complex exercises the patient should be instructed to use the new breathing patterns for short periods multiple times throughout the day while breathing quietly and also while talking, as appropriate.

Facilitators for Increasing Airflow During Phonation

Once an efficient breathing pattern can be replicated, breathing and voicing should be paired together, cueing the patient to produce voicing during exhalation. It is important for the patient to understand that inhalation prior to phonation is as important as releasing air during exhalation to produce phonation. To achieve appropriate airflow during phonation, muscle hyperfunction must be eliminated from the vocal tract by various exercises.

The *yawn-sigh* may be used to promote active inhalation while decreasing muscular tension in the throat in addition to creating increased oral-pharyngeal space by lifting the soft palate. The increased oral-pharyngeal space and the sensation of an open throat should be maintained during exhalation while producing a sigh. The patient may be cued to place the tongue in a relaxed position behind the bottom incisors to maintain oral space. When the targeted yawns-sigh can be replicated consistently, the yawn can then be "downsized" to an open-mouthed inhalation and voicing during exhalation may be shaped into words, phrases, and so forth.

The *stretch and flow* therapy technique, originally developed by R.E. Stone, focuses on increasing ease and quality of voice production by increasing airflow during phonation. The patient is asked to use a strip of tissue, draped over his or her finger, to provide a visual cue for airflow. The patient is instructed to blow a passive airstream onto the tissue. This should feel easy. Confirm this feeling with the patient. Once a consistent, passive airstream is achieved, the patient is instructed to add his or her voice on a /u/ vowel, while maintaining the airstream. The patient should produce a smooth, air-filled, easy voice. This voice may sound slightly more air-filled than "normal." The initial goal is to slightly overexaggerate the airflow during the exercise, so ultimately the ease of voice production is maintained and airflow can be normalized. Each trial should be modified until the targeted voice is achieved. The air-filled, easy /u/ will then be used as a facilitator into words, phrases, sentences, and so forth, through the therapeutic hierarchy. When the patient can produce the targeted voice consistently using the facilitator, its use should be gradually eliminated until the targeted voice can be produced consistently independent of the facilitator.

Lip trills, raspberries, or tongue-out trills are other facilitators to coordinate airflow and phonation. For lip trills, the patient is instructed to expand and produce a raspberry with only airflow. If this is difficult the patient may place his or her index finger on each cheek and slightly press forward to release lip tension. The patient may also be cued not to clench the back molars together. When the patient is consistent with production of the lip trill with air only, they are instructed to add voicing. Consistency should be developed on one pitch and through a range of pitches. Once this is completed the lip trill may be used as a facilitator in initial /br/ words, phrases, and so forth. Similarly with the tongue-out trill, the patient should relax the tongue over the bottom lip, expand during inhalation, and release air to produce a tongue-out trill without voicing. This facilitator requires that the tongue and jaw be relaxed and airflow coordinated to produce the targeted tongue-out trill. When consistency is achieved, voicing should be added and developed at one pitch and through a range of pitches. The tongue out-trill can then be used as a facilitator into open vowels, words, phrases, and so forth. When the targeted voicing is achieved, the use of the facilitator should be faded out.

When evaluating coordination of airflow and phonation, hard glottal attacks (abrupt abductions of the vocal folds on words with an initial vowel) should be addressed. Voicing should be initiated with airflow rather than abrupt adduction of the vocal folds. This can be addressed by targeting coordination of airflow and phonation. Easy onset exercises should be completed beginning with discrimination tasks so the patient is able to identify hard glottal attacks. Minimal pairs

should then be used (ie, hear/ear, hat/at). The patient should be made aware of the abduction of the vocal folds during an /h/ and closure of the vocal folds during the voiced cognate. Prior to each trial, cueing may be required to inhale to ensure vocal fold abduction and gentle adduction of the vocal folds to initiate voicing. The patient in then instructed to maintain the open feeling during the /h/ into the voiced cognate without producing an /h/. Complexity should be increased as appropriate. The above mentioned exercise addresses vowel-initiated words that begin a breath group. When a vowel-initiated word is found within a breath group "linking" should be employed. Linking is used to connect the last sound of the word previous to the vowel-initiated word. For singers or musicians it may be described as tying the words together, just as notes on the staff may be tied.

Facilitators for Oral Resonance

To achieve an optimal balance of oral-nasal resonance, a relaxed vocal tract must be maintained, in addition to maintaining breath support and appropriate airflow during phonation. In many hyperfunctional voice users, it is difficult to achieve forward tone focus secondary to reduced space in the oropharynx which may be caused by increased tongue and/or jaw tension. To increase oral-pharyngeal space, it may be beneficial to increase soft palatal lift, address jaw tension through stretches and massage, and decrease tongue retraction through stretches and tongue relaxation exercises.

Resonance exercises may include the use of a hum to achieve improved balance of oral/nasal resonance. The patient should be cued to maintain oral space. This may be achieved by creating space in between the back molars to release jaw tension and maintaining relaxed tongue placement behind the lower front incisors and away from the roof of the mouth. The patient is instructed to inhale and then exhale while producing a hum, or hum-sigh on a descending glide, with the lips barely touching. The patient's attention should be brought to the targeted frontal tone focus and "buzz" on the lips. This buzz can provide tactile feedback for the patient in working to maintain frontal focus while increasing complexity of trials. If the patient has difficulty achieving a hum without pressing, he or she may be cued to release air through the nose and maintain a consistent airstream. When the targeted hum is achieved consistently, it should be used as a facilitator into vowels, words, phrases, and so forth. Eventually use of the facilitator should be minimized and then eliminated.

"Honking" is used as an effective facilitator for developing awareness and maintenance of balanced oral/nasal resonance. Honking is completed by pinching the nose while phonating on any vowel. The patient is cued to allow the sound to resonate in his or her nose and release airflow through the mouth. Tactile feedback should be provided with vibration or "buzz" at the nasal bridge. When the patient is able to achieve consistent voicing and awareness of the buzzing, words and phrases may be spoken using the honking as a facilitator. The word or phrase may be spoken while occluding the nose and then repeated after releasing the nose, maintaining airflow and frontal focus of the sound production. When consistency of voice production is achieved, the use of the facilitator should be gradually eliminated.

There are multiple other resonance exercises. The last to be discussed is the use of the /f/ and /v/ or /s/ and /z/ sounds. This exercise, as with others mentioned, combines the use of abdominal breathing, use of a continuous airstream, and frontal tone focus. Initially, the /f/ or /s/ sound is used to establish a consistent stream of air coming past the lips. The patient is instructed to expand during inhalation and make an /f/ sound during exhalation with the back molars parted and the top teeth barely touching the bottom lip. Following the trial, confirm the feeling of air past the lips. The patient is then instructed to use the same airflow and breath support with voicing to produce a /v/ sound. A "buzz" should be felt on the lower lip during this trial. This should be confirmed with the patient. If the patient has difficulties achieving the buzz, recheck jaw tension and oral space. Production of a /v/ sound should become consistent and then may be used as a

facilitator into /v/ words, phrases, and so forth. The /v/ may also be used as a facilitator into words and phrases that do not begin with /v/. Use of the facilitator should eventually be faded out.

There are three elements of voice production, respiration, phonation and resonance. There are multiple facilitators that target each element. Choosing an appropriate therapeutic facilitator can be challenging. Clinical judgment should be applied when choosing therapeutic techniques and modifications should be made for patients as needed. When choosing a facilitator, consider the patient's primary complaints, the perceptual and acoustic evaluation of his or her voice, and the physiology of the patient's current voice production versus the targeted efficient voice production. The clinician should be aware of the benefits and limitations of each facilitator and chose appropriately to maximize the patient's voice output and potential for improved voice production

Review Questions

1. What is not within the scope of practice for a speech-language pathologist when treating voice disorders and how does this affect the treatment of the patient?

2. Name and describe the roles of three multidisciplinary team members. Why is it necessary to cultivate professional relationships with team members?

3. Compare history taking for a professional voice user to that for a nonprofessional.

4. How do breath support during phonation and airflow during phonation differ?

5. Name three factors to consider when choosing a therapeutic facilitator.

REFERENCES

1. American Speech-Language Hearing Association. *Scope of Practice in Speech Language Pathology.* Rockville, Md: Author; 2001.
2. Sataloff RT. *Professional Voice: The Science and Art of Clinical Care.* 3rd ed., San Diego, Calif: Plural Publishing; 2005.
3. Sundberg, J. *The Science of the Singing Voice.* DeKalb, Ill: Northern Illinois University Press; 1987:146–156.
4. Smith E, Verdolini K, Gray S, et al. Effects of voice disorders on quality of life. *J Med Speech Lang Pathol.* 1997;4:223–244.

SUGGESTED READING

1. Benninger MS, Jacobson BH, Johnson AF. *Vocal Arts Medicine.* New York, NY: Thieme Medical Publishers, Inc; 1994.
2. Boone DR. *Is Your Voice Telling on You? How to Find and Use Your Natural Voice.* San Diego, Calif: Singular Publishing Group, Inc; 1994.
3. Colton R, Casper J. *Understanding Voice Problems.* Baltimore, Md: Williams & Wilkins; 1990.
4. Rosen DC, Sataloff RT. *The Psychology of Voice Disorders.* San Diego, Calif. Singular Publishing Group, Inc; 1997.
5. Rubin JS, Sataloff RT, Korovin GS. *Diagnosis and Treatment of Voice Disorders.* 3rd ed. San Diego, Calif: Plural Publishing, Inc; 2006.
6. Sataloff, Robert T., *Professional Voice: The Science and Art of Clinical Care.* 3rd ed. San Diego, Calif: Plural Publishing; 2005.
7. Sataloff RT, Castell DO, Katz PO. *Reflux Laryngitis and Other Related Conditions.* 3rd ed. San Diego, Calif: Plural Publishing; 2006.
8. Stemple, JC. *Voice Therapy Clinical Studies.* 2nd ed. San Diego, Calif: Singular Publishing Group, Inc; 2000.
9. Sundburg J. *The Science of the Singing Voice.* DeKalb, Ill: Northern Illinois Press; 1987.
10. Zemlin WR. *Speech and Hearing Science: Anatomy and Physiology.* Englewood Cliffs, NJ: Allyn & Bacon; 1998.

General Principles of Microlaryngeal Surgery

Adam D. Rubin, MD
Robert T. Sataloff, MD, DMA

KEY POINTS

- The surgeon must know *when* and *when not* to operate on the vocal folds.

- Be prepared with the appropriate instrumentation to obtain adequate exposure and perform the surgery.

- Preserve all normal mucosa and superficial lamina propria, and do not traumatize the vocal ligament.

- Excellent postoperative care is essential.

The goal of microlaryngeal surgery (or phono-microsurgery) for benign vocal fold lesions is to improve voice. This is achieved through a complete understanding and respect for the multi-layered structure and function of the vocal folds (see chapter 3, Anatomy of the Larynx and Physiology of Phonation) as well as meticulous surgical technique. Good clinical judgment is paramount when evaluating and planning treatment for the patient with vocal complaints and pathology.

There are four basic principles of microlaryngeal surgery; the key points listed above provide our outline for this chapter.

THE SURGEON MUST KNOW *WHEN* AND *WHEN NOT* TO OPERATE ON THE VOCAL FOLDS

The decision to proceed with surgical excision of a vocal fold mass is complex (Figure 9-1). The mere presence of a mass on the vocal fold is seldom reason enough. Of course, if malignancy is suspected, proceeding with a biopsy is appropriate. Large hemorrhagic polyps, Reinke's edema, and intracordal cysts are likely to need surgical intervention if voice improvement is desired by the patient. However, when considering a small cyst, pseudocyst, or fibrotic mass on the medial edge of the vocal fold, one must weigh the risks of anesthesia—as well as the potential for scarring and making the patient's voice worse—against the chances of voice improvement. Furthermore, there are successful singers and performers who work consistently despite the presence of a vocal fold mass (or masses). Some performers even depend on vocal fold irregularities to provide "character" to their voices. Removing masses that have been present, and perhaps stable for many years, may destroy such a patient's career.

One must be certain that a mass is not only present, but moreover, is the cause of the patient's voice difficulties. In other words, is the mass "*pathologic*"? Voice problems are often multifactorial. Vocal fold vibration and glottic closure problems may be caused by a number of underlying problems such as reflux, allergy, poor technique, and paresis. Such underlying conditions may lead to the development of vocal fold masses. However, sometimes a new insult may occur to a patient with a long-stable vocal fold mass, resulting in new voice symptoms. Recognition of all potentially contributing issues is important for devising the optimal treatment plan. Furthermore, controlling underlying pathology will improve the chances of obtaining an optimal surgical outcome, should surgery become necessary. For example, if a patient's cough from asthma or reflux is not controlled prior to surgery, it will likely lead to trauma to the surgical site and poor healing. Aggressive management of underlying medical issues that may be contributing to a patient's voice problems and impair healing is crucial.

When malignancy is suspected, biopsy should not be delayed excessively. However, recognizing what is a "benign" lesion is important, as this may prevent unnecessary biopsies and consequent scar and dysphonia. Although most often this distinction is not difficult, some pathology is less easy to distinguish. For example, longstanding ulcerative laryngitis and other inflammatory conditions may be mistaken easily for malignancy on clinical examination.[1] Repeated biopsies may reveal only inflammation; it is tempting to sample deeper tissue on subsequent trips to the operating room. A more aggressive approach may result in trauma to the vocal ligament or vocalis muscle, as well as potentially significant scarring and permanent hoarseness. Of course, if there is any doubt, it is better to biopsy than fail to detect an occult malignancy. However, making someone permanently hoarse for a self-limited inflammatory process does not do the patient justice. Rigid stroboscopy with video-documentation is useful for following masses in the office when one is determining whether biopsy is necessary.

Recognizing the patient's goals and motivations is important in the decision-making process, as well. An elderly, retired patient with a large vocal fold polyp may come to clinic with one thought—to make sure that he does not have cancer. He may be less likely to agree to medical or surgical intervention than a schoolteacher with a small cyst on the medial edge of the vocal fold and recurrent hoarseness from phonotrauma.

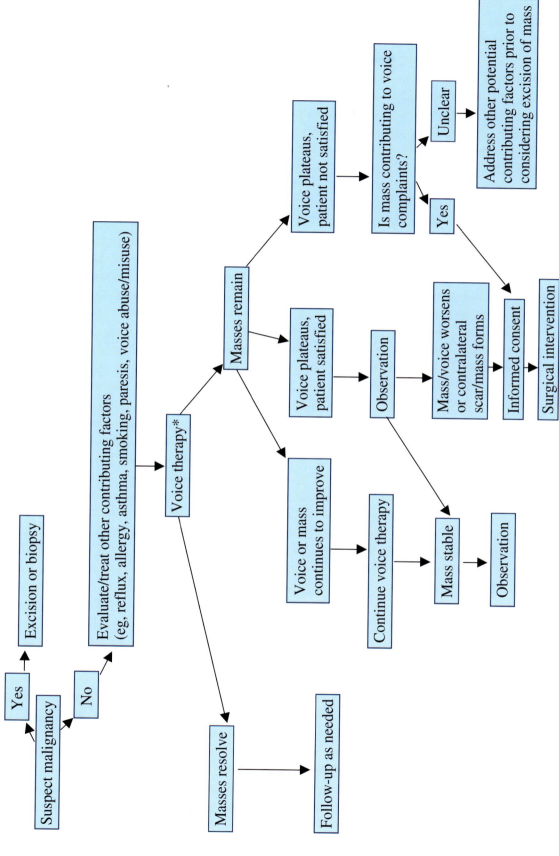

FIGURE 9–1. Voice treatment algorithm.

* Large hemorrhagic polyp, large cysts, and Reinke's edema are unlikely to have significant improvement from voice therapy, although 1 or 2 sessions preoperatively may be useful. Proceeding to surgical intervention may occur sooner than for more subtle lesions, although other underlying issues,

Vocal Paresis and Benign Vocal Masses

Vocal fold paresis has been postulated by some to be involved in the development of benign vocal fold masses. Paresis may involve the superior laryngeal nerve, recurrent laryngeal nerve, or both. The most common etiology is a preceding upper respiratory tract infection. Subtle paresis may be missed on exam, unless it is looked for and the patient is challenged with a series of phonatory tasks. Paresis may be confirmed by laryngeal electromyography.

Supporters of this paradigm believe that a subtle paresis yields a hypofunctional larynx and voice change. Patients try to compensate for the paresis with excessive muscle tension, and become hyperfunctional. Such hyperfunction leads to chronic trauma and the subsequent development of vocal fold masses. For example, a patient with no previous voice problems complains of hoarseness that has not improved since a cold (or perhaps thyroid surgery) 6 months prior. Examination may reveal subtle asymmetry in vocal fold adduction, a small cyst or pseudocyst on the medial edge of one vocal fold, and contact fibrosis on the contralateral fold. LEMG shows reduced recruitment with evidence of chronic denervation when the electrode is inserted in the cricothyroid muscle and the patient asked to do a glissando.

Why is this patient hoarse (let us assume for our purpose that this patient has had a dual-channel pH probe which demonstrated no episodes of reflux at the upper probe)? Was this nerve injury caused by the URI or had it been present years before? The same question could be asked of the mass. If the mass developed after the onset of the URI, how long did it take to develop? Did the patient have a violent coughing fit which led to the development of the mass, or did it result from compensatory hyperfunction?

Of course, it is unlikely that we will able to answer any of the above questions with certainty in most patients. Most people do not have baseline laryngeal examinations when they are healthy with which to compare current examination results. However, it is important to think of all possible scenarios when counseling patients and planning treatment. Say this patient failed voice therapy. What would be the most appropriate surgery? The role of medialization and/or mass excision is not well studied in this clinical scenario. The subtleties and ambiguities of laryngology continue to challenge us and contribute to the "art" of our profession.[42-44]

Furthermore, patients need to be motivated to follow postoperative voice rest and care instructions. It is wise to explain to the patient that his or her treatment requires a team approach involving the patient, the voice therapist, and the surgeon. The patient must be committed to following postoperative instructions, receiving postoperative voice therapy, and complying with follow-up recommendations. Continuance of abusive vocal behavior, particularly in the early postoperative period, may increase the risk of scarring and recurrence.

The surgeon must be aware of the degree of importance of voice quality to each patient's livelihood and quality of life. The physician must weigh the potential medical-legal risks and his or her own comfort level performing this type of surgery. Although every patient's larynx should be treated with the same care and precision as a singer at the Metropolitan Opera, the surgeon with limited experience in microlaryngeal surgery or without the appropriate equipment for thorough evaluation and appropriate surgery, should consider referral to a voice specialist.

Preoperative Evaluation

Understanding a patient's disease and planning treatment begins with a thorough evaluation. A complete medical and voice history should be obtained, and the larynx should be visualized. Flexible laryngoscopy is used to assess the larynx during voice production, to observe gross movement of the vocal folds, to look for hyperfunction, and to detect any sign of paresis or neurologic dysfunction.[2] Videostroboscopy is vital to assess the fine structure of the vocal fold and the mucosal wave. Rigid telescopes currently provide the highest and clearest magnification of instruments available for valuating subtle masses and scar. Flexible laryngoscopes using distal-chip technology are an improvement over traditional fiberoptic flexible laryngoscopes and may be used for videostroboscopy as an alternative to a rigid examination, particularly if the patient is unable to tolerate rigid endoscopy. Although the flexible distal-chip laryngoscopes provide good image quality, they still do not provide the magnification of a rigid scope.

Computerized voice analysis in the voice laboratory is useful in the treatment of voice dis-

orders. Although the "ideal" objective voice measurements do not exist, current measures are useful for documenting severity of dysphonia, and for following and assessing treatment outcomes. Several quality of life instruments exist, including the voice related quality of life instrument (V-RQOL)[3,4] and the Voice Handicap Index (VHI).[5,6] These measures are particularly valuable because they quantify the severity of the effects of a voice problem for each individual patient, which may be the most useful measure in deciding upon treatment and assessing success (see also chapter 8, on perceptual and objective voice assessment).

Preoperative voice therapy is important for both determining whether the patient would be served best by proceeding to the operating room and improving the chances of obtaining a good, long-term surgical result. It relieves the patient of compensatory hyperfunction and helps the patient develop good vocal technique to minimize further trauma to the vocal folds. Some masses, such as nodules, may disappear with voice therapy. Others may not disappear, but the patient may learn to obtain adequate voice despite the mass, without causing further trauma to the mass or the contralateral vocal fold. *If a mass persists despite voice therapy and prevents a patient from meeting his or her vocal needs, if a mass worsens by becoming larger or more fibrotic, or if the patient begins to demonstrate evidence of trauma from the mass on the contralateral vocal fold, surgical excision is warranted in most cases.*

Once the decision to proceed with surgery is made, informed consent must be obtained. In addition to the general risks of endoscopy, such as trauma to oral structures, tongue numbness, tongue weakness, pharyngeal perforation, arytenoid cartilage dislocation/subluxation, and loss of airway, patients, particularly professional voice users, must understand that despite excellent surgical technique, scarring may occur, which can make the voice worse. Although this seldom occurs with good surgical technique, it is important to counsel the patient so that he or she understands the worst of possible circumstances and can make a well-informed decision as to whether to proceed with surgery.

BE PREPARED WITH THE APPROPRIATE INSTRUMENTATION TO OBTAIN ADEQUATE EXPOSURE AND PERFORM THE SURGERY

Performing microlaryngeal surgery well without appropriate instrumentation is difficult, if not impossible. The surgeon must be prepared to obtain adequate exposure even in the most difficult anatomic cases and to handle vocal fold mucosa in a delicate manner. Performing surgery for benign vocal fold masses with a Holinger laryngoscope and large biopsy forceps, for example, is generally inappropriate.

Adequate exposure is paramount to good surgical excision. Surgeons must be prepared to deal with the most unfavorable anatomy. Optimal positioning for laryngeal visualization is the "sniffing" position (Figure 9-2). The neck should be flexed toward the chest, and the head extended. No shoulder roll is required.[7,8] Most operating room tables have a head board that can be flexed to keep the neck flexed against the chest (Figure 9-3). Prior to each procedure, however, the surgeon should check to make sure the head board fasteners are tight, so that the board does not come out of the table while placing it in flexion. Such an event could result in a sudden posterior collapse of the patient's head and potentially result in a catastrophic cervical spine injury.

A suspension system should be used. Many varieties are available. The Lewy system is used most commonly. The arm may be lowered by an assistant; however, the primary surgeon should be holding the laryngoscope in the position he or she wishes to maintain. The system is designed to stabilize a laryngoscope that is already in proper position and should not be used as a lever. The suspension arm should be lowered only until it touches the stand. In other words, one should not use the suspension arm to "crank" the patient's head to try to improve exposure as this will risk traumatizing the patient's teeth. If one arm of the suspension device touches down prior to the other, towels or gauze may be placed

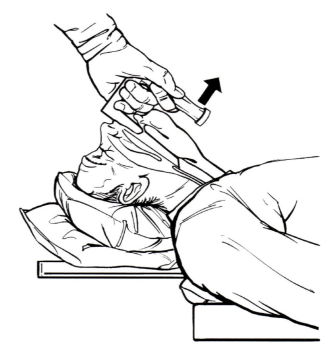

FIGURE 9–2. The "sniffing position" is ideal for visualization during laryngoscopy. Note that the neck is flexed and the head is extended. Often the neck must be flexed considerably more than illustrated. The arrow indicates correct direction of pull during laryngoscopy. (Reprinted with permission from Sataloff R. Voice surgery. In Sataloff R. *Professional Voice: The Science and Art of Professional Care.* 3rd ed. San Diego, Calif: Plural Publishing, Inc; 2005:1146.)

under the hanging footplate to provide support. Other devices, such as the Boston suspension system, are designed to actually help create the exposure. However, this system also works best when optimal exposure is obtained by the surgeon prior to application of the suspension device. Anterior pressure is often useful and can be maintained throughout the case with a broad piece of tape stretched across the neck of the patient from the operating table. It takes very little tension on the tape to effect a change in the laryngeal exposure. In addition to these maneuvers. flexing the neck further usually provides better anterior exposure for difficult cases.

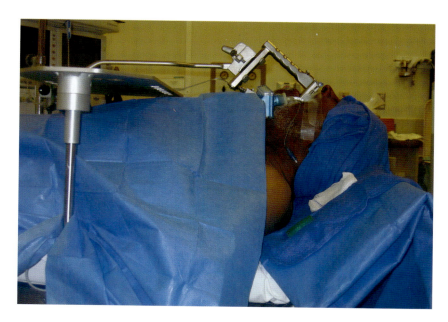

FIGURE 9–3. Patient is in sniffing position with the headboard of the table flexed.

The operating table may be placed in varying degrees of Trendelenburg or reverse Trendelenburg positions to direct the opening of the laryngoscope so that the microscope and surgeon's hands may be positioned ideally. Suspending the laryngoscope from a table which attaches to, and thus moves with, the patient's operating bed will minimize the risk of dental injury and save valuable time.

Having a variety of laryngoscopes to choose from will assist the surgeon in obtaining adequate visualization. One should use the largest laryngoscope that can be inserted safely and expose the entire length of the true vocal folds (Figure 9–4). The laryngoscope should provide internal distention to push the false vocal folds out of the way and provide enough tension on the true vocal folds to ensure precise excision of the mass.

The laryngoscope must be large enough to ensure the ability to operate simultaneously with both hands (Figures 9–5 and 9–6). If exposure cannot be obtained with the largest laryngoscope available, the surgeon should try increasingly smaller scopes, until the largest insertable scope is identified We find the Ossoff-Pilling Large (Teleflex-Pilling 52-2191, Fort Washington,

Pa) laryngoscope to be the smallest scope available currently that will still permit two-handed operating. When even this scope is inadequate, exposure can be obtained in most cases with a subglottiscope (Teleflex-Pilling 52-2245, Fort Washington, Pa) or by using the Ossoff-Pilling laryngoscope and working through it with a 70-degree telescope and angled instruments.

In addition to a sufficient choice of laryngoscopes, one must have appropriate instrumentation to allow surgery on millimeter-sized masses without excessive trauma to surrounding tissue. A number of instrument sets exist with a variety of graspers, microscissors, micropics, hockeysticks, spatulas, ball-dissectors, and microalligator forceps. Disposable knife blades are available with the Medtronic-Xomed Sataloff microlaryngeal set which ensures sharp, fresh knives with each procedure. Having an array of microinstruments to choose from is useful, particularly when raising microflaps and dissecting out difficult intracordal cysts.

Microlaryngeal surgery requires magnification, typically provided by an operating microscope. Surgeons should be familiar and adept with the microscope to avoid long time delays and frustration while making adjustments.

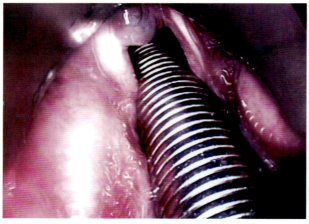
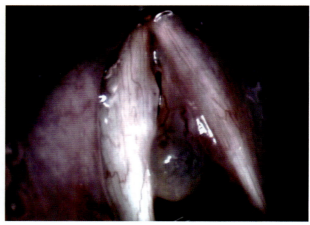

A.   **B.**

FIGURE 9–4. **A.** Inadequate exposure of right vocal fold polyp (0-degree endoscope). **B.** Adequate exposure of right vocal fold polyp and left contact mass. The patient's neck has been flexed more and the laryngoscope adjusted, so that the entire length of the vocal folds is visualized. The extent of the right vocal fold mass cannot be appreciated in *A.* Moreover, the left vocal fold mass was not visualized at all. Of note, the endotracheal tube in *A* is a Mallincrodt. This was placed by anesthesia without discussion with the surgeon. Neither author typically uses these tubes, as they believe the ridges may be traumatic to the vocal folds. Preintubation discussion with the anesthesiologist is critical. Ideally, as small an endotracheal tube as possible for adequate ventilation should be used to leave as much room as possible for instrumentation. The authors prefer a number 5 endotracheal tube if possible. A laser-safe tube need not be used, unless the surgeon plans to operate the laser.

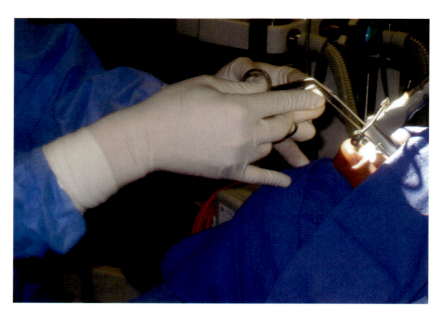

FIGURE 9–5. The fifth digits rest on the patient while performing microsurgery for stability.

Newer microscopes have autofocus and zoom controls, which facilitate procedures. However, older microscopes with knobs for stepwise magnification changes are often sufficient. For laryngologic surgery, a 400-mm lens is used most commonly. Lenses with shorter focal lengths will

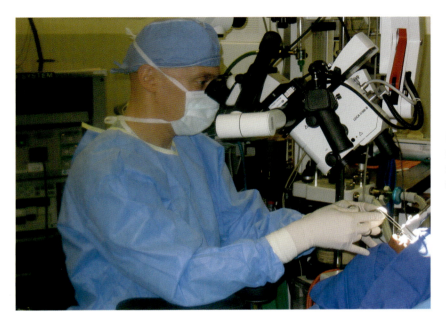

FIGURE 9–6. The surgeon's elbows and fifth digits are stabilized for multipoint stabilization.

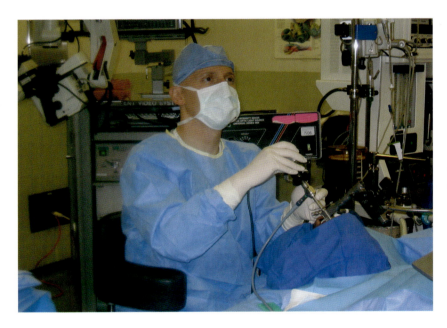

FIGURE 9–7. Surgeon examines lesions with 0- and 70-degree endoscopy. He views images on a monitor.

increase magnification. However, they require the microscope to be too close to the operating field, thereby preventing the insertion of long laryngeal instruments into the laryngoscope.

Laryngeal telescopes are useful to assess the full three-dimensional extent of mass lesions. The authors use 0-degree and 70-degree telescopes in most circumstances (Figure 9–7).[9] Some surgeons use the telescopes during the actual excision.[10] However, someone else must hold the scope to enable the surgeon to operate with both hands. We use this technique only in cases in which good exposure cannot be obtained without a telescope.

The CO_2 laser is useful in the excision of some benign lesions of the larynx, such as amyloid. The use of CO_2 laser on medial edge lesions such as cysts and polyps remains popular, though controversial. The laser offers the advantages of hemostasis (although, hemostasis is usually achievable during cold excision with the application of cotton pledgets soaked in 1:1000 epinephrine) and ease. Many people believe that using a micromanipulator requires less dexterity in the nondominant hand. However, deft control of the "joystick" is essential; an excellent laryngeal laser surgeon generally must be trained as an excellent cold surgeon first.

The depth of tissue injury is less predictable with CO_2 laser and more tissue may be lost through thermal damage than with cold excision.[11] The use of the microspot CO_2 laser in superpulse mode reduces the zone of thermal injury from previous conventional CO_2 lasers.[12] Benninger reported no significant difference in voice outcome comparing microspot CO_2 laser to "cold-knife" excision of benign lesions limited to the medial edge of the vocal fold from a randomized, prospective study.[13]

CO_2 laser is certainly useful in some cases. The excision of malignant lesions of the vocal fold in which muscle must be excised results in bleeding and obscuring of the surgical field with cold instruments, but less trouble with a laser. Laser excision of supraglottic lesions also is appropriate in many cases. Feeding vessels to polyps may be obliterated with low-wattage laser using an unfocused beam. Ultimately, the decision to use cold instrumentation or laser is probably best determined by the individual surgeon, based on what yields his or her best results.

> ## PRESERVE ALL NORMAL EPITHELIUM AND SUPERFICIAL LAMINA PROPRIA AND AVOID TRAUMATIZING THE VOCAL LIGAMENT

A number of techniques have been described for the removal of benign masses. Until 1975, when Hirano described the histology of the vocal fold,[14] *vocal fold stripping* was the most common approach. Although mucosal healing occurs and the vocal fold may appear normal under continuous light, the absence of superficial lamina propria results in loss of vocal fold vibration and voice quality in many patients.

Hirano demonstrated that the vocal fold is a multilayered structure consisting of: an epithelium; superficial, intermediate, and deep layers of the lamina propria; and the thyroarytenoid muscle (Figure 9–8).[14] The superficial lamina propria (Reinke's "space") is composed predominantly of loose fibrous tissue consisting of a network of hyaluronic acid, mucopolysaccharides, decorin, and other extracellular matrix components. It is not a "space," but a layer of the vocal fold that allows for complex vibration. It lies immediately below the epithelium, contains very few fibroblasts, and provides flexibility of the vocal fold cover. The intermediate layer of lamina propria contains mature elastin fibers arranged longitudinally and large quantities of hyaluronic acid which may act as a shock absorber. The deep layer of the lamina propria consists of collagen fibers arranged longitudinally and is rich in fibroblasts.[15] A complete review is presented in

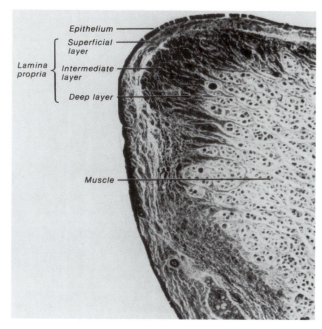

FIGURE 9–8. Structure of the vocal fold. (Reprinted with permission from Hirano M. *Clinical Examination of Voice.* New York, NY: Springer-Verlag; 1981.)

chapter 1, Anatomy of the Larynx and Physiology of Phonation.

These five histologic layers act as three mechanical layers. The epithelium and superficial lamina propria make up the "cover" of the vocal fold; the intermediate and deep layers make up the vocal ligament or the "transition"; and the thyroarytenoid muscle makes up the "body" of the vocal fold. The relationship between these three layers and the gradient of increasing stiffness provide the mechanics for the complex mucosal wave. Understanding this histology is critical when surgically excising benign vocal fold lesions. Respect for these layers is necessary for restoring and preserving the oscillatory properties of the true vocal folds. All normal mucosa and superficial lamina should be preserved, and care must be taken not to traumatize the vocal ligament. Usually it is possible to remove superficial lesions without disturbing the deeper, fibroblast-containing layers.

The classic microflap approach to the excision of vocal fold lesions involves making an incision through the epithelium on the superior surface of the vocal fold lateral to the mass about halfway to the ventricle (Figure 9-9). A plane is then created in the superficial lamina propria until the lesion is identified. The lesion is then separated from the vocal ligament and overlying cover.[16] This technique requires a long incision and is

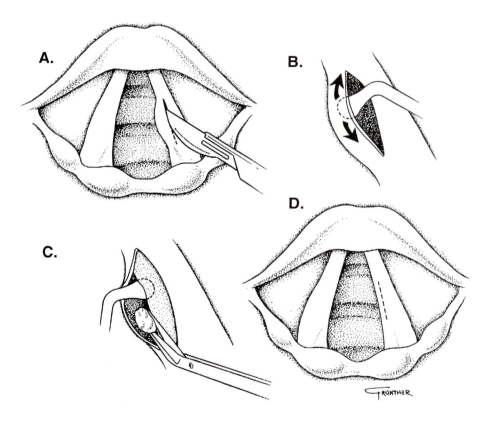

FIGURE 9-9. Microflap procedure, as illustrated by Sataloff in Cummings et al. In this technique, a superficial incision is made in the superior surface of the true vocal fold **A.** Blunt dissection is used to elevate the mucosa from the lesion **B.**, minimizing trauma to the fibroblast-containing layers of the lamina propria. Only pathologic tissue is excised under direct vision **C.** Mucosa is reapproximated **D.** without violating the leading edge. (Reprinted with permission from Sataloff RT. The professional voice. In: Cummings W, et al, eds. *Otolanyngology–Head and Neck Surgery.* Vol. 1. St. Louis, Mo: CV Mosby; 1986:2029–2053.)

difficult technically. It is now reserved for larger lesions (such as diffuse leukoplakia, papilloma, or large intracordal cysts) and for lesions in which identification of the vocal ligament is difficult.[17]

Sataloff et al reapproached the microflap procedure and fashioned the mini-microflap based on

their outcomes assessment of microflap surgery and on Gray's discovery of a complex basement membrane structure between the epithelium and superficial layer of lamina propria (Figures 9-10, 9-11, and 9-12).[18] An intricate series of type VII collagen loops attach the epithelium and

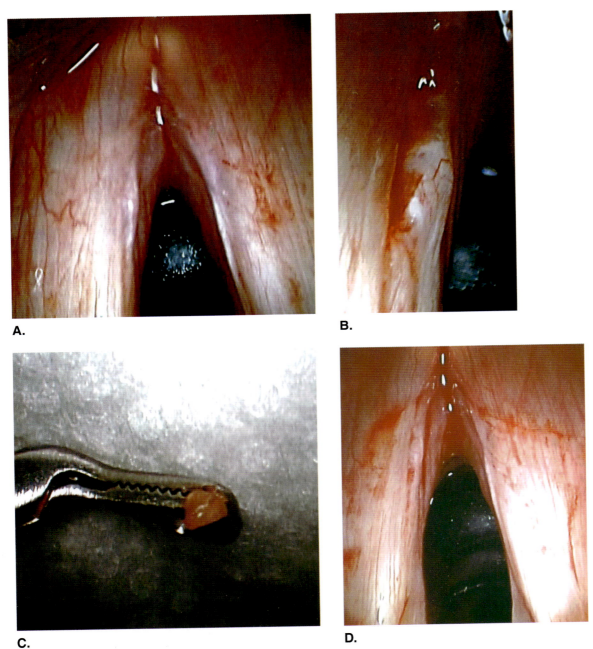

A.

B.

C.

D.

FIGURE 9–10. A. Small submucosal mass in left vocal fold. **B.** Mini-microflap incision made just lateral to the mass. **C.** Fibrovascular mass excised. **D.** Flap redraped with no secondary defect.

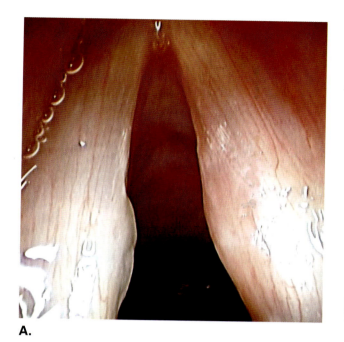
A.

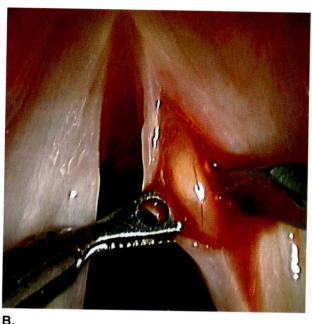
B.

FIGURE 9–11. A. Right submucosal cyst and left contact mass. **B.** Right submucosal cyst exposed after mini-microflap created. Note that the incision was made just lateral to the mass, but was made longer than the previous example to help with exposure of the cyst.

basement membrane to the superficial lamina propria.[15,19] Microflap techniques disturb this arrangement and may lead to hypodynamic segments of mucosa. In creating a mini-microflap, an incision is made at the junction of the mass and normal tissue (Figure 9–13). Small vertical anterior and posterior incisions are made if necessary and the mass is separated by blunt dissection from the superficial layer of the lamina propria. The lesion is excised preserving as much normal adjacent mucosa as possible. A small amount of mucosa directly over the lesion may be removed if necessary. Because the mass often acts as a tissue expander, an inferiorly based "mini-microflap" usually can be created to prevent a significant secondary defect.

Courey et al described the medial microflap technique as a variation of the traditional lateral microflap for submucosal lesions that involve the medial surface exclusively and are covered by atrophic and redundant mucosa. Similar to the mini-microflap, this technique emphasizes sparing all normal lamina propria and overlying mucosa, thereby avoiding any defect along the

medial edge of the vocal fold that would need to heal by secondary intention.[20]

A secondary defect is difficult to avoid in some cases. Some masses, such as broad-based polyps, have significant vertical dimension; and some masses are very difficult to separate from the overlying mucosa. Moreover, leaving redundant or deformed mucosa may result in fluid accumulation and development of a pseudocyst.

Specific Considerations for Common Vocal Fold Lesions

The following section highlights specific approaches and surgical principles for several common phonosurgical procedures. A detailed review of benign vocal fold pathology is found in chapter 18.

Reinke's Edema

Caution must be observed when operating on Reinke's edema. Overaggressive resection may lead to scarring and adherence of the epithelium to

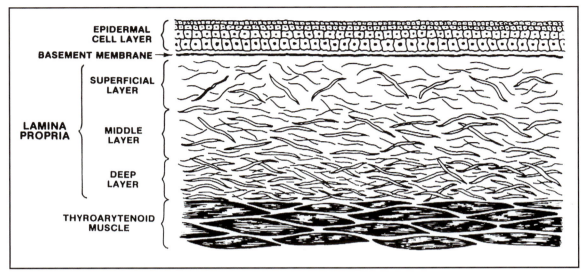

A.

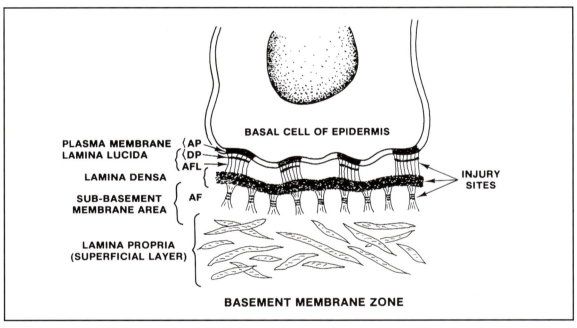

B.

FIGURE 9–12. A. Layers of vocal fold (not drawn to scale). The basement membrane lies between the epithelium and the superficial layer of the lamina propria. **B.** Basement membrane zone. Basal cells are connected to the lamina densa by attachment plax (*AP*) in the plasma membrane of the epidermis. Anchoring filaments (*AF*) extend from the attachment plax through the sub-basal densa plate (*DP*) and attach to the lamina densa (dark single-layer, electron-dense band just beneath the basal cell layer.) The sub-basement membrane zone consists of anchoring fibers (*AF*) that attach to the lamina densa and extend into the superficial layer of the lamina propria. Type VII collagen fibers attach to the network of the lamina propria by looping around Type III collagen fibers. (Reproduced with permission from Gray S. Basement membrane zone injury in vocal nodules. In: Gauffin, J, Hammarberg B, Eds. *Vocal Fold Physiology.* San Diego, Calif: Singular Publishing Group; 1991.)

114

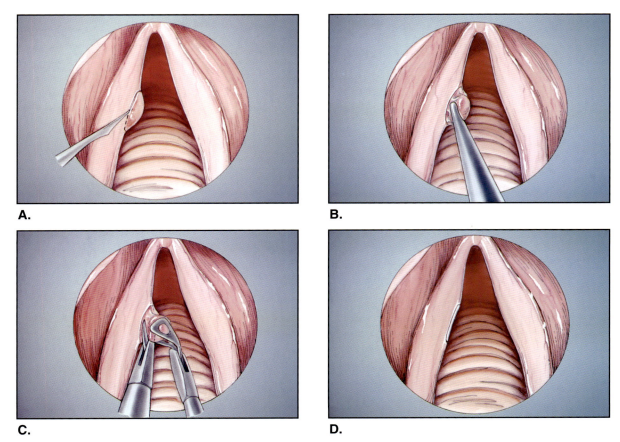

A.

B.

C.

D.

FIGURE 9–13. A. In elevating a mini-microflap, an incision is made with a straight knife at the junction of the mass and normal tissue. Small vertical anterior and posterior incisions may be added at the margins of the mass if necessary, usually using a straight scissors. **B.** The mass is separated by blunt dissection, splitting the superficial layer of the lamina propria and preserving it as much as possible. This dissection can be performed with a spatula, blunt ball dissector (*illustrated*), or scissors (*as illustrated in A*). **C.** The lesion is stabilized and a scissors (straight or curved) is used to excise the lesion, preserving as much adjacent mucosa as possible. The lesion itself acts as a tissue expander, and it is often possible to create an inferiorly based mini-microflap. **D.** The mini-microflap is replaced over the surgical defect, establishing primary closure and acting as a biological dressing. (Reprinted with permission from Sataloff R. Voice surgery. In Sataloff R. *Professional Voice: The Science and Art of Professional Care.* 3rd ed. San Diego, Calif: Plural Publishing, Inc; 2005:1165.)

the underlying vocal ligament. An incision is created along the superior surface and edematous material is removed with suction (Figure 9–14). Not infrequently, some of the fibrous stroma may need to be excised with cold instruments. Redundant mucosa is trimmed and the mucosal edges are reapproximated. This procedure was initially described by Hirano, and replaced the traditional technique of vocal fold stripping for this disease.[21]

There is some controversy as to whether both vocal folds should be operated on at one time.[22] Although bilateral surgery may be performed without an anterior web if care is taken in the anterior commissure, unilateral surgery offers other advantages. If the operated side becomes stiff postoperatively, the contralateral edematous vocal fold will usually compensate well. If a surgeon operates on both sides at once and each side suffers severe scarring, the patient

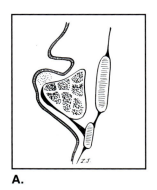
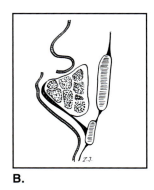
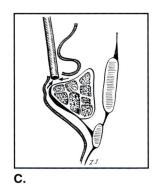
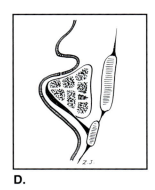

A.   **B.**   **C.**   **D.**

FIGURE 9–14. A. Bulky vocal fold showing Reinke's edema (*small dots*) in the superficial layer of the lamina propria. **B.** Incision in the upper surface opens easily into Reinke's space. **C.** Using a fine-needle suction, the edema fluid is aspirated (*arrows*). **D.** The mucosal edges are reapproximated, trimming redundant mucosa if necessary. (Reprinted with permission from Sataloff R. Voice surgery. In Sataloff R. *Professional Voice: The Science and Art of Professional Care.* 3rd ed. San Diego, Calif: Plural Publishing, Inc; 2005:1170.)

will be left with a hoarse, breathy voice requiring high phonation pressures. This results in strained, effortful phonation, and the patient may be left unhappier than he or she was with the initial low or masculized voice. The patient can return to the operating room for the treatment of the contralateral vocal fold after healing has occurred, if symptoms warrant the additional procedure.

Ectasias and Varicosities

Although often asymptomatic, ectasias and varicosities may lead to dysphonia and/or recurrent vocal fold hemorrhages. Thus, symptomatic lesions require excision. In addition, vocal fold polyps often have a large feeding vessel that may need to be treated. Varices and ectasias may be photocoagulated with low-wattage (1–1.5 watts) CO_2 laser in interrupted single 0.1 second pulses. The beam is defocused to 300 to 400 μm. Low-power density is used to try to avoid thermal injury to the superficial lamina propria and minimize risk of injury to the vocal ligament.[23,24] Cold excision of varices and ectasias is technically more difficult, but potentially safer to the underlying lamina propria; and this procedure eliminates the risk of recanalization, which may occur after laser vaporization. An incision is created adjacent to the vessel, and the vessel is elevated with a 1-mm right-angle vascular knife

(Xomed-Medtronics) (Figure 9–15). The elevated vessel is then retracted gently to provide access to its anterior and posterior limits where it is divided sharply. Bleeding stops spontaneously, although topical 1:1000 epinephrine may be used for hemostasis.[25]

Vocal Process Granulomas

Granulomas usually result from reflux[26] and/or trauma, such as endotracheal intubation. One should resist operating on these lesions until conservative measures, such as antireflux treatment, voice therapy[27] and steroids, have been exhausted. These lesions may take months to resolve. If they do not improve with medical management, surgical excision may be performed. Laser or cold excision may be used. However, care must be taken not to traumatize the underlying perichondrium as this will likely result in recurrent granuloma formation. The authors prefer cold excision of these lesions and injection of decadron (4 mg/cc) into the surgical site. Chemical denervation with botulinum toxin may be useful, particularly in the setting of recurrent granuloma. Pre- and postoperative voice therapy and long-term antireflux therapy also help prevent recurrence. In multiply recurrent cases, mitomycin-C may have a role; and recently, one of the authors (RTS) has had success using pulsed-dye laser therapy.

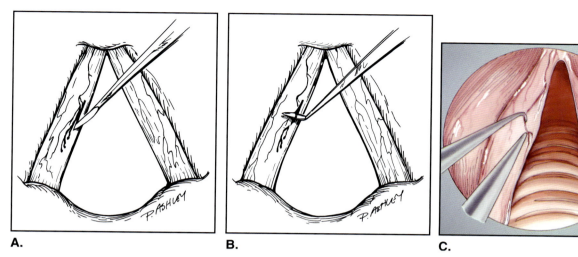

A. **B.** **C.**

FIGURE 9–15. Ectasia. **A.** This figure illustrates the technique for elevating and resecting a varicose vessel. A superficial incision is made in the epithelium adjacent to the vessel using the sharp point of the vascular knife or using a microknife (*illustrated*). **B.** The 1-mm right angle vascular knife is inserted under the vessel and used to elevate it. It may be necessary to make more than one epithelial incision in order to dissect the desired length of the vessel. **C.** Once the pathologic vessel has been elevated, it is retracted gently to provide access to its anterior and posterior limits. These can be divided sharply with a scissors or knife (bleeding stops spontaneously) or divided and cauterized with a laser, as long as there is no thermal injury to the adjacent vocal ligament. (Reprinted with permission from Sataloff R. Voice surgery. In Sataloff R. *Professional Voice: The Science and Art of Professional Care.* 3rd ed. San Diego, Calif: Plural Publishing, Inc; 2005:1169.)

Recurrent Respiratory Papillomatosis

Laryngeal papillomatosis continues to be a difficult problem for the patient and laryngologist. Much of the complexity is a result of the fact that human papilloma virus (HPV) exists in normal epithelial tissue as well as gross papillomas.[28] Recurrence is common, resulting in multiple surgical excisions and subsequent vocal fold scarring and dysphonia.

In addition to numerous medical treatments (none of which is highly effective), a variety of techniques have been described for managing laryngeal papillomatosis surgically including cold excision,[29,30] pulse-dye laser,[31] photodynamic therapy,[32] and the microdebrider or laryngeal shaver.[33,34] Injection of cidofovir is being used adjunct with or in lieu of surgical excision,[35] though concern continues to be raised with regard to the possible transforming effects of this agent.[36] Regardless of the methods used, when excising papillomas of the true vocal fold, the surgeon should remember that this is a disease of epithelium and should preserve all underlying superficial lamina propria and not traumatize the vocal ligament. In addition, the surgeon must remember that surgery is not likely to be curative. Conservative and precise excision should be performed with the hope that the patient's immune response, current adjunctive therapy (eg, cidofovir), or future treatment options (eg, vaccination) will yield complete remission of the disease. Viral subtyping is useful to determine whether there is increased risk for malignant transformation. Anal and genital papilloma data suggest that subtypes 16 and 18 are associated with a higher risk for malignant transformation and may warrant closer follow-up. However, there is evidence that subtype 11 may have a more aggressive course in the larynx than it does at other sites.[37] Otherwise, the decision to proceed to the operating room should be determined on an individualized basis, influenced by patient's desires, risk for airway obstruction, and voice disturbance.

Submucosal Infusion

Submucosal infusion technique arose from anatomic experiments which helped define the connective tissue compartments of the larynx.[38]. The benefits of submucosal infusion include elevation of the mass from the underlying superficial lamina propria and vocal ligament, increasing the tension of the epithelium, and hemostasis. In some cases, however, injection may obscure the mass or the epithelial boundary of normal and abnormal tissue.

A number of substances may be injected including a 1:10,000 dilution of epinephrine (9 cc of sterile saline with 1 cc of epinephrine 1:1000), decadron, and, in selected cases of papilloma, limited amounts of cidofovir. Steroids may be useful particularly when operating on a vocal fold with significant scar and sulcus. However, there is some evidence suggesting that steroids may not be beneficial and, in fact, may delay wound healing.[39]

EXCELLENT POSTOPERATIVE CARE IS ESSENTIAL

Postoperative care and evaluation are critical to obtaining optimal surgical results. The outcomes of voice surgery are unpredictable for any individual. Even with the best surgical technique, voice results can be compromised by postoperative inflammation and scar formation.

The use of postoperative steroids and antibiotics is not universal, but they are used by some surgeons empirically to promote healing. Certainly, underlying medical issues such as reflux and cough should be treated. Aggressive reflux control is especially important. There is little downside to using mucolytics and antitussives in the postoperative period. Patients should be discouraged from taking medications that may be irritating or otherwise harmful to the vocal folds, such as steroid inhalers, aspirin, ibuprofen, and antihistamines.

The issue of voice rest is controversial. There is no consensus as to the application of voice rest postoperatively. A recent survey suggested that, although the majority of otolaryngologists performing microlaryngeal surgery recommend voice rest postoperatively, there is lack of agreement as to duration and type of voice rest (absolute vs relative). The most common recommendation was 7 days of absolute or relative voice rest.[40] There are no adequate prospective trials comparing surgery with and without voice rest. However, it seems likely that reducing traumatic forces at the surgical site would reduce the risk of scar formation. Certainly, when we make an incision elsewhere on the body, we discourage traumatizing it while it is healing.

Phonation should probably be avoided until the epithelium has healed and can provide protection for the underlying lamina propria. The authors recommend 1 week of absolute voice rest in most cases, followed by strobovideolaryngoscopic evaluation. If resection has been very limited, reepithelization may occur within 2 or 3 days and short periods of voice rest may be acceptable in carefully selected patients. The findings of the postoperative evaluation determine how rapidly a patient may increase voice use. Useful parameters include return of mucosal wave (favorable), and the development of early postoperative complications such as hemorrhage or early scar or granuloma formation. If such complications arise, one should consider restricting voice use longer and using steroids (either systemically or by local injection). The authors typically gradually increase voice use over the following 2 to 6 weeks, under supervision of the voice team. Additional voice therapy is important in the postoperative period to prevent the development of hyperfunctional compensatory techniques, and consequent phonotrauma, and to optimize surgical outcome.

After about 6 weeks, strobovideolaryngoscopy should be repeated. If there has been good return of mucosal wave and no additional injuries, the patient should be permitted to speak freely.

Emerging Concepts

Although microsurgical techniques for removing benign vocal fold lesions have improved since the days of vocal fold stripping, there is still much room for improvement. Innovations in the treatment of papilloma, such as intralesional cidofovir injections, the careful use of the laryngeal microdebrider, and pulsed-dye laser are good examples of innovations achieved through people thinking "beyond-the-box" to improve treatment of a very difficult and often frustrating disease process. Time and well-controlled studies will determine the efficacy of these novel ideas. Current surgical treatment of other benign lesions also still leaves something to be desired. Although we can minimize scar formation in most situations by using meticulous technique, we cannot eliminate it. In addition, many patients have scar present preoperatively, that, to date, we cannot treat as well as we would like. Fat, hyaluronic acid, and collagen have all been used to try to treat scar, although the ideal injectable does not exist. Eventually, genetic screening may be able to identify people at high risk for scar formation, and genetic engineering may allow us to grow new superficial lamina propria to repair scar. We should not be satisfied until we are able to obtain maximal voice improvement in every microsurgical case.

The patient should be advised that any worsening of the voice should prompt an urgent evaluation and return to more voice restrictions. In general, singing should not be started until about 6 weeks postoperatively. Return of mucosal wave is desirable prior to return to singing. Performers should be advised that surgical results are variable, and some patients may not be able to get back to full capabilities until after 6 months to a year of rehabilitation.[41] Occasionally, full recovery does not occur at all, usually due to scar formation.

Microlaryngeal surgery for benign vocal fold lesions is a challenging and important part of care for the voice patient. The otolaryngologist must exercise good judgment before, during, and after surgery. A thorough understanding of the anatomy and physiology of the voice, as well as access to and familiarity with appropriate instrumentation, is critical to provide quality surgical care for the laryngeal surgery patient.

Review Questions

1. Optimal positioning for viewing the entire length of the vocal folds during microdirect laryngoscopy includes:
   a. Head extension, neck extension
   b. Head flexion, neck flexion
   c. Head flexion, neck extension
   d. Head extension, neck flexion
   e. None of the above

2. A young professional soprano presents to you with mild hoarseness, loss of upper range, and increased vocal fatigue since an upper respiratory tract infection 3 months ago. Her voice is becoming progressively worse. She complains of globus sensation and the

need to clear her throat frequently. Visualization of the larynx with both flexible and rigid videostroboscopy demonstrates symmetrical vocal fold adduction and abduction, posterior inflammatory changes, bilateral vocal fold edema, a small cyst on the medial edge within the left vocal fold striking zone, contralateral fibrosis, and an hourglass deformity. Which of the following would be the most appropriate initial course of action?

a. Surgical excision of the cyst and steroid injection into the contralateral vocal fold
b. Treatment of reflux followed by surgical excision of the cyst.
c. Treatment of reflux and voice therapy
d. Treatment of reflux, voice therapy, then surgical excision of the cyst.
e. Bilateral thyroplasty

3. The medial microflap and mini-microflap are similar in that they both:
a. Try to reduce scarring
b. Try to preserve as much superficial lamina propria as possible
c. Try to preserve normal overlying epithelium
d. Are useful for masses along the medial edge of the vocal fold
e. All of the above

4. Potential advantages of cold excision of benign vocal fold lesions over CO_2 laser include all of the following except:
a. Cold excision provides more control of depth of injury
b. CO^2 laser introduces a risk of airway fire
c. CO^2 laser provides better hemostasis
d. CO^2 laser requires less surgical skill
e. In the right hands, either technique can yield good results.

5. A severely dysphonic, breathy patient presents to you 6 months after having "smokers' polyps" removed. Which of the following are you most likely to see with videostroboscopy?
a. Severe scarring bilaterally
b. Bilateral hemorrhage
c. Recurrent polyposis
d. Vocal fold immobility
e. Function dysphonia

REFERENCES

1. Rakel B, Spiegel JR, Sataloff RT. Prolonged ulcerative laryngitis. *J Voice*. 2002;16(3):433–438.
2. Merati AL, Heman-Ackah Y, Abaza M, Altman KW, Bielamowicz S. Common movement disorders of the larynx: a report of the Neurolaryngology Subcommittee. *Otolaryngol Head and Neck Surg*. 2005; 133(5):654–665.
3. Hogikyan ND, Sethuraman G. Validation of an instrument to measure voice-related quality of life (V-RQOL). *J Voice*. 1999;13(4):557–569.
4. Rubin AD, Wodchis WP, Spak C, Kileny PR, Hogikyan ND. Longitudinal effects of Botox injections on voice-related quality of life (V-RQOL) for patients with adductory spasmodic dysphonia: part II. *Arch Otolaryngol Head and Neck Surg*. 2004;130(4):415–420.
5. Benninger MS, Ahuja AS, Gardner G, Grywalski C. Assessing outcomes for dysphonic patients. *J Voice*. 1998;12(4):540–550.
6. Rosen CA, Lee AS, Osborne J, Zullo T, Murry T. Development and validation of the voice handicap index–10. *Laryngoscope*. 2004; 114(9):1549–1556.
7. Zeitels SM, Vaughan CW. "External counterpressure" and "internal distension" for optimal laryngoscopic exposure of the anterior glottal commissure. *Ann Otol Rhinol Laryngol*. 1994; 103:669–676.
8. Hochman II, Zeitels SM, Heaton JT. Analysis of the forces and position required for direct laryngoscopic exposure of the anterior vocal folds. *Ann Otol Rhinol Laryngol*. 1999;108(8):715–724.
9. Anderson TD, Sataloff RT. Value of the 70 degrees telelaryngoscope in microlaryngoscopy for benign

pathology. *Ear Nose Throat J.* 2002;81(12): 821–822.

10. Yeh AR, Huang HM, Chen YL. Telescopic video microlaryngeal surgery. *Ann Otol Rhinol Laryngol.* 1999;108:165–168.

11. Zeitels SM. Laser versus cold instruments for microlaryngologic surgery. *Laryngoscope.* 1996; 106(5):545–552.

12. Garrett G, Reinisch L. New generation pulsed CO_2 laser: comparative effects on vocal fold wound healing. *Ann Otol Rhinol Laryngol.* 2002;111(6): 471–476.

13. Benninger MS. Microdissection or microspot laser for limited vocal fold benign lesions: a prospective randomized trial. *Laryngoscope.* 2000;110 (2 pt 2, suppl 92):1–17.

14. Hirano M. Phonosurgery. Basic and clinical investigations. *Otologia Fukuoka.* 1975;21:239–442.

15. Gray SD. Cellular Physiology of the vocal folds. *Otolaryngol Clin North Am.* 2000;33(4) 679–697.

16. Courey MS, Gardner GM, Stone RE, Ossoff RH. Endoscopic vocal fold microflap: a three-year experience. *Ann Otol Rhinol Laryngol.* 1995;104 (4 pt 1):267–273.

17. Ford CN. Adavances and refinements in phonosurgery. *Laryngoscope.* 1999;109(12):1891–1900.

18. Sataloff RT, Spiegel JR, Heuer RJ, et al. Laryngeal mini-microflap: a new technique and reassessment of the microflap saga. *J Voice.* 1995;9(2):198–204.

19. Gray S. Basement membrane zone injury I vocal nodules. In: Gauffin J, Hammarberg B, eds. *Vocal Fold Physiology: Acoustic, Perceptual and Physiologic Aspects of Voice Mechanics.* San Diego, Calif: Singular Publishing Group; 1991:21–27.

20. Courey MS, Garrett CG, Ossoff RH. Medial microflap for excision of benign vocal fold lesions. *Laryngoscope.* 1997;107:340–344.

21. Hirano M, Shin T, Morio M, et al. An improvement in surgical treatment for polypoid vocal cord: sucking technique. *Otologia (Fukuoka).* 1976; 22:583–589.

22. Zeitels S, Casiano R, Gardner G, Hogikyan N, Koufman J, Rosen C. Management of common voice problems: committee report. *Otolaryngol Head Neck Surg.* 2002;126(4):323–348.

23. Postma, GM, Courey, MS, Ossoff, RH. Microvascular lesions of the true vocal fold. *Ann Otol Rhinol Laryngol.* 1998;107(6):472–476.

24. Garrett G, Reinisch L. New generation pulsed CO_2 laser: comparative effects on vocal fold wound healing. *Ann Otol Rhinol Laryngol.* 2002;111(6):471–476.

25. Hochman I, Sataloff RT, Hillman R, Zeitels S. Ectasias and varices of the vocal fold: clearing the striking zone: *Ann Otol Rhinol Laryngol.* 1999; 108(1)10–16.

26. Ylitalo R, Ramel S. Extraesophageal reflux in patients with contact granuloma: a prospective controlled study. *Ann Otol Rhinol Laryngol.* 2002;111(5 pt 1):441–446.

27. Leonard R, Kendall K. Effects of voice therapy on vocal process granuloma: a phonoscopic approach. *Am J Otolaryngol.* 2005;26(2):101–107.

28. Rihkanen H, Aaltonen LM, Syrjanen SM. Human papillomavirus in laryngeal papillomas and in adjacent normal epithelium. *Clin Otolaryngol Allied Sci.* 1993;18(6):470–474.

29. Zeitels SM, Sataloff RT. Phonomicrosurgical resection of glottal papillomatosis. *J Voice.* 1999;13(1): 123–127.

30. Courey MS, Ossoff RH. Laser applications in adult laryngeal surgery. *Otolaryngol Clin North Am.* 1996;29(6):973–986.

31. Franco RA Jr, Zeitels SM, Farinelli WA, Anderson RR. 585-nm pulsed dye laser treatment of glottal papillomatosis. *Ann Otol Rhinol Laryngol.* 2002; 111(6):486–92.

32. Shikowitz MJ, Abramson AL, Freeman K, Steinberg BM, Nouri M. Efficacy of DHE photodynamic therapy for respiratory papillomatosis: immediate and long-term results. *Laryngoscope* 1998;108:962–967.

33. Patel N, Rowe M, Tunkel D. Treatment of recurrent respiratory papillomatosis in children with the microdebrider. *Ann Otol Rhinol Laryngol.* 2003;112(1):7–10.

34. Patel RS, MacKenzie K. Powered laryngeal shavers and laryngeal papillomatosis: a preliminary report *Clin Otolaryngol Allied Sci.* 2000;25(5):358–360.

35. Bielamowicz S, Villagomez V, Stager SV, Wilson WR. Intralesional cidofovir therapy for laryngeal papilloma in an adult cohort. *Laryngoscope.* 2002;112(4):696–699.

36. Wemer RD, Lee JH, Hoffman HT, Robinson RA, Smith RJ. Case of progressive dysplasia concomitant with intralesional cidofovir administration for recurrent respiratory papillomatosis. *Ann Otol Rhinol Laryngol.* 2005;114(11):836–839.

37. Gerein V, Rastorguev E, Gerein J, Draf W, Schirren J, Incidence, age at onset, and potential reasons of malignant transformation in recurrent respiratory papillomatosis patients: 20 years experience. *Otolaryngol Head Neck Surg.* 2005;132(3):392–394.

38. Kass ES, Hillman RE, Zeitels SM. Vocal fold submucosal infusion technique in phonomicrosurgery. *Ann Otol Rhinol Laryngol.* 1996;105(5):341–347.

39. Coleman JR Jr, Smith S, Reinisch L, Billante CR, Ossoff JP, Deriso W, Garrett CG. Histomorphometric

and laryngeal videostroboscopic analysis of the effects of corticosteroids on microflap healing in the dog larynx. *Ann Otol Rhinol Laryngol.* 1999;108(2):119–127.

40. Behrman A, Sulica L. Voice rest after microlaryngoscopy: current opinion and practice. *Laryngoscope.* 2003;113:2182–2186.

41. Emerich KA, Spiegel JR, Sataloff RT. Phonomicrosurgery III: pre- and postoperative care. *Otolaryngol Clin North Am.* 2000;33(5):1071–1080.

42. Dursun G, Sataloff RT, Spiegel JR, Mandel S, Heuer RJ, Rosen DC. Superior laryngeal nerve paresis and paralysis. *J Voice.* 1996;10(2):206–211.

43. Amin MR, Koufman JA. Vagal neuropathy after upper respiratory infection: a viral etiology? *Am J Otolaryngol.* 2001;22(4):251–256.

44. Rubin AD, Praneetvatakul V, Heman-Ackah Y, Moyer C, Mandel S, Sataloff RT. Repetitive phonatory tasks for identifying vocal fold paresis. *J Voice.* 2005;19(4)702–706.

PART IV

Disorders of the Voice
A. Neurologic Disorders

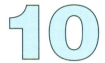

10

Voice and Speech Abnormalities in Systemic Neurodegenerative Disorders

Ted Mau, MD, PhD
Mark S. Courey, MD

KEY POINTS

■ Lesions in different parts of the nervous system produce characteristic signs. The key to neurologic diagnosis is to infer the location of the lesion or the neurosystem involved from specific findings on the physical examination.

■ The possibility of a treatable, unrelated voice disorder in a dysarthric neurodegenerative patient should not be overlooked.

■ The addition of speech tasks to a standard head and neck examination can aid in pinpointing deficits in specific muscle groups involved in articulation.

■ Patients with a breathy voice as the result of a neurodegenerative process may benefit from vocal fold augmentation if they demonstrate a glottal gap on laryngoscopic examination and have breathy dysphonia as a major contributing factor to their decreased intelligibility.

■ A significant number of patients with undiagnosed systemic neurologic disorders are seen initially by otolaryngologists for voice and speech complaints. A familiarity with neurodegenerative disorders and heightened clinical suspicion may avoid a delay in diagnosis.

Voice and speech difficulties are common in patients with neurodegenerative syndromes. More than 70% of patients with Parkinson's disease experience problems with voice and speech, and 30% of them describe these abnormalities as the most debilitating aspect of their disease.[1] Given the prevalence of these problems in this patient population, it is all the more puzzling that these disorders traditionally have received little attention in the otolaryngology literature. There are several reasons for this neglect. First, the neurodegenerative processes that underlie the voice and speech difficulties are progressive and typically not amenable to current surgical or medical intervention. Second, the patients and the medical professionals who care for them are largely unaware of the possible role of the otolaryngologists in carrying out interventions that can potentially improve, albeit temporarily, the quality of life of the patients. This chapter aims to discuss the classification of the neurodegenerative syndromes, review pertinent physical findings, and summarize the available interventions. The discussion is limited to voice and speech abnormalities as part of generalized neurologic disorders. Localized laryngeal disorders with a neurologic origin, such as spasmodic dysphonia, are mentioned for comparison here (see also chapters 12, The Larynx in Parkinson's Disease; 14, Spasmodic Dysphonia, and 13, Laryngeal Tremor).

VOICE AND SPEECH

We begin with a clarification of the distinction between voice and speech. Voice is the sound produced by the vibration of the vocal folds. A voice disorder has its origin in the sound-generating structures, the true vocal folds. Physical lesions of the vocal folds can produce an abnormal voice. Central or peripheral neurologic lesions that affect the innervation of laryngeal muscles can also produce a voice disorder. For example, spasmodic dysphonia, a focal dystonia of the larynx with a presumed origin in the basal ganglia, is a disorder of the voice.

Speech, on the other hand, requires four components for production: a pulmonary power supply, a vibratory source for phonation, a resonance chamber for amplification, and an articulatory system. In the source-filter model of speech production, the larynx is the source of sound production. Airflow from the pulmonary system moves past the vocal folds causing the tissue to vibrate. Vibration of the vocal folds creates local disturbances in air pressure equilibrium. These changes in air pressure equilibrium are interpreted as sound by the receiving auditory system. Sounds produced by vocal fold vibration are termed "voiced." An example of the difference between a voiced and unvoiced sound can be heard when comparing an "s" (voiceless) to a "z" (voiced). This is also true for the voiceless "f" sound and the voiced "v" sound. Vocal fold vibration creates a complex sound with a characteristic fundamental frequency of vibration related to the actual vibratory rate of vocal folds and a harmonic spectrum. As this sound is propagated through the tube created by the pharynx and oral cavity, some frequencies of the harmonic spectrum are amplified and others suppressed. The modulation of the phonated sound by the vocal tract is known as resonance and is determined by the length, shape, and openings of the vocal tract. The sound generated by the vocal folds and resonating cavity is then shaped into words by movement of the lips, tongue, palate, and pharynx through the process of articulation. It is this final product that is perceived as speech.

Motor speech disorders include both apraxia and dysarthria. *Apraxia* is the inability to execute (coordinate) a skilled motor act. Apraxia of speech is a deficit in the ability to smoothly sequence the speech-producing movements of the tongue, lips, palate, and pharynx. Apraxia of speech affects articulation, the shaping of the sounds of speech, and prosody, the patterns of stress and intonation in a language. Speech apraxia is largely due to cortical lesions. On the other hand, apraxia of voice refers to the inability to properly time the onset of voicing with vocal fold adduction. The intensity or volume of speech is often poorly coordinated with prosody, making the vocal product inappropriately loud and/or soft.

Dysarthria is the impaired production of speech due to disturbed motor control of the speech mechanism. This can originate from disturbances in the central or peripheral nervous system and manifests as a deficit in articulation. The voice in terms of intensity and pitch is usually well preserved. In generalized neurologic disorders, dysarthria can be secondary to lesions in both central and peripheral structures. Central lesions or lesions of the upper motor neuron produce slowing in speech with relatively preserved articulation, whereas lesions in the peripheral nervous system (lower motor neurons) or in the end organ muscle produce imprecise articulation with relatively well preserved rate of speech.

NEUROANATOMY OF SPEECH PRODUCTION

To understand how neurodegenerative processes produce voice and speech abnormalities, it is necessary to review the neuroanatomic pathways that lead to speech production[2] (Figure 10–1). The motor control of speech originates from the cerebral cortex and descends through the internal capsule in the corticobulbar tract. The motor outputs are modulated by the basal ganglia and the cerebellum. The basal ganglia modulates the rate of motor contractions, whereas the cerebellum is thought to coordinate the actions of the multiple muscle groups to produce speech. The "fine-tuned" motor signals arrive in the brain stem via the corticobulbar tracts, which synapse onto the motor nuclei of the respective cranial nerves. Fibers of the corticobulbar tracts are upper motor neurons (UMN), whereas the motor component of the cranial nerves is the lower motor neurons (LMN). Lesions that affect the upper motor neurons cause different physical signs than those that affect the lower motor neurons and this distinction should be noted on the physical examination. Finally, the motor signals

arrive at the neuromuscular junction. This is the site of action of botulinum toxin, a mainstay in the symptomatic treatment of the neurodegenerative patient. The anatomy and physiology of phonation and airway regulation are reviewed in chapters 1 and 2.

Anatomically, it is useful to think of specific locations of disease involvement: UMN, LMN, basal ganglia, cerebellum, and the neuromuscular junction. Because many neurodegenerative syndromes involve multiple structures, it is also useful to think in terms of functional groups. Although a comprehensive classification of neurologic voice disorders has been proposed,[2] for the purpose of the current discussion, three groups of diseases will be considered. The first include the extrapyramidal and cerebellar disorders, which classically are thought to be due to lesions in the basal ganglia and/or the cerebellum. The second are the motor neuron diseases with lesions in the UMN and/or the LMN. The third are diseases of the neuromuscular junction. The key to neurologic diagnosis is to infer the location of the lesion or the neurologic system involved based on characteristic signs on physical examination (Table 10–1). Before introducing specific disease entities, terms used to describe examination findings are reviewed first.

DEFINITION OF TERMS

Spasticity and flaccidity are descriptors of muscle tone. *Spasticity*, or chronically increased muscle tone, originates from lesions in the central nervous system and is specifically associated with lesions of UMN in the descending corticospinal tracts of axial nerves and/or descending corticobulbar tracts of the cranial nerves. As otolaryngologists, we are most often called to deal with symptoms affecting the bulbar musculature innervated by the cranial nerves. Examples include a strained voice as a result of a corticobulbar lesion in patients with primary lateral sclerosis and spasticity of the facial muscles contributing to labored speech in pseudobulbar palsy.

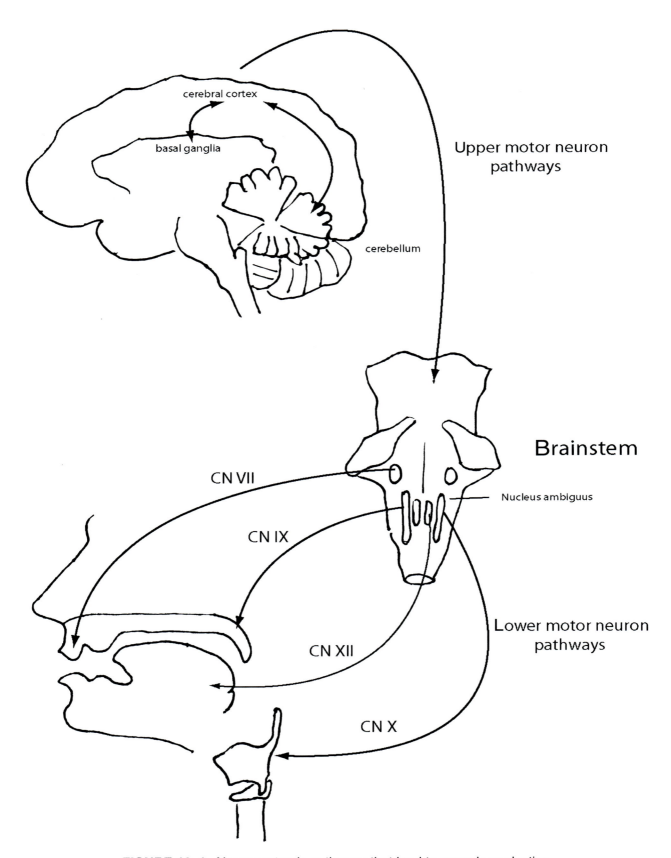

FIGURE 10–1. Neuroanatomic pathways that lead to speech production.

TABLE 10–1. Neuroanatomic Systems Involved in Voice and Speech Production

Neurologic System Involved	Examination Findings
Extrapyramidal system	Tremor
	Spasmodic contractions (eg, pitch instability)
	Excessive tension (eg, vocal strain)
	Irregular rhythm of repetition
	Hyperkinesia/hypokinesia
	Rigidity
Upper motor neuron (UMN)	Spasticity (eg, vocal strain)
	Slow but regular rhythm of repetition
	Hyperreflexia
	Myoclonus
Lower motor neuron (LMN)	Flaccidity
	Weakness
	Atrophy
	Fasciculations
	Hyporeflexia
Neuromuscular junction	Fatigue with repetitive use

Flaccidity, or chronically decreased muscle tone, is associated with lesions of the LMN. Flaccidity manifests as weakness, atrophy, and/or fasciculations. Examples include a weak voice and atrophy of the vocal folds secondary to a high vagal lesion or flaccidity of the tongue with fasciculations, known as "bag of worms," seen in patients with amyotrophic lateral sclerosis (ALS).

Tremor, dystonia, and myoclonus are terms used to describe movement disorders. *Tremors* are rhythmic oscillatory movements that occur at rest or with action. Tremors result from alternating contractions of opposing muscle groups. Pathologic resting tremor is usually in the range of 3 to 6 Hz and is exemplified by the tremor seen in Parkinson's disease. It is associated with basal ganglia lesions. *Intention tremor* occurs with action and is associated with cerebellar lesions. Intention tremor occurs at a rate between 2 and 5 Hz. The oscillations are coarse and increase in amplitude as the movement target is approached. In its most severe form, intention or kinetic tremors are present at rest and then increase in severity as the body part is activated. Multiple sclerosis is the most common cause of this cerebellar postural tremor. Other causes of this tremor include tumors and strokes, as well as neural degeneration in the cerebellum. *Essential tremor* is typically a postural tremor that occurs with sustained posture or during movement but in severe forms may also occur at rest. Essential tremor exhibits a frequency between 8 to 12 Hz and is thought to result from overactivity of the cerebellum. It most commonly affects the hands but can also affect the legs, head, tongue, or the larynx. Essential tremor of the voice is further discussed later in this chapter and in chapter 13.

Dystonia is broadly defined as a deviation of posture caused by involuntary sustained or spasmodic muscular contractions. It is attributed to dysfunction of the extrapyramidal system. Dystonia that occurs only during voluntary movement or is worsened by movement is called *action* dystonia. Action dystonia that occurs only with specific actions (eg, writer's cramp) is a task-specific dystonia. As a dystonic condition progresses, dystonia may occur even at rest, causing *rest* dystonia. Dystonias are also classified by the body regions affected. *Focal* dystonias affect one area of the body, *segmental* dystonias affect two or more adjacent areas, *multifocal* dystonias affect two or more nonadjacent areas, and *generalized* dystonias involve several areas on both sides of the body. Blepharospasm and oromandibular dystonia are examples of focal dystonias. The presence of both constitutes oral facial dystonia, also known as Meige's syndrome. Spasmodic dysphonia is generally thought of as a focal dystonia of the larynx. Patients with adductor spasmodic dysphonia exhibit abrupt initiation and termination of vocal production during speech caused by irregular hyperadduction of the vocal folds, whereas patients with abductor spasmodic dysphonia have aphonic, segmented speech due to irregular abduction of the vocal folds.

Myoclonus describes periodic, jerky contractions of 1 to 2 Hz that are typically multifocal. It can be associated with UMN lesions. Myoclonus is distinguished from tremor in that the former is monophasic while the latter is biphasic, involving opposing muscle groups. Myoclonus is not suppressible with conscious effort.

Tics are intermittent, nonrhythmic, patterned movements associated with an irresistible urge to perform them. Motor tics manifest as visible movements or twitches. Phonic or vocal tics can manifest as unwanted vocalizations such as throat clearing, coughing, barking, or yelling. Complex vocal tics may involve repeated words or phrases, including profanities. Unlike myoclonus, tics are suppressible with effort, and a postsuppression train of tics is characteristic. *Tourette's syndrome* is a chronic tic disorder characterized by both motor and vocal tics with onset in childhood. The disorder begins with simple tics and progresses to more complex tics. The tics have a migrating pattern, with one tic replaced by another. This distinguishes tics from dystonic movements, which do not migrate.

PHYSICAL EXAMINATION

The physical examination plays a pivotal role in the evaluation of patients with neurodegenerative disorders. Although a typical otolaryngologic office visit may not allow the type of comprehensive assessment possible during a neurology or speech pathology consultation, the diagnostic yield of a routine head and neck examination can be increased by careful, targeted observation. Even before starting a standard head and neck examination, the examiner gains valuable clues about the disease state from observing the overall appearance of the patient. Abnormal posture should be noted. Spontaneous limb or truncal movements such as tremor suggest the possibility of synchronous movements in the pharyngeal or laryngeal musculature.

The patient's speech and voice offer more insights. The rate, prosody, articulation, and resonance should be noted. Slow but fluent speech can result from a problem with rate control (eg,

basal ganglia or UMN lesion), with muscular coordination (eg, cerebellar lesion), and/or with muscular contraction (eg, UMN lesion). A flat, expressionless voice suggests the lack of fine motor control of the intrinsic laryngeal musculature needed to produce normal inflections in pitch and tone. Difficulty with articulation can result from weakness and/or incoordination. A test word such as "butterfly" can elicit deficiency in facial muscle (/b/), the tongue (/t/, /l/), or the lip (/f/). Rapid repetition of the syllables "pa-ta-ga" tests lip closure, tongue tip motion, and tongue base motion, respectively. A hypernasal quality suggests palatal weakness, and tremor in the voice cues the examiner to pay special attention to tremors of the pharyngeal and laryngeal musculature during the head and neck examination. Voice evaluation with perceptual techniques usually reveals strained sounds in UMN disease and breathy/asthenic patterns in LMN disorders. The voice is variable in extrapyramidal disorders, but typically becomes breathy and asthenic in the later stages of the disease.

The face is examined next. Involuntary facial twitches or blepharospasm should be noted. A limited range of facial expression may point to an extrapyramidal defect. Spasticity of facial movements suggests a disorder of UMNs whereas flaccidity of the facial muscles suggests an LMN disorder. The presence of either should alert the examiner to look for the same in other muscle groups controlled by the cranial nerves important in speech and swallow.

Examination of the oral cavity and oral pharynx should note symmetry and strength of tongue movement, symmetry and strength of palatal elevation, symmetry and strength of lateral pharyngeal wall motion, and any abnormal movements such as myoclonus or fasciculations. Isolated palatal myoclonus is a specific disorder associated with lesion in the Guillain-Molaret triangle in the brainstem. Tongue fasciculations imply weakness secondary to lesion in the LMN. Tongue strength can be assessed by asking the patient to push the tongue into the cheek while the examiner applies opposing digital pressure externally, by asking the patient to push the tongue out against a tongue depressor, or it can be formally measured by a pressure transducer connected to a bulb placed in the oral cavity.[3] Palatal strength should be assessed by asking the patient to say "ah" repetitively while upward and lateral motion are observed.

The evaluation continues with endoscopic examination of the nasopharynx, the posterior oropharynx, hypopharynx, and larynx. Palatal closure is assessed best with a flexible endoscope by placing the tip of the scope in the nasopharynx. Completeness of palatal closure can be visualized during production of non-voiced consonants such as sustained /ss/ or the word "popeye." A flexible scope can then be advanced into the oropharynx, or alternatively a rigid endoscope or a mirror can be used through the oral cavity. The examiner should first look for the presence of secretions or food residue in the vallecula. Retained secretions in the vallecula implies weakness of tongue base, whereas retained secretions or food in the piriform sinus suggests weakness of lateral pharyngeal wall contraction, poor laryngeal elevation, and/or the failure of the cricopharyngeal sphincter to relax completely during swallow. Tongue base strength can be assessed with words such as "ball" or "mall." In patients with normal strength of tongue base musculature, the tongue base will nearly contact the posterior pharyngeal wall during each of these tasks. Lateral pharyngeal wall strength and symmetry of motion are best evaluated during sustained high pitched /i/ or glides up in pitch. The lateral pharyngeal walls should contract symmetrically as the posterior pillars contract toward the midline. Unilateral weakness suggests LMN lesion because most pharyngeal muscles receive bilateral UMN innervation.

Finally, examination of the vocal folds and arytenoids during phonation should yield an assessment of strength and symmetry of movement. The vocal folds should abduct and adduct fairly symmetrically and briskly. Significant unilateral asymmetry usually suggests an LMN lesion such as paralysis or paresis. Bilateral slowing or motion and/or sphincteric closure patterns can be suggestive of UMN. If there are any voice complaints, then stroboscopy is required to assess the adequacy of laryngeal tissue vibratory patterns and completeness of laryngeal closure during vibration. Often atrophic vocal folds as seen

in extrapyramidal disorders, late stage UMN disease, or early LMN disease can result in asymmetric vibratory patterns and failure of com-plete closure of the glottis during phonation. This is often visualized during stroboscopy as a spindle-shaped glottic gap anterior to the vocal process.

EVALUATION OF SWALLOWING

Patients who present with dysphagia should undergo fluoroscopic and/or endoscopic swallowing evaluation. The modified barium swallow (MBS), or videofluorographic swallow study, is usually carried out jointly by a speech-language pathologist (SLP) and a radiologist. The patient ingests barium-coated boluses or liquid barium of varying consistencies while the oral, oropharyngeal, and hypopharyngeal phases of swallowing are observed fluoroscopically with the patient in a sitting or standing position. Abnormal tongue movement, barium pooling in the vallecula or piriform sinus, and aspiration can be easily observed. Bolus transit through the pharyngeal phases of swallow is also assessed. Opening of the cricopharyngeus muscle is best observed with barium swallow. Failure of opening is often seen as an indentation in the posterior aspect of the esophagus and cannot be well visualized by either methods of swallow evaluation. MBS provides objective evidence of swallow function and helps to identify specific functional deficits. Based on the study, recommendations for maneuvers to minimize aspiration and on food consistencies can be made.

Although the MBS provides a global view of the oral and pharyngeal structures during the swallow, endoscopic evaluation shows selected details of the swallowing process and allows simultaneous assessment of laryngeal competence. Fiberoptic endoscopic evaluation of swallowing (FEES) is performed either by an SLP or an otolaryngologist with a fiberoptic laryngoscope. Patients ingest food boluses with varying consistencies treated with food dye as the pharynx is observed before and after the pharyngeal swallow. FEES directly observes premature spillage of food into the pharynx or larynx during the oral phase, assesses airway closure during the swallow, and localizes food residue. If aspiration is present, flexible endoscopic evaluation of swallowing with sensory testing (FEESST) should be performed. FEESST delivers controlled air pulses to determine the sensory threshold in various parts of the laryngopharynx. This method of airway protection assessment is gaining popularity and has been applied to patients with neurodegenerative syndromes.[4]

Whether MBS, FEES/FEESST, or both should be performed for a particular patient depends on several factors.[5] In general, FEES is preferred over MBS when access to fluoroscopy is limited, when the patient requires a bedside examination, or when the test is also used to determine therapeutic options. Most patients will tolerate the flexible endoscope for an extended period of time as different food consistencies and therapeutic maneuvers are attempted. Radiation exposure during MBS limits its usefulness for repeated swallows with different maneuvers. FEES/FEESST is also favored when there is laryngeal involvement of the disease. In addition, sensory testing is only possible with FEESST. On the other hand, MBS is indicated when the oral phase, the oral-pharyngeal transition, hyoid and laryngeal elevation, or cricopharyngeal relaxation needs to be examined. These are some of the areas not observed during FEES/FEESST. MBS is also preferred as a screening examination when the patient complaint is vague and global assessment is needed. Either the fluoroscopic or the endoscopic examination should suffice for most patients.

CATEGORIES OF NEUROGENIC DISEASES

Extrapyramidal and Cerebellar Disorders

Extrapyramidal disorders include Parkinson's disease and Parkinson-related disorders. Parkinsonism is a syndrome consisting of resting tremor, rigidity, bradykinesia, and gait disturbance. Parkinson's disease (PD) is idiopathic parkinsonism without more widespread neurologic involvement. PD results from lesion in the substantia nigra of the basal ganglia. PD patients have characteristic hypokinetic dysarthria and vocal tremor. Speech is poorly articulated and patients may be described as mumbling. There is a typical festination pattern with delayed onset then an increased rate. The voice is usually hypophonic, but some patients have a strained voice with aphonic breaks, reflecting the rigidity component of the disease. On laryngoscopic examination, PD patients have good vocal fold mobility and usually demonstrate normal vocal process excursion.[6] However, the vocal folds have a typical atrophic appearance. The vocal process is unusually prominent. During stroboscopic assessment, the mucosal membranes do not vibrate to closure as the prephonatory gap is too wide, due to muscle atrophy that precludes the vocal folds from being placed in an adequate prephonatory position. In addition to the phonatory glottal gap, bradykinesia of the intrinsic laryngeal musculature may also contribute to Parkinson dysphonia. Delayed adduction of the "rigid" vocal folds relative to expiration allows premature air leakage, resulting in lower subglottic pressure when the vocal folds are finally brought to the phonatory position. This further aggravates the hypophonia and decreases phonation time. In terms of swallowing, patients with PD usually do not have prominent dysphagia, reflecting the brainstem mediation of most of the swallowing process. A complete review of Parkinson's disease and its effect on the larynx is presented in chapter 12.

When patients with parkinsonism do not respond to standard dopaminergic treatment and have additional signs and symptoms, other Parkinson-related disorders need to be considered. One such syndrome is *multiple system atrophy* (MSA).[7] The dominant features of MSA are parkinsonism, ataxia, and autonomic failure. MSA encompasses three previously described central nervous system degenerative syndromes that differ in the predominant neurosystem involved but have overlapping clinical manifestations.

Direct Electrical Stimulation of Denervated Laryngeal Muscles: Is It Possible?

In the future, some patients with laryngeal symptoms due to systemic neurodegenerative disorders, such as multisystem atrophy and motor neuron diseases, may benefit from a laryngeal pacemaker designed to bypass degenerated nerves and stimulate the target muscles directly. In the past, laryngeal pacing with direct electrical stimulation has been explored as a means to restore oral ventilation in patients with bilateral vocal fold paralysis who are tracheotomy-dependent. The premise of laryngeal pacing lies in the ability of the posterior cricoarytenoid (PCA) muscle to be stimulated by an external electrical signal delivered by an implanted electrode. In 1996 the first report of electrical pacing of a unilaterally paralyzed human vocal fold showed it was possible to produce stimulated abduction of the paralyzed fold of a magnitude comparable to the normal side using impulses synchronized with inspiratory effort generated by a plethysmographic transducer.[30] Subsequent studies in patients with bilateral vocal fold paralysis showed it was possible to produce sufficient increase in airflow with unilateral laryngeal electrical stimulation to achieve decannulation.[31,32] The later studies were carried out with a device that delivered programmed impulses rather than impulses synchronized with inspiration. Certain technical issues limited the clinical outcome. For example, size and spacing of the electrode channels on existing electrode devices were suboptimal for PCA stimulation, and the implanted electrode was susceptible to corrosion. Nevertheless, this innovative technology holds great promise not only for patients with paralyzed vocal folds but also for those with impaired neurologic function of the larynx.

One group of patients who may benefit from laryngeal pacing are patients with multiple system atrophy (MSA) with nocturnal stridor. These patients have inappropriate inspiratory vocal fold adduction and abductor paresis during sleep. This problem seems ideally suited for laryngeal pacing. An electrode array implanted in the PCA can be connected to an impulse generator synchronized to a chest wall sensor[30] or diaphragmatic contraction. With an external switch, the device can be turned on at night when the patients go to sleep and be turned off when the patients wake up in the morning. The additional stimulus for abduction from the pacer during inspiration can potentially reverse the unfavorable adduction-abduction balance and eliminate stridor. A more advanced design could incorporate simultaneous blocking of adductor muscles. One challenge is to implant the stimulating electrode in the PCA without jeopardizing native recurrent laryngeal nerve function.

A second group of patients who may benefit from this technology are patients with motor neuron disease (MND) who are at increased risk of aspiration due to degeneration of motor neurons that control the pharyngeal and laryngeal musculature. It may be possible to produce stimulated laryngeal closure, namely, true vocal fold abduction and false vocal fold approximation, that is triggered by swallowing. This may reduce the likelihood of aspiration. Another possibility is to synchronize glottic closure with cough. This would enable patients to generate larger subglottic pressures and produce stronger coughs to clear airway secretions or aspirated material.

Technical hurdles obviously exist, but advances in microarray technology, electronics design, and surgical implantation should make these therapeutic concepts into reality one day and produce laryngeal pacers that can benefit selected patients with generalized neurodegenerative disorders.

Patients with *striatonigral degeneration* have predominantly parkinsonism features. Patients with *olivopontocerebellar atrophy* have prominent cerebellar dysfunction. *Shy-Drager syndrome* is characterized by autonomic instability, urinary and rectal incontinence, and orthostatic hypotension. Patients with MSA may have a mixed dysarthria with variable hypokinetic, ataxic, and spastic components depending on the predominant neurosystem affected.[8] Sixteen percent of patients with MSA, particularly those with Shy-Drager, have inspiratory stridor during sleep,[9] and rarely this can be the initial manifestation of MSA.[10] The etiology of inspiratory stridor is thought to be a combination of bilateral abductor paresis and inappropriate inspiratory adduction.[11-12] Patients with Parkinsonism who are evaluated for hypophonia should be carefully questioned for the presence of stridor during sleep. If the history is positive and abductor paresis or paradoxic vocal fold movement is seen on laryngoscopy, the diagnosis of MSA should be entertained, and a polysomnograph should be obtained.[13] Such patients often demonstrate obstructive sleep apnea, presumably due to obstruction at the glottic level. Although continuous positive airway pressure (CPAP) does not usually provide relief of fixed glottal obstruction

or bilateral vocal fold paralysis due to LMN injury, some MSA patients have benefitted from CPAP for treatment of nocturnal stridor.[14] One sleep physiology study showed the application of CPAP reduced the inspiratory activity of the TA muscle.[11] The authors speculate that the inspiratory TA activation in MSA patients is an inappropriate response to negative airway pressure during sleep and that CPAP suppresses TA activation by reducing the negative airway pressure. They caution that further studies are necessary before CPAP is routinely applied to patients with MSA.

Progressive supranuclear palsy (PSP) is another Parkinson-related syndrome. In addition to bradykinesia and rigidity, patients with PSP have characteristic vertical gaze paresis, frequent falls, and blepharospasm. There may be facial weakness, dysarthria, and dysphagia. The diagnosis is usually suspected due to gait instability.

Essential tremor is a disorder characterized by tremor that occurs with sustained action and is suppressed by alcohol intake. It is thought to result from overactivity of the cerebellum. Although it is not considered a neurodegenerative disorder, it is included here for comparison. A type of essential tremor familiar to otolaryngologists is essential tremor of the voice, which involves the periodic contraction of antagonistic adductor-abductor and/or superior-inferior laryngeal muscles in an alternating or synchronous fashion resulting in a periodic tremulous voice.[15] The thyrohyoid muscle is most commonly involved, followed by the thyroarytenoid, sternothyroid, and cricothyroid.[16] Most patients with essential tremor of the voice also have tremors elsewhere in the body, most notably the upper extremity.[17] Essential tremor is detailed further in chapter 14.

Motor Neuron Diseases

Motor neuron diseases result in progressive weakness of voluntary muscles throughout the body due to degeneration and eventual loss of the cell bodies of UMNs and/or LMNs. The weakness usually starts in one muscle group then progressively involves others. Motor neuron diseases are classified according to the type of motor neurons involved. Disease in which the UMNs alone are affected is termed primary lateral sclerosis (PLS). The motor neuron deficit can primarily be limited to the LMNs, for example in progressive bulbar palsy (PBP). Finally, when both UMNs and LMNs are affected, the disease is called amyotrophic lateral sclerosis (ALS), or *Lou Gehrig's disease.*

Primary lateral sclerosis (PLS) involves predominantly the UMNs. It results from the selective loss of large pyramidal cells in the precentral gyrus and degeneration of corticobulbar projections. PLS typically presents with gradual onset lower extremity stiffness and pain due to spasticity, which may lead to imbalance. As the disease progresses, upper extremities and bulbar muscles become involved. Spasticity of the lip, tongue, pharyngeal, and laryngeal musculature results in slow, labored articulation and dysphagia. The voice is typically harsh and strained and may sound like patients with spasmodic dysphonia. Botox injection may provide some benefit. The rate of progression is usually slow, and the disease does not significantly shorten life expectancy. In most cases, the disease does progress to involve the LMNs and develop into ALS, in which flaccid weakness becomes the predominant symptom.

Patients with *pseudobulbar palsy* have prominent UMN symptoms in the bulbar muscles. Unlike PLS, pseudobulbar palsy is not a distinct disease entity. It results from bilateral corticobulbar tract lesions that can be produced by stroke, encephalitis, multiple sclerosis, or neoplasm. Spasticity of the muscles of mastication, facial expression, and speech result in characteristic difficulty with chewing, expressionless facies, hyperactive gag reflex, and inability to protrude the tongue. Patients may also demonstrate emotional lability.

Progressive bulbar palsy (PBP) involves the motor nuclei of the LMNs, predominantly the lower cranial nerves IX, X, and XII. Weakness of the pharyngeal musculature leads to nasal regurgitation, slurred, hypernasal speech, poor cough and gag reflex, and aspiration. The tongue is usually affected first and may be atrophic and show fasciculations. Facial muscles, starting with the orbicularis oris, may be affected as well. Patients with adult-onset symptoms have a variable disease course and eventually progress to ALS. PBP of childhood, or Fazio-Londe disease, is a rare entity that shows rapid progression leading to death within 1 to 3 years of diagnosis from respiratory compromise.

Amyotrophic lateral sclerosis (ALS) affects both UMN and LMN. Although patients with ALS commonly present with movement complaints involving their extremities, as many as 25% have initial speech and swallowing symptoms,[18] and a significant number of these patients are initially seen by an otolaryngologist before the neurologic diagnosis is made.[19] In ALS, idiopathic progressive degeneration of both UMN and LMN results in spasticity, weakness, atrophy, and fasciculations. Palatal weakness results in hypernasal speech and nasopharyngeal regurgitation, and tongue weakness produces dysarthria. A characteristic finding on physical examination is the "bag of worms" appearance of the tongue fasciculations. About half the patients demonstrate a glottal gap on videostroboscopic examination.[20] As the disease progresses, patients with ALS often need tracheotomy for pulmonary toilet and eventually depend on mechanical ventilation.

Swallowing difficulties in patients with motor neuron diseases manifest differently according to the site of lesion. Patients with UMN involvement may have difficulty initiating the swallow in the oral phase, a voluntary action that requires input from the corticobulbar tract. The pharyngeal and esophageal phases of swallow, which entail involuntary actions mediated by the brainstem, are relatively unaffected in early stages of the disease. The dysphagia is a consequence of predominantly incoordination rather than weakness. Therefore, in patients with PLS, swallowing is usually well preserved. On the other hand, patients with LMN disease tend to have more severe dysphagia because all phases of the swallow are affected. Swallowing difficulty can often be one of the symptoms first noted in patients with PBP or ALS and PLS presenting with initial bulbar symptoms. Some ALS patients are candidates for laryngotracheal separation, thus completely preventing aspiration at the cost of any phonation. These patients typically do not have intelligible speech due to derangement of tongue function. The procedure does not allow for efficient swallowing, but it does remove the risk of aspiration of secretions (Figure 10–2).

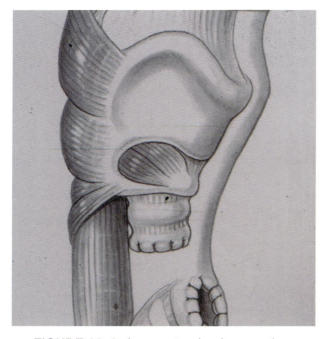

FIGURE 10–2. Laryngotracheal separation.

Diseases of the Neuromuscular Junction

The best example of a disease in this category is *myasthenia gravis*. Although it is not generally considered a neurodegenerative disorder, myasthenia gravis is included here as an example of a systemic neurologic disorder where undiagnosed patients may present with vocal complaints to an otolaryngologist. The pathophysiology underlying myasthenia gravis is the production of autoantibodies to the acetylcholine receptor, which results in easy fatigue with repetitive use. The hallmark of myasthenia gravis is the fluctuating nature of the weakness. Ocular muscles and eyelids are affected first in 40% of patients, resulting in ptosis and diplopia. Facial and oropharyngeal muscles are next commonly involved. Patients may complain of fluctuating hoarseness, and laryngeal complaints can be the presenting symptom.[21] The fatigue may be elicited by asking the patient to repeat the vocalization of "ee-ee-ee." Patients with more severe disease may demonstrate dysarthria, dysphagia, aspiration, and even stridor, although stridor as the presenting symptom is unusual and tends to be due to delayed diagnosis. Response to anticholinesterase (eg, Tensilon), establishes the diagnosis. Myasthenia gravis is most common in women between the second and fourth decades. It must be ruled out in women in this age group who present with fluctuating hoarseness.

ROLE OF THE OTOLARYNGOLOGIST

Patients with neurodegenerative disorders present significant challenges in management. Their primary disease process is irreversible, and they deteriorate over time despite the physician's best efforts. The otolaryngologist participates in their care in several ways. Patients are sent to otolaryngologists for assessment of their voice, speech, and swallowing abnormalities. Sometimes a neurologic diagnosis has already been made based on systemic symptoms. For patients who aspirate, the neurologist may seek assistance in evaluating airway protection mechanisms and the need for tracheotomy. For patients with predominantly voice and speech complaints, speech therapy may be beneficial. Not uncommonly, patients who do not carry a neurologic diagnosis are referred to a laryngologist or voice and swallowing center for management of what was perceived by the referring center as an isolated voice, speech, or swallowing abnormality. In these cases, a familiarity with the neurodegenerative disorders enables the otolaryngologist to suspect or establish the diagnosis. Timely referral for neurologic consultation is especially critical if symptoms are advanced and progressing, as sometimes seen in ALS.[22]

Although otolaryngologists traditionally have not played a major role in the management of patients with neurodegenerative disorders, interventions that already exist in the otolaryngologic armamentarium for other disorders can improve the quality of life in selected patients.

Botulinum toxin (Botox, Allergan) injection, which has an established role in the treatment of spasmodic dysphonia, has been applied to patients with essential tremor of the voice. Warrick et al reported a crossover study of unilateral versus bilateral injection of Botox for 10 patients.[15] They found that, although most patients did not have a significant improvement in objective acoustic measures, most benefitted from a subjective reduction in vocal effort, which may be attributed to reduced laryngeal airway resistance from decreased adduction. Most patients reported satisfaction with the procedure.

Botox injection may also have a role in the treatment of dysphagia in patients with neurodegenerative disorders. The cricopharyngeus (CP) muscle is tonically active at rest and relaxes during swallow. Failure of the CP muscle to relax or hypertonicity can contribute to dysphagia in patients with systemic neurodegenerative disorders. Both percutaneous[23] and endoscopic[24] injection of the CP muscle have been described, although no report specifically addresses the treatment of dysphagia in the context of neurodegenerative disorders. Of the 12 patients reported by

Parameswaran and Soliman,[24] one suffered from ALS, and another had Parkinson's disease. Both patients reported only modest improvement in their swallowing function. The limited gain from CP injection is not surprising as the dysphagia results from global pharyngeal dysfunction rather than isolated CP involvement. The use of Botox as a therapeutic and diagnostic modality in these patients, therefore, was beneficial in evaluating the potential effects of CP myotomy. If the Botox is minimally effective, then it is unlikely that myotomy will help and the patient can avoid the morbidity of the more invasive procedure. Overall, the utility of Botox injection of the CP muscle in the neurodegenerative patient requires further investigation. For patients who may be hesitant to undergo botulinum toxin injection, a "test" injection of lidocaine into the UES may provide similar diagnostic information. This is an embraceable but not well-studied approach (Figure 10–3). The test injection may be performed in the clinic or in the fluoroscopy suite. In the clinic, the patient may be asked to eat different consistencies and subjectively report any impact of the injection on his or her dysphagia. In the fluoroscopy, the patient may be imaged immediately before and after injection to more objectively determine any change on swallowing function.

Botox can also be used to treat spasticity and sialorrhea in patients with diseases of the UMN including pseudobulbar palsy and PLS. In patients with symptoms of pseudobulbar palsy, Botox injection into facial muscles may ameliorate spasticity which will lessen dysarthria and oral incompetence associated with the disorder. In one case report, Botox injection into the thyroarytenoid muscles was also found to reduce spastic vocal symptoms.[25] Clinically, Botox can be beneficial in reducing dysarthria and vocal strain in patients with PLS. In this group of patients, Botox must be used with caution. EMG of the muscles considered for injection, either facial or laryngeal, should be undertaken to document the absence of LMN findings. If there are no signs of LMN loss, then injection of Botox in small increments can result in a reduction of

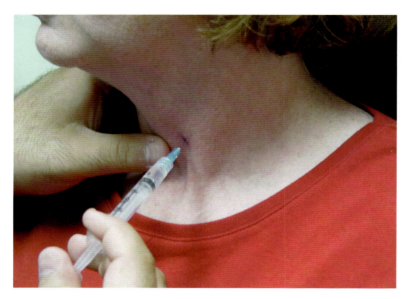

FIGURE 10–3. Percutaneous injection of lidocaine along cricoid cartilage into the UES. The left hand is on the patient's neck with the thumb on the cricoid. Lidocaine 2% without epinephrine is used.

spasticity. For reduction of laryngeal spasticity and vocal strain, Botox injections in the range of 0.3 to 0.6 mouse units into one thyroaryntenoid muscle are usually effective. Vocal and often speech fluency improves and the patients report less effort required to speak. Reduction in sialorrhea in patients with ALS after salivary gland Botox injection has been reported also, but its efficacy has yet to be proven.

Parkinson's dysphonia is traditionally treated with speech therapy (see chapter 12).[26] However, when vocal training in itself is ineffective due to excessive vocal fold atrophy, augmentation of vocal fold mass with either injection laryngoplasty or bilateral type I thyroplasty may provide additional vocal improvement. Berke et al reported a series of 35 Parkinson patients with hypophonic dysphonia who underwent percutaneous injection of cross-linked collagen.[27] These patients were selected based on the finding of persistent glottic aperture on videostroboscopic examination. Parkinson patients with dysphonia but with normal glottal closure were excluded. After injection, 75% of the patients reported satisfaction with the procedure. Kim et al reported a series of 18 patients with similar findings.[28] More recently, the use of calcium hydroxylapatite as a vocal fold augmentation material for Parkinson patients has also been reported.[29] In the senior author's clinical experience, bilateral

type I thyroplasty (medialization laryngoplasty) works well in this select group of patients. The goal is to medialize the membranous portion of the vocal folds so they remain in an adducted position even during inspiration. The airway in the posterior cartilaginous portion of the glottis is preserved. Therefore, patients do not report a significant alteration in breathing and usually notice that the voice is louder with the sensation of less phonatory effort. Pre- and postoperative measures of vocal intensity can be used to objectively evaluate these changes.

Selection of Parkinson patients for any type of vocal fold augmentation must take into consideration the severity of the disease. As discussed previously, the dysphonia in patients with PD has multiple contributing factors, only one of which is addressed by vocal fold augmentation or medialization. Patients with large phonatory glottal apertures as the predominant factor for their dysphonia are more likely to benefit from augmentation than those with severe bradykinesia. Patients with advanced disease, aphonia, difficulty with speech initiation, or dysphagia are likely to have more significant bradykinesia and are less likely to benefit from augmentation.[28]

Finally, otolaryngologists are often involved in airway management in patients with motor neuron disease, although the options are largely palliative. Intractable aspiration may be managed with tracheotomy with limited efficacy. Laryngeal diversion or laryngectomy are alternatives that are rarely indicated.[22] The most common indication for tracheotomy in motor neuron disease is for mechanical ventilation as the respiratory apparatus weakens.

CONCLUSIONS

Voice and speech abnormalities are common in patients with neurodegenerative disorders. Evaluation of these patients is facilitated by an understanding of the anatomic location of the neurologic lesion and the neurologic system affected by the particular disorder. The care of the patient with neurodegenerative disorder is multidisciplinary. The neurologists are the specialists of the primary disease process and direct the medical therapies. The speech pathologists perform detailed functional assessments of voice, speech, and swallowing functions and carry out behavioral therapies. The otolaryngologists have the potential to improve the quality of life in selected patients with interventions already familiar to them. A familiarity with the neurodegenerative disorders will enable the otolaryngologist to potentially make the initial diagnosis in patients with isolated voice and speech complaints.

Review Questions

1. A 33-year-old business consultant presents with a 2-month history of intermittent hoarseness. She complains that she often "loses her voice" during meetings. On examination, her voice is mildly asthenic but otherwise normal. Videostroboscopic examination shows vocal folds without lesions and apparent normal mobility. What disease entity should you consider, and what other diagnostic maneuver would you perform?

2. Which of the following findings on laryngoscopic examination of a patient with Parkinson's disease indicates possible benefit from vocal fold augmentation?
   a. Atrophic, bowed vocal folds
   b. Vocal cord paresis
   c. Glottal gap
   d. Laryngeal tremor

3. Which of the following is not a sign of LMN lesion?
   a. Tongue fasciculations
   b. Voice strain
   c. Hypernasality
   d. Vocal cord paresis

4. A patient with parkinsonism is sent to you for the evaluation of dysphonia. Laryngoscopic examination shows limited abduction of bilateral vocal cords. What specific history should you query, and what disease entity should you consider?

5. Botox injection of vocal cords has been found to be beneficial for some patients with which of the following conditions?
   a. Parkinson's disease
   b. ALS
   c. Shy-Drager
   d. Essential tremor of the voice

REFERENCES

1. Hartelius L, Svensson P. Speech and swallowing symptoms associated with Parkinson's disease and multiple sclerosis: a survey. *Folia Phoniatr Logop.* 994;46:9–17.
2. Hanson DG. Neuromuscular disorders of the larynx. *Otolaryngol Clin North Am.* 1991;24:1035–1051.
3. Robin DA, Goel A, Somodi LB, et al. Tongue strength and endurance: relation to highly skilled movements. *J Speech Hear Res.* 1992;35: 1239–1245.

4. Aviv JE, Murry T, Zschommler A, et al. Flexible endoscopic evaluation of swallowing with sensory testing: patient characteristics and analysis of safety in 1,340 consecutive examinations. *Ann Otol Rhinol Laryngol.* 2005;114:173-176.

5. Langmore SE, Aviv JE. Endoscopic procedures to evaluate oropharyngeal swallowing. In: Langmore SE, ed. *Endoscopic Evaluation and Treatment of Swallowing Disorders.* New York, NY: Thieme; 2001: chap 5.

6. Perez KS, Ramig LO, Smith ME, Dromey C. The Parkinson larynx: tremor and videostroboscopic findings. *J Voice.* 1996;10:354-361.

7. Siemers E. Multiple system atrophy. *Med Clin North Am.* 1999;83:381-392.

8. Kluin KJ, Gilman S, Lohman M, Junck L. Characteristics of the dysarthria of multiple system atrophy. *Arch Neurol.* 1996;53:545-548.

9. Wenning GK, Tison F, Shlomo YB, et al. Multiple system atrophy: a review of 203 pathologically proven cases. *Mov Disord.* 1997;12:133-147.

10. Hughes RG, Gibbin KP, Lowe J. Vocal fold abductor paralysis as a solitary and fatal manifestation of multiple system atrophy. *J Laryngol Otol.* 1998; 112:177-178.

11. Isono S, Shiba K, Yamaguchi M, et al. Pathogenesis of laryngeal narrowing in patients with multiple system atrophy. *J Physiol.* 2001;536:237-249.

12. Merlo IM, Occhini A, Pacchetti C, et al. Not paralysis, but dystonia causes stridor in multiple system atrophy. *Neurology.* 2002;58:649-652.

13. Blumin JH, Berke GS. Bilateral vocal fold paresis and multiple system atrophy. *Arch Otolaryngol Head Neck Surg.* 2002;128:1404-1407.

14. Iranzo A, Santamaria J, Tolosa E, et al. Long-term effect of CPAP in the treatment of nocturnal stridor in multiple system atrophy. *Neurology.* 2004; 63:930-932.

15. Warrick P, Dromey C, Irish JC, et al. Botulinum toxin for essential tremor of the voice with multiple anatomical sites of tremor: a crossover design study of unilateral versus bilateral injection. *Laryngoscope.* 2000;110:1366-1374.

16. Koda J, Ludlow CL. An evaluation of laryngeal muscle activation in patients with vocal tremor. *Otolaryngol Head Neck Surg.* 1992;107:684-696.

17. Brown JR, Simonson J. Organic voice tremor: a tremor of phonation. *Neurology.* 1963;13:520-525.

18. Kent RD, Kent JF, Weismer G, et al. Impairment of speech intelligibility in men with amyotrophic lateral sclerosis. *J Speech Hear Disord.* 1990;55: 721-728.

19. McGuirt WF, Blalock D. The otolaryngologist's role in the diagnosis and treatment of amyotrophic lateral sclerosis. *Laryngoscope.* 1980;90: 1496-1501.

20. Chen A, Garrett CG. Otolaryngologic presentations of amyotrophic lateralsclerosis. *Otolaryngol Head Neck Surg.* 2005;132:500-504.

21. Mao VH, Abaza M, Spiegel JR, et al. Laryngeal myasthenia gravis: report of 40 cases. *J Voice.* 2001;15:122-130.

22. Hillel A, Dray T, Miller R, et al. Presentation of ALS to the otolaryngologist/head and neck surgeon: getting to the neurologist. *Neurology.* 1999;53 (8 suppl 5):S22-S25.

23. Blitzer A, Brin M. Use of botulinum toxin for diagnosis and management of cricopharygeal achalasia. *Otolaryngol Head Neck Surg.* 1997;116: 328-329.

24. Parameswaran MS, Soliman AM. Endoscopic botulinum toxin injection for cricopharygeal dysphagia. *Ann Otol Rhinol Laryngol.* 2002;111:871-874.

25. McHenry M, Whatman J, Pou A. The effect of botulinum toxin A on the vocal symptoms of spastic dysarthria: a case study. *J Voice.* 2002;16:124-131.

26. Ramig LO, Fox C, Sapir C. Parkinson's disease: speech and voice disorders and their treatment with the Lee Silverman Voice Treatment. *Semin Speech Lang.* 2004;25:169-180.

27. Berke GS, Gerratt B, Kreiman J, et al. Treatment of Parkinson hypophonia with percutaneous collagen augmentation. *Laryngoscope.* 1999;109: 1295-1299.

28. Kim SH, Kearney JJ, Atkins JP. Percutaneous laryngeal collagen augmentation for treatment of parkinsonian hypophonia. *Otolaryngol Head Neck Surg.* 2002;126:653-656.

29. Belafsky PC, Postma GN. Vocal fold augmentation with calcium hydroxylapatite. *Otolaryngol Head Neck Surg.* 2004;131:351-354.

30. Zealear DL, Rainey CL, Netterville JL, et al. Electrical pacing of the paralyzed human larynx. *Ann Otol Rhinol Laryngol.* 1996;105:689-693.

31. Zealear DL, Billante CR, Courey MS, et al. Electrically stimulated glottal opening combined with adductor muscle Botox blockade restores both ventilation and voice in a patient with bilateral laryngeal paralysis. *Ann Otol Rhinol Laryngol.* 2002;111:500-506.

32. Zealear DL, Billante CR, Courey MS, et al. Reanimation of the paralyzed human larynx with an implantable electrical stimulation device. *Laryngoscope.* 2003;113:1149-1156.

11

Vocal Fold Paralysis

Tanya Meyer, MD
Lucian Sulica, MD
Andrew Blitzer, MD

KEY POINTS

■ Vocal fold paralysis implies immobility as a result of injury to the vagus or the recurrent laryngeal nerve. Although nerve injury is usually the cause of immobility, it is important to consider potential causes of mechanical fixation in the differential.

■ Laryngeal EMG can help differentiate neurogenic from mechanical immobility and can help prognosticate return of function.

■ The *need* for the treatment of glottic insufficiency resulting from a vocal fold paralysis is determined by symptomatology: adequacy of cough, presence of dysphagia, and defects in phonatory function. The *type* of treatment offered to the patient is determined by the patient's overall prognosis, the potential for spontaneous return of glottic function, and the glottic configuration.

■ Most patients are well served by medialization of the vocal fold; an arytenoid adduction suture is often needed for individuals with a large posterior glottic gap and flaccid arytenoid.

■ Reinnervation procedures can enhance the tone of the paralyzed vocal fold, but will not recover meaningful vocal fold motion.

As a dynamic organ, the larynx and associated structures are responsible for regulating the major functions of the upper aerodigestive tract. Proper laryngeal valving is therefore essential in voice, breathing, swallowing, coughing, as well as stabilization of the thorax (*Valsalva*) during upper limb activity. When the proper function of the larynx is disturbed, any or all of these domains may be affected.

This chapter provides a summary of the clinical evaluation and management of vocal fold paralysis, focusing on adult unilateral vocal fold paralysis. In the final sections of the chapter, key issues related to bilateral vocal fold paralysis, isolated superior laryngeal nerve dysfunction, and pediatric issues are reviewed.

TERMINOLOGY

In common parlance, "vocal fold paralysis" is used to describe the *sign* of vocal fold motion impairment, regardless of cause. More precise usage would restrict the term to compromised mobility due to loss of motor innervation. Although paralysis is by far the most common cause, "vocal fold immobility" is a more accurate term until the etiology of the motion impairment has been determined. For example, although a patient with acute voice changes and "paralysis" following a carotid enarterectomy very likely has suffered a neuropathic injury, the proper descriptor is "immobility" until nerve damage can be confirmed by laryngeal electromyography (see chapter 9) fold excursion due to the neuropathy could properly be called "vocal paralysis."

"Recurrent laryngeal nerve paralysis" is often used interchangeably with "vocal fold paralysis"; although the recurrent nerve is almost always involved, vocal fold paralysis may or may not also involve the superior laryngeal nerve. "Paresis" is used clinically to refer to a vocal fold that retains some mobility despite partial dysfunction.

CAUSES OF VOCAL PARALYSIS

Vocal fold immobility may be broadly categorized as neurogenic or mechanical in nature. Unilateral immobility is usually the result of nerve dysfunction, the causes of which fall into four broad categories: neoplastic (compression or infiltration by tumor), trauma (surgical and nonsurgical trauma), medical disease, and those that are idiopathic in nature (Table 11–1).

Neoplasms along the course of the cervical or thoracic vagus and recurrent laryngeal nerve may cause paralysis. Mediastinal tumors, often metastases from primary lung malignancies, account for the majority of paralyses from neoplastic causes. The roster of surgical procedures that place the laryngeal nerves at particular risk includes thyroidectomy and a variety of skull base, cervical, and thoracic procedures. Historically, thyroid procedures have been the most common cause of iatrogenic paralyses; this may be changing as the anterior approach to cervical spine surgery becomes more widely performed.[1] This has also affected the "sidedness" of vocal paralysis due to the preference for right-sided approaches and the risk for paralysis in these cases.[2]

Despite appropriate evaluation (see below), a significant proportion of cases has continued to defy diagnosis. These are usually designated as "idiopathic" neuropathies. It has been suggested that viral neuritis may be responsible, based on analogies to other cranial palsies and occasional suggestive serologic associations.

Mechanical causes may be due to fixation of the joint from fibrosis or arthritis, posterior glottic stenosis, or neoplastic invasion of the vocal fold muscle. Arytenoid dislocation has been reported as a cause of immobility; the majority of laryngologists believe that this entity is rare, although the clinical history may be compelling in certain cases.[6]

Overall, however, the frequency of vocal fold paralysis by etiology varies considerably from study to study (Table 11–2).

TABLE 11–1. Causes of Vocal Fold Paralysis

1. TRAUMA

Iatrogenic Trauma
- Cervical surgery
  - eg, thyroidectomy, anterior approach to the cervical spine (ACD)
- Thoracic procedures
  - eg, repair of thoracic aortic anuerysm
- Skull base surgery
- Other medical procedures
  - Endotracheal intubation
  - Central venous catheterization
  - Forceps delivery

Noniatrogenic Trauma

2. TUMOR, MALIGNANT OR BENIGN

Brain or Skull Base

Cervical
- Thyroid
- Metastatic lymphadenopathy
- Parapharyngeal space masses
- Vagal neuroma

Thoracic
- Esophageal
- Mediastinal lymphadenopathy
- Thymoma

3. MEDICAL DISEASE

Cardiovascular Disease
- Left heart failure (Ortner's syndrome)
- Aortic arch aneurysm

Neurologic Disease
- Stroke—Wallenberg's syndrome
- Amyotrophic lateral sclerosis
- Postpolio syndrome
- Charcot-Marie-Tooth disease (hereditary peripheral nerve palsy)
- Bulbar palsies

Developmental Abnormalities
- Arnold-Chiari malformation

Drug Neurotoxicity
- Vinca alkaloids (vincristine/vinblastine)
- Organophosphates

Granulomatous disease
- Tuberculosis
- Sarcoid

4. IDIOPATHIC

TABLE 11–2. Etiology of Unilateral Vocal Fold Immobility

Etiology	Terris 1992[3]	Maisel 1974[4]	Benninger 1998[5]
Malignancy	40.5	25.2	24.7
Iatrogenic	34.5	15.7	23.9
Idiopathic	10.7	26.8	19.6
Trauma	1.2	10.2	11.1
Intubation	7.1	3.1	7.5
CNS tumors	2.4	7.9	7.9
Thoracic disease	—	6.3	5.4
Other	3.6	4.7	—

EVALUATION

The clinician evaluating the patient with vocal fold immobility is faced with two separate issues—the workup of the etiology of the vocal fold immobility and the management of the patient's symptoms related to the subsequent glottic insufficiency. It is paramount that the clinician conduct a rigorous search for the underlying etiology, such as malignancy, infection, or granulomatous disease, and not be distracted from the completion of this investigation by the management of the patient's voice or swallowing symptoms. Although the exact nature of the evaluation beyond history and physical examination is not widely agreed on, most practitioners routinely order computed tomography (CT) along the course of the recurrent laryngeal nerve. This is described in further detail below.

History

Patients with unilateral vocal fold immobility complain of a weak (asthenic), breathy, and hoarse voice, the severity of which is generally proportional to the gap between the vocal folds at adduction. Patients are particularly bothered by the increased *effort* of phonation and report progression of

Pathophysiology of Paralysis

"Paralysis" creates a mental image of a completely denervated, perfectly immobile vocal fold. The reality is considerably more complex and variable; vocal fold paralysis is not an all-or-none phenomenon as it has been commonly conceptualized. As the nervous system attempts to regenerate from a given nerve injury, reinnervation occurs at variable degrees and effectiveness. Nerve fibers must not only regenerate in sufficient number, but also return to their correct original target to enable recovery of meaningful motion. For the recurrent laryngeal nerve, both adductor and abductor fibers are intermingled and consequently varying degrees of dysfunctional (crossed or *synkinetic*) reinnervation is common. Such dysfunctional reinnervation may yield simultaneous excitation of adductor and abductor musculature resulting in minimal *net* vocal fold movement.

In the ideal scenario, presumably following neuropraxic lesions, there is appropriate and complete regeneration of neural input and resulting motor function. On the other end of the spectrum, some individuals appear to have little to no return of nervous inputs as evidenced by a flaccid and atrophied vocal fold. In most cases where there is persistent motion impairment, recovery probably occurs somewhere between the extremes, such that there is a certain degree of reinnervation but with variable adequacy and accuracy.

Both human and animal studies have shown that a paralyzed vocal fold is only sometimes a denervated fold,[7-9] and even in cases of deliberate recurrent nerve section for spasmodic dysphonia,[10] reinnervation is the rule. This robust tendency for the vocal musculature to become reinnervated over time may account for the return of acceptable voice in the absence of vocal fold motion in certain cases of paralysis, through restoration of muscular bulk and tone by nerve regrowth inadequate and/or inappropriate to restore motion.[11]

these symptoms over the day (vocal fatigue). Challenging acoustic situations, such as speaking over background noise or using a telephone, will exacerbate these complaints.

Complaints of mild or moderate dysphagia, particularly for liquids, are fairly common in cases of paralysis. Whatever degree of aspiration that may be present will be exacerbated by the attendant weak cough. Frank aspiration is rare with isolated recurrent nerve injury, but more common with so-called "high-vagal" injuries, which impair both motor and sensory innervation to the larynx. Pooling of secretions in the piriform sinuses may be observed on the affected side. Because the recurrent laryngeal nerve also contributes to innervation of the cricopharyngeus muscle, delay in relaxation and opening of the upper esophageal sphincter may contribute to this problem.

Individuals may report breathlessness during speech due to rapid escape of air during phonation. Dyspnea with exertion may reflect different aspect of paralysis and requires careful consideration. Individuals at the extremes of fitness, such as the young athlete exercising to maximum capacity or the medically compromised aging patient, may symptomatically recognize partial obstruction of the glottis from failure of complete purposeful adduction. In most cases, however, the dyspnea represents a compromise of thoracic fixation during the Valsalva maneuver, which aids in a wide variety of everyday physical tasks like lifting objects, using the arms to assist in climbing stairs or rising from the sitting position, and defecation. Unfamiliarity with laryngeal biomechanics may lead the physician directly away from steps necessary to restore appropriate glottic competence.

In cases of paresis, the dysphonia may be subtle, particularly in the relatively quiet environment of the examination room, and the physician may have to rely on patient reports of fatigue, neck discomfort, and an intermittently poor voice.

Physical Examination

The clinician should assess the voice during both normal conversation and a variety of speech tasks. A breathy, diplophonic voice can occur because each vocal fold is at a different tension and will therefore vibrate at a different frequency for a given level of subglottic pressure. With a dense paralysis, patients will be unable to yell due to the flaccidity of the dysfunctional vocal fold. Simple bedside tests may approximately quantify the degree of glottic insufficiency, although they depend heavily on patient effort. Maximum phonation time (MPT) measures the duration that a patient can phonate the voiced vowel /i/. Normal values are greater than 21 seconds, although many individuals, especially singers, may have much longer phonation times.[12] The s/z ratio compares maximum phonation time between an unvoiced (/s/) and a voiced sound (/z/). In glottic insufficiency, this ratio increases as the phonation time for the voiced sound /z/ decreases (see chapter 5, Clinical and Instrumental Evaluation of the Voice Patient).

Prior to endoscopy, the patient should undergo a complete neurologic evaluation of the head and neck.[13] Signs such as a unilateral palatal weakness, tongue deviation, Horner's syndrome, and dysarthria may indicate the site of the lesion and suggest an underlying neurologic disease.

In most individuals, frank vocal paralysis will be readily detectable by flexible or rigid laryngoscopy. Slight vocal fold movement may occur due to cricothyroid, interarytenoid, and extralaryngeal muscle function, which may cause some diagnostic confusion. In such an individual, alternating sustained vowel phonation and sniffing (/i/-sniff) will highlight the inability of the paralyzed vocal fold to abduct.

The apex of the affected arytenoid may sag anteriomedially (Figure 11-1) due to a loss of active muscle stabilization (especially posterior cricoarytenoid) of the arytenoid cartilage on the crest of the cricoid. In this scenario, the vocal process is displaced caudally, and the paralyzed fold appears shortened and lower than its partner. Some patients may be able to approximate the vocal folds with low intensity phonation, but upon attempts to increase volume through raising subglottic pressure, a denervated fold tends to luff away from the midline due to flaccidity. Thus, one symptom that can differentiate a patient with paralysis from other causes of hoarseness is an inability to yell.

Often, the mobile arytenoid may "bump" the arytenoid on the denervated side and displace it laterally. The displacement of the muscular process of the paralyzed arytenoid under the mucosa of the piriform sinus is usually the most noticeable feature of this motion. This "jostle sign" was first described by Chevalier Jackson[14] and may serve as conclusive clinical evidence of a mobile arytenoid in cases where ankylosis or other fixation is suspected.

Ventricular fold hyperadduction may obscure the view of the vocal fold in some cases. This type of hyperfunction is in fact a common compensatory mechanism for glottic insufficiency[15] and should by itself direct the examiner's attention to glottal closure. In cases of paresis, it may be the only clue to the underlying problem (Figure 11-2).

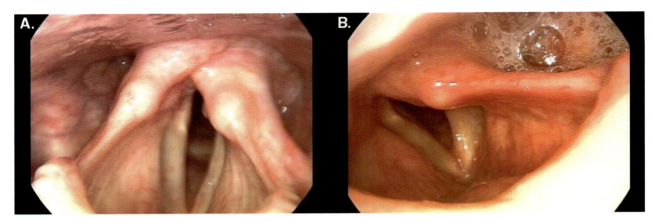

FIGURE 11–1. Left vocal fold paralysis. The individuals in both **A.** and **B.** have left vocal fold paralysis from metastatic mediastinal lymphadenopathy. They both have breathy diplophonic voices, and complain of extreme fatigue with prolonged speaking. The individual in **A.** has a fairly upright arytenoid with minimal flaccidity of the vocal fold, although atrophy is apparent. The individual in **B.** has an anteriorly prolapsed arytenoid, marked vocal fold flaccidity with bowing, and obvious pooling of secretions in the ipsilateral piriform sinus. These images illustrate the variability in presentation of vocal fold paralysis.

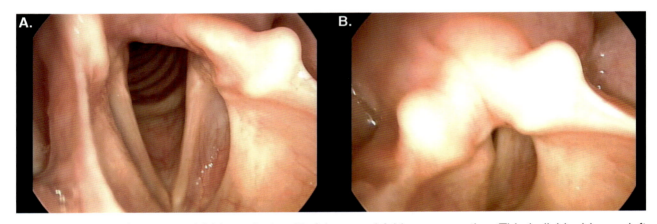

FIGURE 11–2. Left true vocal fold paralysis with false vocal fold compensation. This individual has a left vocal fold paralysis following a thoracic aneurysm repair. **A.** shows the vocal fold during abduction and **B.** during adduction. Note that the right hemilarynx attempts to compensate for the glottic insufficiency caused by paralysis of the left recurrent laryngeal nerve by recruiting the right false vocal (ventricular) fold during adduction to improve glottal closure. The reason for this behavior is obvious in this case, but false vocal fold hyperadduction may be the only clue to a subtle glottic insufficiency or paresis in other cases.

A detailed analysis of glottic configuration is important for planning surgical intervention. Vocal fold position must be assessed in both the coronal (rostral/caudal) and axial (abduction/adduction) planes. *Vertical height mismatches* are more likely to require an arytenoid procedure. Many studies also speak of posterior and anterior glottic closure. Posterior closure generally refers to contact at the vocal process, whereas anterior closure refers to contact between the vibrating edge of the membranous vocal folds. This distinction is also important in the selection of medialization approaches.

Further Investigations

If the cause of the vocal fold mobility is not evident, such as immediately following neck surgery or other trauma, further workup should include a complete medical history to identify possible causes and imaging of the course of the vagus from skull base *through* the mediastinum. Although most practitioners obtain a CT scan, MRI of the brain and skull base should also be considered when high vagal or central lesions are suspected.

Several studies[16] have suggested that chest radiography (CXR) may be adequate, particularly if the paralysis is right-sided. This is in contrast to the findings from the CT literature. In one study,[17] 13 of 18 (72%) cases with *left*-sided aortopulmonary masses on CT scan had a *normal* appearing mediastinum on CXR; the mean size of these chest masses was 2.3 cm. The smallest mass detected in this paper by CXR group was 3.8 cm. This controversy has not been resolved scientifically, with equal percentages of practitioners in a recent national survey choosing CT and CXR.[13] An evidence-based medicine review of the existing literature failed to reveal any support for one over the other.[13] It is important to note that plain film will neither evaluate the skull base nor the cervical course of the vagus and recurrent laryngeal nerves.

Serologies are generally not revealing, and have no role unless there is strong suspicion based on clinical history.[3,13] Direct laryngoscopy, once considered a standard part of evaluation, has largely been supplanted by improved imaging and should be reserved for cases in which ankylosis or posterior glottic stenosis is considered. Laryngeal electromyography can also give important information regarding cause and prognosis of vocal fold immobility, as outlined in chapter 9. Coughing, "wet" voice quality, or other symptoms which suggest dysphagia should prompt a formal evaluation of swallowing.

MANAGEMENT

Decisions regarding treatment in cases of vocal fold paralysis are guided by the severity of voice, swallowing, and airway symptoms balanced against expectations for spontaneous recovery. In cases where there is potential for spontaneous return of movement, and the patient has an acceptable voice, minimal dysphagia, and an adequate cough, it may be reasonable to defer intervention. Alternatively, for the symptomatic patient in the same scenario, a temporary vocal fold augmentation procedure may provide immediate airway stabilization while awaiting recovery. In other cases where there is little hope of functional return, a permanent procedure can be considered.

Although poor voice may be the most obvious symptom to the casual observer, significant dysphagia, aspiration, and poor cough are the symptoms that clinically mandate early intervention. Aspiration has been identified in 18 to 38% of patients with unilateral vocal fold paralysis of all causes.[18-20] It is probably more likely in high vagal injuries[21] (lesion of the vagus proximal to the branching of the superior laryngeal nerve) and of more concern in the face of pulmonary dysfunction or additional cranial nerve deficits. For this reason, algorithms featuring prompt medialization have been proposed after skull base surgery[22-23] and thoracic surgery.[24-27] Although any type of vocal fold medialization (temporary or permanent) appears to be equally effective in improving swallowing dysfunction,[19] it is worth noting that a significant proportion of patients remain troubled by aspiration after medialization.[22,27]

There are no studies that provide clear information regarding the natural history of vocal fold paralysis, and existing clinical series offer variable data. Willatt and Stell[21] published a series in 1989 in which only idiopathic paralyses were followed prospectively; of the 42 patients, although half returned to normal or "near-normal" function, only a fraction of them had return of vocal fold motion. None returned after being immobile for 12 months. Despite the lack of data for all etiologies, a clinical consensus has arisen, which states that prognosis is poor for return of vocal fold movement after a prescribed time interval of 6 to 12 months. For symptomatic treatment before the paralysis has reached this watershed, temporary medialization, usually synonymous with injection augmentation, is recommended. After this time period, medialization thyroplasty (framework surgery) is preferred, as the vocal fold is felt to have reached a condition that will remain stable over the long term. It is important to understand that these practices should not be applied uniformly without regard to the specific clinical circumstance. Requiring a person vocally disabled by a paralysis of overwhelmingly poor prognosis, such as that due to mediastinal metastases, to wait 6 months for rehabilitation is suboptimal management. An additional note requires vigilance; Stell[28] and Ward[29] have independently noted the small but real incidence of delayed presentation of causative neoplasms in patients previously thought to have "idiopathic" vocal paralysis. As many as 10% of cases may eventually be discovered to be due to a vagal schwannoma or other indolent but treatable cause.

Many investigators have attempted to determine prognostic indicators in various cases of paralysis to allow more expeditious rehabilitation of these individuals. To date, laryngeal electromyography has provided the best, although imperfect, information in this regard, largely because reinnervation is not synonymous with recovery. Thus, the appearance of unambiguous signs of reinnervation does not always lead to return of motion. In cases of less than 6 months duration, accurate prediction of unilateral vocal fold motion recovery ranges from 13% to 80%.[30-35] As a general rule, the LEMG features that indicate a good prognosis are the same as those predicted by the basic electrophysiology of muscle: preservation of normal MUAP waveforms, activation during an appropriate voluntary task, preservation of brisk recruitment, and absence of spontaneous activity. Factors suggestive of poor outcome are the converse of these. It should be noted that LEMG is a more reliable predictor of poor prognosis (75% to 100%), which stands to reason, as there is little ambiguity regarding findings such as fibrillation potentials several months following injury. Time elapsed since injury is important, insofar as the earlier favorable signs are present, the more likely it is that spontaneous recovery will take place. An extremely early EMG assessment (3 weeks or less after injury) may exaggerate the degree of injury, and beyond 6 months, LEMG is of limited use, as prognosis is uniformly poor.[35]

SURGICAL OPTIONS

Injection Laryngoplasty (See Table 11–3)

Injection augmentation techniques improve glottic closure by augmentation of the paraglottic space with a biocompatible substance, thereby adding bulk to the vocal fold and medializing the free edge. Injection augmentation is usually considered a temporary measure because most available injection substances (autologous fat, Gelfoam, collagen preparations [Zyderm, Zyplast, others], micronized dermis [Cymetra], hyaluronic acid [Hylaform, Restylane, others]) are resorbed over time. As a general rule, the collagen preparations are felt to persist in the tissue approximately 3 to 6 months, and the hyaluronic acid probably lasts longer, although there is marked interpatient variability. The bovine collagen preparations (Zyderm, Zyplast) do require prior skin testing to ensure no allergic reaction to the injectate; human collagen preparations (Cymetra), hyaluronic acid, and the permanent injectables mentioned below do not require formal allergy testing although there are rare reports of adverse tissue reactions.

Polytetrafluoroethylene paste (Teflon, Polytef) and calcium hydroxylapatite paste (Radiesse) are permanent synthetic injectables. Teflon was used extensively in the past but has fallen out of favor due to the delayed formation of granulomas requiring surgical resection (see chapter 15). Calcium hydroxylapatite (Radiesse) paste has been shown effective in several preliminary studies,[37] but long-term data regarding safety and efficacy are not yet available at the time of this writing.

Injection augmentation may be performed perorally (Figure 11–3) or transcutaenously in the office under topical or local anesthetic, or by suspension laryngoscopy in the operative suite. Injection augmentation is generally felt to be more suitable in cases where the glottic closure is only mildly compromised and predominantly affecting the membranous vocal fold; it will not effectively reposition the arytenoid to rectify a

TABLE 11–3. Overview of Materials for Glottic Injection

Material	Ease of Use	Duration	Drawbacks
Fat	+	6 to 9 months	Requires donor site, general anesthesia
Teflon	+++	Permanent	Granuloma formation
Gelfoam	++	1 to 2 months	Difficult in the awake patient, large needle
Calcium Hydroxylapatite	+++	Permanent?	Irreversible
Collagen			
Bovine (*Zyplast, Zyderm*)	+++	4 to 6 months	Requires pretesting and waiting period
Human donor (*Cymetra*)	++	4 to 6 months	Preparation, short shelf life
Human tissue culture (*Cosmoplast*)	+++	Unknown	No track record in laryngology
Human autologous	+	Unknown	Requires skin harvest
Radiesse Voice Gel	+++	Unknown	No track record; made for vocal fold
Hyaluronic Acid	+++	6 to 12 months	Good rheology, supportive studies

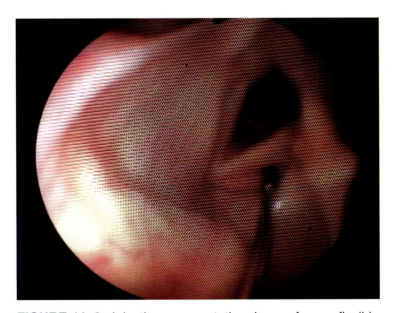

FIGURE 11–3. Injection augmentation. Image from a flexible nasolaryngoscope during a transoral injection laryngoplasty.

height discrepancy or close a posterior glottal gap. Most injection substances require overinjection to allow for resorption, rendering fine adjustments to vocal fold position virtually impossible. In addition, should the injectate infiltrate into an unintended site—typically and most distressingly, into the superficial layers of the vocal fold, impairing mucosal vibration—corrective intervention is challenging, and patients may have to await natural resolution over weeks to months. Some patients retain acceptable voice quality over time despite the use of a temporary injectable material, but it is not possible to definitively attribute these to injection alone (despite some assertions in the literature), given the tendency of paralytic dysphonia to improve over time.

Medialization Thyroplasty

Medialization thyroplasty is a precise, effective, permanent procedure that forms the mainstay of surgical management of vocal fold paralysis. This procedure involves creation of a window in the thyroid cartilage through which the paraglottic space can be accessed. An implant is then placed into the paraglottic space displacing the true vocal fold medially. Typically performed under local anesthesia, this procedure allows fine-tuning of the position, shape, and size of the implant guided by the immediate feedback of the patient's voice with each repositioning maneuver.

Initially introduced by Erwin Payr in 1915,[38] medialization thyroplasty was handicapped in its early iterations by the unpredictable durability of cartilage and bone used as medialization implants. This difficulty was solved with the introduction of the Silastic implant by Isshiki.[39] Since then, several additional medialization materials have been described. Solid prefabricated implants are available in a variety of materials (Silastic, hydroxyapatite, and bioimplantable metal). Due to ease of implant placement, many authors advocate the use of expanded polytetrafluoroethylene (Gore-Tex) ribbon, which can be layered into the paraglottic space through a small thyroplasty window until adequate voicing is achieved. Others prefer to hand carve individual implants out of Silastic

block, which allows custom variation of the height, depth, and width of each implant.

For the most part, the procedure is similar regardless of the implant used (Figure 11–4). Local anesthesia with epinephrine is injected into the skin and subcutaneous tissues of the anterior neck and along the thyroid cartilage. A modest incision just above the CT membrane extending just across the midline is created and subplatysmal flaps are elevated. The strap muscles are separated in the midline and retracted to expose the lateral aspect of the thyroid cartilage—some surgeons divide the medial 2 cm of the sternohyoid muscle to facilitate exposure.

The critical anatomic task is to identify the level of the vocal fold in relation to the thyroid lamina so that the thyroid cartilage window can be placed appropriately. In general, the vocal fold lies closer to the lower border of the thyroid cartilage than is generally believed. A lower cartilage strut is carefully preserved to stabilize the implant. The final dimensions and location of the window depend on the implant choice. The vocal fold is then medialized to yield a satisfactory voice (Figure 11–5). Visual feedback via a flexible fiberoptic laryngoscope intraoperatively is essential to ensure adequate medialization and accurate contact between the vibrating edges of the vocal folds.

During implant manipulation, some patients may not achieve optimal voicing due to persistence of hyperfunctional compensation. For this reason, some surgeons advocate preop voice therapy for "unloading" although others feel that these vocal patterns will "break" intraoperatively when physiologic vocal fold approximation is achieved.

When satisfactory placement has been achieved, and the surgeon is satisfied with the patient's voice and endoscopic view of the extent of medialization, the implant is secured with a permanent stitch, the strap muscles are reapproximated, and a small drain is placed. The patient is monitored overnight in the hospital for airway compromise. Voice rest is encouraged for 3 to 7 days and the patient is allowed to resume a regular diet although asked to refrain from heavy activity.

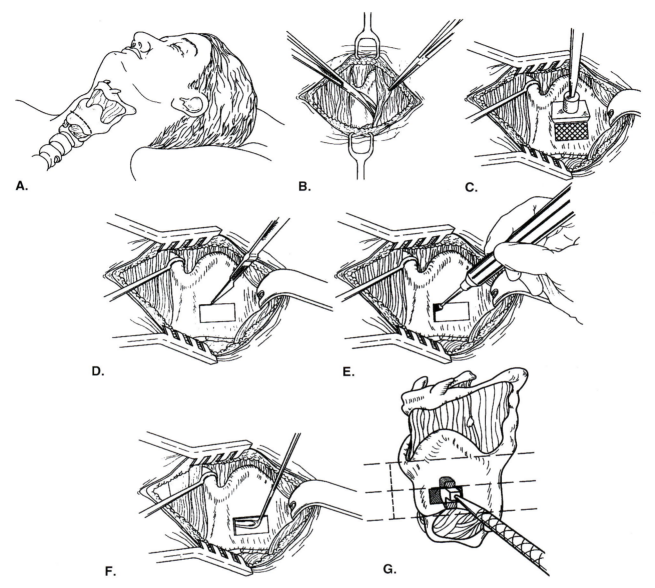

FIGURE 11–4. Thyroplasty technique. This series of drawings illustrates the technique for placing the VoCoM thyroplasty implant. The basic principles are the same for any implant technique. **A.** A 5- to 6-cm skin incision is planned horizontally at the level of the cricoid cartilage. **B.** After elevation of subplatysmal flaps, the strap muscles are divided and retracted laterally. **C.** The larynx is rotated using a single hook and the location of the thyroplasty window is marked—this kit uses a specialized template tool. **D.** and **E.** The window can be fashioned using a scalpel, Kerrison punch, or an otologic drill. **F.** The paraglottic tissues are freed from the inner table of the thyroid cartilage. **G.** A series of trial implants are placed to determine the optimum implant size and position, after which the final implant is placed and secured. The position of the vocal fold relative to external landmarks is shown. (Images courtesy of Gyrus-ENT.)

Principal complications include airway obstruction and perforation into the laryngeal lumen. Necessarily, medialization narrows the airway, and in combination with postoperative edema and hematoma, this can cause airway obstruction. For this reason, many surgeons prefer

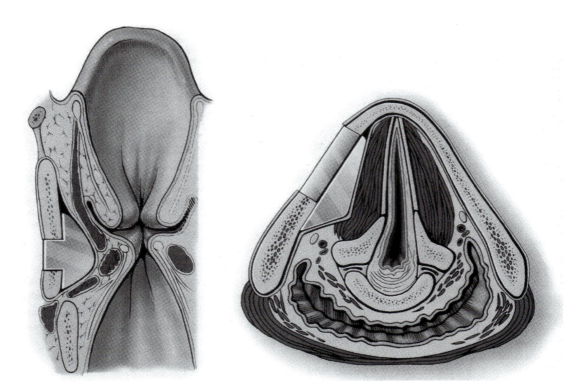

FIGURE 11–5. Coronal (*left*) and axial (*right*) views of final implant placement. (Reprinted from Ossoff R, *The Larynx.* Baltimore, Md: Lippincott Williams & Wilkins; 2003:292 with permission. Copyright 2003 Lippincott, Williams & Wilkins.)

to observe these patients in the hospital for one night following the procedure. Approximately 0.6% to 11% of patient undergoing medialization laryngoplasty, and 2.2% to 3.5% undergoing medialization plus arytenoid adduction, required intubation or tracheotomy in the immediate postoperative period.[40,41] The incidence of airway emergencies and implant extrusion have dropped in the years since the introduction of these procedures.

Violation of the laryngeal mucosa is significant because of the likelihood of infection and subsequent extrusion of implanted material. Perforation typically takes place in the delicate ventricular mucosa, which lies close to the thyroid lamina, or anteriorly, where there is little soft tissue cover; surgeons should use special care when undermining the paraglottic tissues in these areas. Mucosal tears are not always obvious, but any blood seen intralumenally via the endoscope should prompt a careful inspection. Flooding the operative field with irrigation and looking for

bubbles during a Valsalva maneuver is also useful, and may be performed in all cases prior to implant placement.

Dissatisfaction with the medialization procedure does not typically arise because of complications, but because of suboptimal voice results. These are typically due to technical factors, and revision rates have been reported to range from 5.4%[41] to 14%,[40] to as high as 33%[42] when adjunctive procedures such as fat injection are included. Certain causes of poor voice result occur with greater frequency, including a persistent posterior gap, undermedialization, and implant malposition, generally in too anterior or superior a position.

Persistent posterior glottic gap can account for as many as 50% of revisions in cases where arytenoid adduction has not been performed.[43] Revision medialization alone is generally ineffective in shifting arytenoid position. Even when the implant can displace the vocal process of the arytenoid medially, it cannot remedy a height mismatch, nor can it readily correct a mismatch in vocal fold tension, which is commonly found in cases of paralysis.

Undercorrection is another relatively frequent cause of poor results,[44] and may be especially likely to occur in cases that last longer than usual and allow the accumulation of intraoperative edema to mislead the surgeon regarding the degree of medialization required. In these cases, the initial voice result is satisfactory, but deteriorates with time as swelling resolves.

Netterville and Billante[45] have reported placing the implant too far superior as the most common cause for revision in their series, an error that probably arises from misconceptions regarding position of the vibratory margin of the fold in relation to the profile of the thyroid lamina. Too anterior an implant placement, on the other hand, likely arises from a poor appreciation of the overall length of the thyroid lamina and yields early mucosal contact during adduction, damping of phonatory oscillation, and a characteristic strained or pressed voice quality.

Arytenoid Repositioning Procedures

Although injection laryngoplasty and medialization thyroplasty provide excellent results and may be adequate treatment in many patients, some individuals require repositioning of the arytenoid to achieve optimal voicing. The typical clinical scenario involves an arytenoid that is tipped anteriorly into the airway and externally rotated, resulting in a flaccid foreshortened vocal fold with a lateralized vocal process. Despite successful medialization of the anterior membranous vocal fold, the vocal processes do not approximate, leaving a posterior gap and a vertical mismatch of the vocal fold level.

Several procedures to manipulate the arytenoid are described. The most common procedure is the placement of an *arytenoid adduction* suture (Figure 11-6). This suture theoretically mimics the action of the thyroarytenoid-lateral cricoarytenoid (TA-LCA) muscle complex and achieves glottal closure by internal rotation of the vocal process. Although some debate continues regarding the physiologic effect of arytenoid adduction, most surgeons agree that this procedure rotates the arytenoid cartilage medially, displaces the vocal process caudally and medially, and stabilizes the vocal process.[46,47] This effectively aids in closing a posterior gap and re-establishes vocal fold tension, which in turn improves glottic performance during phonation, particularly at increased vocal intensity.

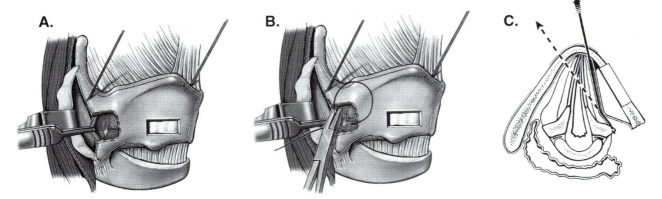

FIGURE 11-6. Arytenoid adduction suture. **A.** The arytenoid can be approached through exposure of the posterior edge of the thyroid lamina after the attachments of the inferior constrictor are dissected free. The mucosa of the piriform sinus is elevated from the internal surface of the cartilage, and a posterior fenestra can be created using a Kerrison punch. **B.** A stitch is placed through the muscular process of the arytenoid, mimicking the action of the lateral-cricoarytenoid muscle by bringing the free ends of the stitch through the thyroplasty window. **C.** An axial view showing the vector of pull of the arytenoid adduction stitch with a thyroplasty implant in place. (Reprinted from Ossoff R, *The Larynx.* Baltimore, Md: Lippincott Williams & Wilkins; 2003:296-297 with permission. Copyright, 2003 Lippincott, Williams & Wilkins.)

Exposure of the arytenoid requires approach around or through the posterior margin of the thyroid lamina, elevation of the piriform sinus mucosa, and identification of the muscular process. Most surgeons facilitate exposure by removing the posterior portion of the thyroid cartilage overlying the arytenoid and piriform with a rongeur. A nonabsorbable suture is passed through the muscular process of the arytenoid and tension placed anterolaterally to approximate the action of the thyroarytenoid-lateral cricoarytenoid (TA-LCA) muscle complex. Once rotation is judged adequate, the suture is secured to the thyroid cartilage. Very little tension is required on the arytenoid adduction suture.

Regardless of the exact technique chosen, arytenoid repositioning procedures are designed to internally rotate and/or suspend the arytenoid in the physiologic phonatory position. These procedures are technically challenging, time consuming, and have a higher rate of complications than simple medialization.[48] Elevation of the piriform sinus mucosa is a delicate task and presents an additional opportunity for perforation. Airway complications are more frequent due to additional manipulation and resultant edema. Despite these concerns, for the accomplished phonosurgeon, these procedures are an essential adjunct to medialization thyroplasty to achieve an optimal vocal outcome.

Laryngeal Reinnervation

Restoration of physiologic adductor and abductor function is the idealized goal of reinnervation procedures. Many methods of selective reinnervation have been described, including neuromuscular transfer, selective neural anastomosis, and direct nerve implantation, but reliable restoration of physiologic function has not been realized to date. Additionally there are no alternative donor nerves that will provide the complex respiratory and phonatory neural signals required. Thus, current reinnervation techniques restore neural input to the intrinsic laryngeal muscles to mimic the natural reinnervation process, thereby restor-

ing the bulk and tone of the vocal fold and arytenoid musculature.

In cases of obvious nerve transection, primary nerve reanastomosis is probably worthwhile and beneficial, providing that sufficient length exists for tension-free approximation. When the procedure is performed for an intact nerve, the recurrent laryngeal nerve can be anastomosed to an alternative donor nerve, similar to facial reanimation techniques utilizing the XII to VII jump graft, in the hope that the number of functional axonal connections after reinnervation will exceed the existing quantity of functional axonal connections. Both the ansa cervicalis[49] and hypoglossal[50,51] have been proposed for this role, although in the second case, the surgeon must weigh carefully the added morbidity of hemitongue denervation.

The neuromuscular pedicle (NMP) technique involves transfer of a nerve with a small block of muscle (ansa cercicalis with omohyoid) into a denervated laryngeal muscle bed to encourage graft implantation with eventual arborization of the donor nerve into the host muscle. Again, the goal is to maintain bulk and tone of the thyroarytenoid muscle over time. These procedures can be combined with a medialization thyroplasty.

SPECIAL ISSUES IN PARALYSIS

Isolated SLN Paresis

Superior laryngeal nerve paresis manifests as sensory loss from the internal branch with motor weakness of the cricothyroideus muscle innervated from the external branch. Several authors have demonstrated a high association between SLN injury and dysfunction of the cricopharyngeus muscle, thus contributing to dysphagia.[52] This can occur independently of recurrent nerve injury and can be iatrogenic (thyroidectomy, neck dissection) or idiopathic. The sensory loss can cause throat clearing, coughing, and a globus sensation. Bilateral sensory loss can lead to aspiration. The vocal characteristics are due to loss of

Vocal Fold Position in Paralysis

Historically, it was felt that topographic information regarding the location of a neurologic insult along the course of the vagal nerve could be gained through evaluation of laryngeal and vocal fold position. Thus, a lesion of the recurrent nerve in isolation would theoretically give a vocal fold in the paramedian position, a lesion of the superior laryngeal nerve would be demonstrated by rotation of the laryngeal posterior commisure toward the side of nerve dysfunction, and a lesion of the vagal trunk would give a vocal fold in the cadaveric or lateral position. Theories such as the Wagner-Grossman hypothesis attempted to explain vocal fold position based on the presence or absence of cricothyroid muscle activity; Semon's law held that there was a differential vulnerability of nerve fibers to injury with the abductors affected first, followed by the adductors.[6] These theories, although prevalent in historical literature, have been successfully challenged by contemporary investigators. It is currently accepted that laryngeal and vocal fold position does not reliably correlate with the site of vagal nerve injury.[7,53,54]

symmetric cricothyroideus function. Although individuals without complicated vocal demands may not notice any vocal defect, singers will complain of a ceiling effect—inability to reach their highest registers. Additionally, individuals may complain of voice fatigue and diplophonia. On exam, pooling in the piriform on the affected side reflects the sensory defect, and rotation of the posterior commissure toward the side of the paralysis may occur during phonatory effort. The diagnosis can be confirmed by LEMG. Unfortunately, in the absence of spontaneous recovery, there are no unique medical or surgical interventions available for this process.

Bilateral Vocal Fold Immobility

Bilateral vocal fold immobility has a similar legion of etiologies, although with a differing incidence as compared to unilateral vocal fold immobility. Bilateral vocal fold paralysis is most often a result of surgical misadventure, with thyroidectomy accounting for the majority of cases. Fixation

from posterior glottic stenosis after prolonged intubation, radiation-induced fibrosis, and infiltrative disorders (amyloid and granulomatous diseases) may mimic bilateral nerve injury. Esophageal malignancy extending to the tracheoesophageal groove may account for up to half of neoplastic causes.[5] The voice is usually close to normal, but patients may develop significant airway compromise from inability to abduct the vocal folds. Interestingly, even after bilateral injury, patients may tolerate the restricted airway for days to years before developing symptoms, which may then be misdiagnosed as asthma or bronchitis before the airway is examined. If the airway compromise is severe, an emergency tracheotomy may be required. This is best done awake as it may not be absolutely evident if the embarrassment is due to nerve injury or laryngeal fixation.

Once the nature and cause of the bilateral immobility is established, treatment should be determined by symptomatology. Although the best function is often obtained with tracheotomy, many patients are reluctant to accept this option. Vocal fold lateralization procedures for decannulation, such as a laser posterior cordotomy[55] and arytenoidectomy,[56] are destructive and irreversible. These procedures are designed to maintain approximation of the anterior membranous vocal folds for phonation but increase the posterior aperture for improved airflow. The Lichtenberger tech-nique of suture lateralization can be performed as a reversible or permanent method of opening the airway in these cases.[57,58] Bilateral vocal fold immobility is one of the greatest challenges in the treatment of benign laryngeal disorders.

Pediatric Laryngeal Nerve Paralysis

The symptoms and etiology of vocal fold immobility in children is different from adults and varies with the age of the patient population. Causes include surgical trauma (cardiac and thoracic), neurologic disease (Arnold-Chiari malformation and other neurologic defects), birth trauma, and idiopathic. Paralysis is the predominant cause of immobility, the second-most common cause of neonatal stridor (laryngomalacia being the first), and may account for 10% of congenital anomalies of the larynx.[59] Daya in 2000[60] reported a series from Great Ormond Street in which the percentage of bilateral immobility was approximately equal to that of unilateral immobility. As opposed to adults, unilateral immobility often causes stridor in addition to a weak cry, feeding difficulties, and aspiration. Also in contrast to adults, children with bilateral vocal fold paralysis may not require tracheotomy and may have a higher rate of spontaneous recovery.[60] Evaluation includes a complete neurologic exam, magnetic resonance imaging of the brain, neck, and mediastinum, fiberoptic laryngoscopy, and rigid endoscopy under anesthesia, as up to half of patients may have an associated upper airway anomaly. In the past, treatment is conservative as patients have shown a propensity to compensate over a number of years. The rate of actual vocal fold motion recovery is not known.

In most cases, vocal fold immobility or hypomobility is neurogenic, caused by disease of or traumatic insult to the laryngeal nerves. Mechanical factors may result in cricoarytenoid fixation,

usually after prolonged intubation or other trauma. Some cases of paralysis resolve, or at least improve symptomatically, without intervention; others require treatment. Distinguishing between these two groups remains a challenge, and many otolaryngologists consequently choose to delay treatment, sometimes despite considerable patient disability. In cases of unilateral paralysis, a broad armamentarium of procedures is available to alleviate symptoms including temporary and permanent injection laryngoplasty, medialization thyroplasty, arytenoid repositioning, and reinnervation procedures.

Review Questions

1. Describe in detail the types of laryngeal injectables, their duration, and potential complications.

2. Why do some individuals with a vocal fold paralysis have an adequate voice, and other individuals suffer extreme glottic insufficiency?

3. What findings on LEMG predict a favorable prognosis for return of function?
   a. Activation of motor unit potentials during an appropriate task, absence of fibrillation potentials, preservation of motor unit morphology
   b. Polyphasic motor unit potentials and decreased recruitment pattern
   c. Fibrillation potentials and positive sharp waves (spontaneous activity)
   d. Bilateral mildly diminished recruitment
   e. Electrical silence

4. Does reinnervation correlate with return of motion?

5. What are the treatment options for bilateral vocal fold immobility? What are the risks and benefits of each option?

6. A 45-year-old female undergoes a right thyroid lobectomy for benign disease and has a breathy voice postoperatively. Right vocal fold immobility is confirmed by endoscopy. LEMG at 1 month shows polyphasic potentials and absence of fibrillation potentials. She would like a better voice and has no swallowing complaints. What treatment option would you offer her?
   a. None as she has a good chance of spontaneous recovery
   b. Injection laryngoplasty with a permanent material
   c. Injection laryngoplasty with a temporary material with an option for future type I thyroplasty if there is inadequate return of function
   d. Type I thyroplasty and arytenoid adduction

REFERENCES

1. Merati AL, Shemirani N, Smith TL, Toohill RJ. Changing trends in the nature of vocal fold motion impairment. *Am J Otolaryngol.* 2006; 27(2):106-108.
2. Weisberg NK, Spengler DM, Netterville JL. Stretch-induced nerve injury as a cause of paralysis secondary to the anterior cervical approach. *Otolaryngol Head Neck Surg.* 1997;116(3):317-326.
3. Terris, DJ, Arnstein D, Nguyen HH, Contemporary evaluation of unilateral vocal cord paralysis. *Otolaryngol Head Neck Surg.* 1992;107(1):84-90.
4. Maisel RH, Ogura JH. Evaluation of vocal cord paralysis. *Laryngoscope.* 1974;84(2):302-316.
5. Benninger MS, Gillen JB, Altman JS. Changing etiology of vocal fold immobility. *Laryngoscope.* 1998;108(9):1346-1350.
6. Rubin AD, et al. Arytenoid cartilage dislocation: a 20-year experience. *J Voice.* 2005;19(4):687-701.
7. Blitzer A, Jahn AF, Keidar A, Semon's law revisited: an electromyographic analysis of laryngeal synki-

nesis. *Ann Otol Rhinol Laryngol.* 1996;105(10): 764-769.
8. Crumley RL, McCabe BF. Regeneration of the recurrent laryngeal nerve. *Otolaryngol Head Neck Surg.* 1982;90(4):442-447.
9. Zealear DL, Hamdan AL, Rainey CL, Effects of denervation on posterior cricoarytenoid muscle physiology and histochemistry. *Ann Otol Rhinol Laryngol.* 1994;103(10):780-788.
10. Netterville JL, Stone RE, Rainey C, Zealear DL, Ossoff RH. Recurrent laryngeal nerve avulsion for treatment of spastic dysphonia. *Ann Otol Rhinol Laryngol.* 1991;100(1):10-14.
11. Crumley RL, Laryngeal synkinesis revisited. *Ann Otol Rhinol Laryngol.* 2000;109(4):365-371.
12. Kent RD, Kent JF, Rosenbek JC, Maximum performance tests of speech production. *J Speech Hear Disord.* 1987;52(4):367-387.
13. Merati AL, Halum S, Smith TL. Diagnostic testing for vocal paralysis: A survey of contemporary practice and evidence-based medicine review. In press.
14. Jackson C. Jackson CL. *The Larynx and Its Diseases.* Philadelphia, Pa: WB Saunders; 1937.
15. Belafsky PC, Postma GN, Reulbach TR, Holland BW, Koufman JA. Muscle tension dysphonia as a sign of underlying glottal insufficiency. *Otolaryngol Head Neck Surg.* 2002;127(5):448-451.
16. Altman, JS, Benninger MS, The evaluation of unilateral vocal fold immobility: is chest X-ray enough? *J Voice.* 1997;11(3):364-367.
17. Glazer, H.S., et al., Extralaryngeal causes of vocal cord paralysis: CT evaluation. *Am J Roentgenol.* 1983;141(3):527-531.
18. Tabaee A, et al., Flexible endoscopic evaluation of swallowing with sensory testing in patients with unilateral vocal fold immobility: incidence and pathophysiology of aspiration. *Laryngoscope.* 2005;115(4):565-569.
19. Bhattacharyya N, Kotz T, and Shapiro J, Dysphagia and aspiration with unilateral vocal cord immobility: incidence, characterization, and response to surgical treatment. *Ann Otol Rhinol Laryngol.* 2002;111(8):672-679.
20. Heitmiller RF, Tseng E, Jones B. Prevalence of aspiration and laryngeal penetration in patients with unilateral vocal fold motion impairment. *Dysphagia.* 2000;15(4):184-187.
21. Flint, PW, Purcell LL, Cummings CW, Pathophysiology and indications for medialization thyroplasty in patients with dysphagia and aspiration. *Otolaryngol Head Neck Surg.* 1997;116(3):349-354.

22   Bielamowicz S. Gupta A, Sekhar LN, Early arytenoid adduction for vagal paralysis after skull base surgery. *Laryngoscope.* 2000;110(3 pt 1):346-351.

23. Netterville JL. Civantos FJ. Rehabilitation of cranial nerve deficits after neurotologic skull base surgery. *Laryngoscope.* 1993;103(11 pt 2 suppl 60): 45-54.

24. Bhattacharyya N, Batirel H, Swanson SJ, Improved outcomes with early vocal fold medialization for vocal fold paralysis after thoracic surgery. *Auris Nasus Larynx.* 2003;30(1):71-75.

25. Mom T., Filaire M, Advenier D, et al. Concomitant type I thyroplasty and thoracic operations for lung cancer: preventing respiratory complications associated with vagus or recurrent laryngeal nerve injury. *J Thorac Cardiovasc Surg.* 2001; 121(4): 642-648.

26. Abraham MT, Bains MS, Downey RJ, Korst RJ, Kraus DH. Type I thyroplasty for acute unilateral vocal fold paralysis following intrathoracic surgery. *Ann Otol Rhinol Laryngol.* 2002;111(8): 667-671.

27. Nayak VK, Bhattacharyya N, Kotz T, Shapiro J. Patterns of swallowing failure following medialization in unilateral vocal fold immobility. *Laryngoscope.* 2002;112(10):1840-1844.

28. Willatt DJ Stell PM. The prognosis and management of idiopathic vocal cord paralysis. *Clin Otolaryngol Allied Sci.* 1989;14(3):247-250.

29. Ward PH. Berci G. Observations on so-called idiopathic vocal cord paralysis. *Ann Otol Rhinol Laryngol.* 1982;91(6 pt 1):558-563.

30. Hirano M, et al. Electromyography for laryngeal paralysis. In: Hirano M, Kirchner JA, Bless DM, eds. *Neurolaryngology: Recent Advances.* San Diego, Calif: Singular Publishing; 1991:232-248.

31. Sittel C. et al. Prognostic value of laryngeal electromyography in vocal fold paralysis. *Arch Otolaryngol Head Neck Surg.* 2001;127(2):155-160.

32. Parnes SM, Satya-Murti S. Predictive value of laryngeal electromyography in patients with vocal cord paralysis of neurogenic origin. *Laryngoscope.* 1985;95(11):1323-1326.

33. Munin MC,Rosen CA, Zullo T. Utility of laryngeal electromyography in predicting recovery after vocal fold paralysis. *Arch Phys Med Rehabil.* 2003;84(8):1150-1153.

34. Mostafa BE, Gadallah NA, Nassar NM, Al Ibiary HM, Fahmy HA, Fouda NM. The role of laryngeal electromyography in vocal fold immobility. *J Otorhinolaryngol Relat Spec.* 2004;66(1):5-10.

35. Gupta SR, Bastian RW. Use of laryngeal electromyography in prediction of recovery after vocal cord paralysis. *Muscle Nerve.* 1993;16(9):977-978.

36. Hollinger LD, Hollinger PC, Hollinger PH. Etiology of bilateral abductor vocal cord parlaysis: a review of 389 cases. *Ann Otol Rhinol Laryngol.* 1976; 85(4 pt 1):428-436

37   Rosen CA, Thekdi AA. Vocal fold augmentation with injectable calcium hydroxylapatite: short-term results. *J Voice.* 2004;18(3):387-391.

38. Payr E. Plastik am Schildknorpel zur Behebung der Folgen einseitiger Stimmbandlähmung. *Deutsche Med Wochenshr.* 1915;41:1265.

39. Isshiki N, Morita H, Okamura H, Hiramoto M. Thyroplasty as a new phonosurgical technique. *Acta Otolaryngol.* 1974;78(5-6):451-477.

40. Weinman EC, Maragos NE, Airway compromise in thyroplasty surgery. *Laryngoscope.* 2000;110(7): 1082-1085.

41. Rosen CA. Complications of phonosurgery: results of a national survey. *Laryngoscope.* 1998; 108(11 pt 1):1697-1703.

42. Anderson TD, Spiegel JR, Sataloff RT. Thyroplasty revisions: frequency and predictive factors. *J Voice.* 2003;17(3): 442-448.

43. Woo P, et al. Failed medialization laryngoplasty: management by revision surgery. *Otolaryngol Head Neck Surg.* 2001;124(6):615-621.

44. Cohen JT, Bates DD, Postma GN. Revision Gore-Tex medialization laryngoplasty. *Otolaryngol Head Neck Surg.* 2004;131(3):236-240.

45. Netterville JL, Billante CR. The immobile vocal fold. In: Ossoff RH, Shapshay SM, Woodson GE, Netterville JL. eds. *The Larynx.* Philadelphia, Pa: Lippincott, Williams & Wilkins, 2004:269-305.

46. Woodson G. Cricopharyngeal myotomy and arytenoid adduction in the management of combined laryngeal and pharyngeal paralysis. *Otolaryngol Head Neck Surg.* 1997;116(3):339-343.

47. Woodson GE, et al. Arytenoid adduction: controlling vertical position. *Ann Otol Rhinol Laryngol.* 2000;109(4):360-364.

48. Abraham MT, Gonen M, Kraus DH. Complications of type I thyroplasty and arytenoid adduction. *Laryngoscope.* 2001;111(8):1322-1329.

49. Crumley RL, Update: ansa cervicalis to recurrent laryngeal nerve anastomosis for unilateral laryngeal paralysis. *Laryngoscope.* 1991;101(4 pt 1): 384-387. Discussion, 388.

50. Paniello RC. Lee P, Dahm JD. Hypoglossal nerve transfer for laryngeal reinnervation: a preliminary

study. *Ann Otol Rhinol Laryngol.* 1999. 108(3): 239-244.

51. Paniello RC, West SE, Lee P, Laryngeal reinnervation with the hypoglossal nerve. I. Physiology, histochemistry, electromyography, and retrograde labeling in a canine model. *Ann Otol Rhinol Laryngol.* 2001;110(6):532-542.

52. Halum S. et al. Electromyography findings of the cricopharyngeus in association with ipsilateral pharyngeal and laryngeal muscles. *Ann Otol Rhinol Laryngol.* In press.

53. Koufman JA, Walker FO, Joharji GM. The cricothyroid muscle does not influence vocal fold position in laryngeal paralysis. *Laryngoscope.* 1995; 105(4 pt 1):368-372.

54. Woodson GE. Configuration of the glottis in laryngeal paralysis. I: Clinical study. *Laryngoscope.* 1993;103(11 pt 1):1227-1234.

55. Kashima HK. Bilateral vocal fold motion impairment: pathophysiology and management by transverse cordotomy. *Ann Otol Rhinol Laryngol.* 1991;100(9 pt 1):717-721.

56. Ossoff RH, Sisson GA, Duncavage JA, Moselle HI, Andrews PE, McMillan WG. Endoscopic laser arytenoidectomy for the treatment of bilateral vocal cord paralysis. *Laryngoscope.* 1984;94(10): 1293-1297.

57. Lichtenberger G. Reversible lateralization of the paralyzed vocal cord without tracheostomy. *Ann Otol Rhinol Laryngol.* 2002;111(1):21-26.

58. Lichtenberger G. Comparison of endoscopic glottis-dilating operations. *Eur Arch Otorhinolaryngol.* 2003;260(2):57-61.

59. Holinger PH, Brown WT. Congenital webs, cysts, laryngoceles and other anomalies of the larynx. *Ann Otol Rhinol Laryngol* 1967; 76(4):744-752.

60. Daya H, Hosni A, Bejar-Solar I, Evans JN, Bailey CN. Pediatric vocal fold paralysis: a long-term retrospective study. *Arch Otolaryngol Head Neck Surg,* 2000;126(1):21-25.

61. Vilensky JA, Sinish PR. Semon and Semon's law. *Clin Anal.* 2004;17(8):605-606.

12

The Larynx in Parkinson's Disease

Mona M. Abaza, MD
Jennifer Spielman, MA, CCC-SLP

KEY POINTS

■ Parkinson's disease is a common progressive degenerative neurologic disorder in which significant dysphonia is present in at least 70% of cases.

■ A soft, breathy, monotone voice with or without a tremor is typical. The dysphonia can be associated with poor articulation, difficulty initiating speech, stutteringlike quality, and "flat" affect. Videostroboscopic examination of the larynx can provide helpful diagnostic characteristics such as glottal incompetence and decreased vocal fold vibration.

■ Parkinson's plus syndrome, a more severe and rapidly degenerating process, demonstrates more significant changes such as vocal fold paralysis and more significant tremor.

■ Systemic treatments of the disease, although often helping limb motion abnormalities, do not always help with vocal issues, whereas the Lee Silverman Voice Therapy (LSVT) has been shown to improve the dysphonia.

■ Dysphagia is a common complaint associated with the disorder and oropharyngeal abnormalities are present in almost all patients.

Parkinson's disease (PD), the most common movement disorder in patients over 55 years of age, affects an estimated 1.5 million people in the United States. It is a degenerative process of the brainstem nuclei significantly affecting the *substantia nigra*, creating decreased dopamine availability as the fundamental deficiency. Characteristic physical changes include resting tremors of the arms and legs, pill-rolling tremor movements at rest, overall rigidity, a festinating gait, reduced arm swing, and a slow initiation of movement. Approximately 70 to 89% of all patients demonstrate vocal difficulties with the disease, and over 30% of these patients find it the most disabling part of the disorder for them.[1] Dysphagia has been reported in most patients with oropharyngeal abnormalities seen on videofluoroscopy in almost all patients. Choking, piecemeal deglutition, regurgitation, and aspiration (silent and known) can all be present.[2] Postural abnormalities, olfactory dysfunction, depression, and micrographia are also reported as systemic components of PD.

The most characteristic voice in PD patients is soft, breathy, and monotonal. The voice is perceived by the patient as normal in loudness and quality, although it is not. A resting vocal tremor is also a common component, present in 55% of patients with idiopathic PD.[3] Vertical laryngeal movement secondary to tremor of the strap muscles is evident even at rest. The tremor occurs when the affected body part is at repose and completely supported. In general, it occurs at a rate of 4 to 10 Hz, whereas physiologic tremors occur at faster rates, 8 to 12 Hz, and cerebellar tremors are slower, 2 to 5 Hz.[4-6] Other components of the speech abnormalities include poor articulation, a variable rate speech, a stuttering-like voice quality, difficulty initiating speech, reduced facial expression, and overall "flat" affects. The speech of PD, although often breathy and of low intensity, does not always demonstrate the changes in a typical rhythmic fashion. Rather, the hypophonia is constant, with exacerbation by the articulatory difficulties and the cognitive problems associated with the disease.

The diagnosis of Parkinson's disease is often made by a neurologist, but dysphonia may be the first presentation, and the otolaryngologist may be the first to recognize the disorder. Assessing the fluidity of the voice, the quality of articulation, and the quality of the voice signal itself are easily accomplished by active listening during the patient history. As the differentiation of abnormal fluidity from poor articulation is important in differentiating PD from other movement disorders affecting the voice, such as essential tremors and stroke, an oral mechanism evaluation can be useful in these situations. Assessment of voice quality should include an assessment of the overall degree of dysphonia and the presence of raspiness, breathiness, and/or strain, which can be indications of other vocal pathology. Flexible fiberoptic and videostroboscopic examination findings are helpful in the diagnosis of PD. The examination of the larynx should be performed at rest and during a variety of phonatory tasks. Typically both a flexible fiberoptic scope and a rigid laryngoscope, each providing different information, are used in a complete exam. Whereas rigid stroboscopy allows one to assess the vibratory function and detailed anatomic structure of the vocal folds, portions of the neurolaryngeal examination are best performed with a flexible transnasal endoscope. Lingual traction, required for a transoral examinations, does not allow for connected speech evaluations, and the change in tongue position may suppress characteristic diagnostic signs.

Vocal fold bowing, midfold opening of the glottis during phonation, and a slowed vibration are considered characteristic of PD. Glottal incompetence is one of the most consistent findings described. Detected more commonly during rigid examination of the larynx, bowing may be overcalled (due to distortion of the laryngeal anatomy by the rigid scoping procedure. The hypophonia of PD is considered a manifestation of incomplete glottic closure and poor breath support resulting from the chest wall rigidity. A paralyzed vocal fold can be a sign of Parkinson's plus syndromes. PPS includes multisystem degeneration,

Shy-Drager syndrome, basal ganglia degeneration, and progressive supranuclear palsy. These disorders show a more rapid progressive deterioration of motor functions, with significantly worse speech deficits. Vocal tremor is found in 55% of idiopathic Parkinson's patients, but 64% of Parkinson's plus patients. Stroboscopy findings of open phase closure and asymmetric vibration are more commonly found in general PD than in PPS.[2] Other findings on laryngeal exam include pooled hypopharyngeal secretions, decreased sensation, diminished cough reflex, and aspiration.

Diagnostic studies such as EMG and objective voice measures may provide some information in patients with PD. Single motor unit laryngeal EMG studies have been investigated in younger and older patients with PD of both sexes. A decreased firing rate and increased variability are seen in older patients and males only.[7] Objective instrumental measures of voice have revealed elevated jitter and shimmer and decreased harmonic-to-noise ratio, s/z ratio, and maximum phonation time in tremulous voices, abnormalities shared with other conditions of glottic insufficiency.[8] In addition, a brief generalized neurologic examination encompassing the upper extremities and gait can identify and reveal other characteristic signs of PD such as bradykinesia and cogwheeling.

TREATMENT

In addition to studying treatment of the overall disease process and its effect on communication, several treatments directed at the dysphonia of PD have been attempted, Collagen augmentation of the vocal folds has demonstrated temporary effectiveness (11/18 patients showing improvements lasting >2 months). No improvement of the articulatory function has been seen and often repeat procedures are required. It is also not as effective in severely affected patients.[9,10] Thalamic deep brain stimulation (DBS) by means of implanted electrodes, a neurosurgical intervention, is an evolving means of treating disabling, medication-resistant tremor and PD. Initial reports of postoperative dysarthria, particularly after bilateral procedures, created reservations about its utility in voice tremor, as speech and voice require a high degree of coordination. The procedure shows limited improvements to voice and speech function in PD, despite significant changes in limb movements.[11] Evidence does suggest DBS may be practical and useful in the treatment of the voice tremor component.[12-15] Standard Parkinson's treatment with L-dopa has had mixed results in PD dysphonia. Decreased jitter and increased fundamental frequency in a mildly affected population are shown by some, but not others.[16]

Despite the many forms of therapies tried, only behaviorally based intervention has been shown to have an effect on the voice and speech functions of patients with PD. Lee Silverman Voice Treatment (LSVT), an intensive rehabilitative program, is designed to increase intensity by increasing phonatory effort and maximum adductory vocal tasks. This approach depends on a behaviorally based system to generalize the increased effort by the patient toward audibly louder speech. LSVT should be administered by a speech pathologist certified in the therapy, as the program relies on carefully defined processes. Numerous studies have shown a sustained or improved vocal intensity over pretreatment levels.[17] Laryngeal examinations show a decrease in glottal incompetence without a significant change in supraglottal hyperfunctioning.[18] Swallowing function appears to be improved after treatment as well. Changes in tongue movement, both in the oral (lateral movement) and pharyngeal phase (tongue base retraction), are reduced post-therapy and appear to be a significant component of the noted decreased oral and pharyngeal transit time.[19] More research is underway to confirm and elaborate on these findings. Preliminary studies, using PET scans, show reduced activity in the globus pallidus, an effect similar to pallidotomy.[19] Initial data show that improvement in the overall affect and facial expression of the patient may be improved by this therapy as well.[20]

The Effects of the Lee Silverman Voice Therapy (LSVT) on Emotional Expression in PD

Impaired emotional expression is a common consequence of PD, marked by reduction of both vocal[21] and facial[22] mobility and variability. Despite the potentially serious social and medical consequences of decreased expressivity[24] efforts to improve expression in PD have been few, and the success limited.[24-26]

As described in this chapter, the LSVT was developed to specifically treat the speech and voice deficits associated with PD[28] and is considered among the most efficacious speech treatments for PD.[28,29] It is showing unexpected and far-reaching effects beyond the improvement of voice and speech. One such improvement appears to be an increase in facial expressivity. In a recent prospective, randomized pilot study,[30] 36 individuals with PD received either respiratory therapy (n = 14) or LSVT (n = 22) and were videotaped before and after treatment. Twenty-second video samples were judged by inexperienced observers on "expressivity," defined as *meaningful* and *communicative* facial movement. The data revealed a positive trend ($p = 0.067$) in the direction of the LSVT group.

A more detailed study using the same group of subjects was done with six trained female raters[31] These raters were trained to examine multiple variables for facial expression, including *mobility*, *engagement*, and *positive emotion*. Results indicate that members of the LSVT group were perceived as having increased their facial *mobility* ($p = 0.036$) and *engagement* ($p = 0.056$) following treatment relative to members of the respiratory group. Additionally, the LSVT group demonstrated a greater extent of change for facial *mobility* after treatment compared to the respiratory group ($p = 0.05$) (see Figure 12–1)

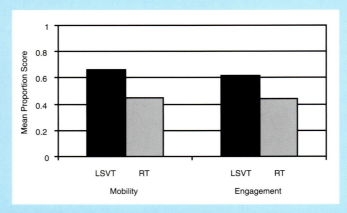

FIGURE 12–1. Mean ratings for facial mobility and engagement

Ongoing research is underway to examine facial expression using more detailed protocols, and to evaluate the effects of the LSVT on specific areas of vocal expressivity. A quick look at the speech of one subject receiving LSVT shows the extent of change in voice variability and quality during spontaneous speech that is typical following treatment (Figure 12–2).

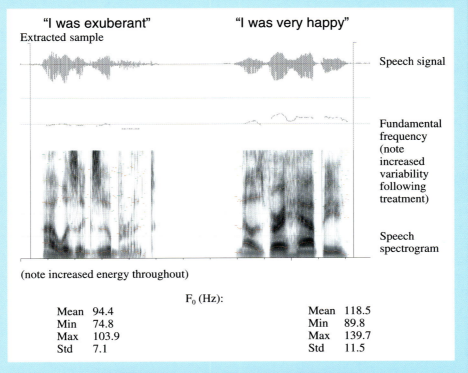

FIGURE 12–2. Pre- versus post-LSVT therapy.

Further evaluation is necessary to quantify the type and extent of change, and determine whether these quantitative results reflect functional improvements in expression and communication for individuals with PD. Ideally, this programmatic approach to the study of communicative disorders will yield benefit beyond the voice and speech

Parkinson's disease is a very common motor disorder with significant voice and speech, and swallowing components. The otolaryngologist and trained speech pathologist, particularly through the Lee Silverman Voice Treatment, can play a large role in the rehabilitation of these patients by both identification of the disorder in its early stages and in provision of treatment.

Review Questions

1. Vocal complaints are present in approximately what percentage of Parkinson's disease patients?
   a. 20%
   b. 40%
   c. 60%
   d. 80%
   e. 100%

2. Parkinson's tremor occurs at which frequency range?
   a. 1 to 2 Hz
   b. 4 to 10 Hz
   c. 10 to 20 Hz
   d. It cannot be measured

3. The best established treatment for patients with dysphonia related to Parkinson's disease is:
   a. Vocal resonance therapy
   b. Lee Silverman Voice Treatment
   c. Collagen injection laryngoplasty
   d. Deep brain stimulation
   e. Pallidotomy

4. According to estimates, Parkinson's affects approximately what number of persons in the United States?
   a. 500,000
   b. 1,000,000
   c. 1,500,000
   d. 2,000,000
   e. 2,500,000

REFERENCES

1. Hartelius L, Svensson P. Speech and swallowing symptoms associated with Parkinson's disease and multiple sclerosis: a survey. *Folia Phoniatr Logoped.* 1994;46:9–17.

2. Monte FS, da Silva-Junior FP, Braga-Neto P, Nobre e Souza MA, Sales de Bruin VM. Swallowing abnor-malities and dyskinesia in Parkinson's disease. *Mov Disord.* 2005;20(4):457–462.

3. Perez KS, Ramig LO, Smith ME, Dromey C. The Parkinson larynx: tremor and videostroboscopic findings. *J Voice.* 1996;10:354–361.

4. Elble RJ. Diagnostic criteria for essential tremor and differential diagnosis. *Neurology.* 2000;54 (suppl 4):S2–S6.

5. Fahn S, Greene PE, Ford B, Bressman SB. *Handbook of Movement Disorders.* Philadelphia, Pa; Current Medicine, Inc, 1998.

6. Findley LJ. Epidemiology and genetics of essential tremor. *Neurology.* 2000;54(suppl 4):S8–S13.

7. Luschei ES, Ramig LO, Baker KL, et al. Discharge characteristics of laryngeal single motor units during phonation in younger and older adults and in persons with Parkinson's disease. *J Neurophysiol.* 1999;81:2131–2139.

8. Gamboa J, Jimenez-Jimenez FJ, Nieto A, et al. Acoustic voice analysis in patients with essential tremor. *J Voice.* 1998;12:444–452.

9. Kim SH, Kearney JJ, Atkins JP. Percutaneous laryngeal augmentation for treatment of Parkinsonian hypophonia. *Otolaryngol Head Neck Surg.* 2002;126:653–656.

10. Berke GS, Gerratt B, Kreiman J, et al. Treatment of Parkinson's hypophonia with percutaneous collagen augmentation. *Laryngoscope.* 1999;109: 1295–1299.

11. Gentil M, Chauvin P, Pinto S, et al. Effect of bilateral stimulation of the subthalamic nucleus on Parkinsonian voice. *Brain Lang..* 2001;78: 233–240.

12. Carpenter MA, Pahwa R, Miyawaki KL, Wilkinson SB, Send JP, Koller WC. Reduction in voice tremor under thalamic stimulation. *Neurology.* 1998;50: 796–798.

13. Yoon MS, Munz M, Sataloff RT, Spiegel JR, Heuer RJ. Vocal tremor reduction with deep brain stimulation. *Stereotact Funct Neurosurg.* 1999;72: 241–244.

14. Pahwa R, Lyons K, Koller WC. Surgical treatment of essential tremor. *Neurology.* 2000;54 (suppl 4): S39–S44.

15. Taha JM, Janszen MA, Favre J. Thalamic deep brain stimulation for the treatment of head, voice and bilateral limb tremor. *J Neurosurg.* 1999;91:68–72.

16. Dedo HH. Recurrent laryngeal nerve section for spastic dysphonia. *Ann Otol Rhinol Laryngol.* 1976;85:451–459.

17. Poluha PC, Euling HL, Brookshire RH. Handwriting and speech changes across the levodopa cycle

in Parkinson's disease. *Acta Psychol*. 1998;100: 71–84.

18. Ramig LO, Sapir S, Countryman S, et al. Intensive voice treatment (LSVT) for patients with Parkinson's disease: a two year follow up. *J Neurol*. 2001;71:493–498.

19. Liotti M, Ramig LO, Vogel D, et al. Hypophonia in Parkinson's patients:neural correlates of voice treatment revealed by PET. *Neurology*. 2003;60: 432–440.

20. Sharkawi AE, Ramig LO, Logemann JA, et al. Swallowing and voice effects of Lee Silverman Voice Treatment (LSVT): a pilot study. *J Neurology Neurosurg Psychiatry*. 2002;72:31–36.

21. Stewart C, Winfield L, Hunt A. Bressman S. Fahn, S. Blitzer A. Brin M. Speech dysfunction in early Parkinson's disease. *Mov Disord*. 1995;10(5):1995: 562–565.

22. Madeley P, Ellis A, Mindham R. Facial expressions and Parkinson's disease. *Behav Neurol*. 1995;8: 115–119.

23. Pentland B, Gray, JM, Riddle, WJR, Pitcairn, TK. The effects of reduced nonverbal communication in Parkinson's disease. *Br J Disord Commun*. 1988;23:31–34.

24. Katsikitis, M, Pilowsky I.. A controlled study of facial mobility treatment in Parkinson's disease. *J Psychosom Res*. 1996;40(4):387–396.

25. Scott S, Caird FI, Williams BO. *Communication in Parkinson's Disease*. Rockville, Md: Aspen; 1985.

26. Robertson S, Thomson F. Speech therapy in Parkinson's disease: a study of the efficacy and long term effects of intensive treatment. *Br J Disord Commun*. 1984;19:213–224.

27. Ramig LO, Countryman S, Thompson LL, Horii Y. Comparison of two forms of intensive speech treatment for Parkinson disease. *J Speech Hear Res*. 1995;38:1232–1251.

28. Schulz G. The effects of speech therapy and pharmacological treatments on voice and speech in Parkinson s disease: a review of the literature. *Curr Med Chem*. 2002;9(14):1359–1366.

29. Yorkston K, Spencer K, and Duffy J. Behavioral management of respiratory/phonatory dysfunction from dysarthria: a systematic review of the evidence. *J Med Speech Lang Pathol*. 2003;11(2): xiii–xxxviii.

30. Spielman J, Ramig LO, Borod J. Preliminary effects of voice therapy on facial expression in Parkinson's disease. *J Int Neuropsycholog Assn*. 2001; 7(2):244.

31. Spielman J, Borod J, Ramig L. The effects of intensive voice treatment on facial expressiveness in Parkinson disease: preliminary data. *Cog Behav Neurol*. 2003;16(3):177–188.

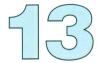

Essential Voice Tremor

Lucian Sulica, MD
Elan Louis, MD, MS

KEY POINTS

■ Essential tremor is an age-related disease of involuntary movement. Voice is affected in some 25 to 30% of patients.

■ Essential voice tremor usually affects pharyngeal, palatal, and extrinsic laryngeal muscles in addition to intrinsic laryngeal muscles.

■ Essential voice tremor usually produces rhythmic oscillatory motion of both vocal folds, and may be present during quiet breathing in addition to phonation.

■ There are no pharmacologic agents of documented benefit in essential voice tremor.

■ Botulinum toxin injections may be helpful in carefully selected patients with essential voice tremor.

The phonatory apparatus may be involved in 25 to 30% of patients with essential tremor.[1,2] Voice tremor may be the only manifestation of essential tremor,[3] but usually it is associated with tremor in other parts of the body, including the upper extremities or head. In order to recognize and treat the symptoms of essential voice tremor, an understanding of essential tremor as a diagnostic entity must be combined with knowledge of phonatory biomechanics.

ESSENTIAL TREMOR

Essential tremor is an age-related disease of involuntary movement. Although generally acknowledged to be the most common adult-onset movement disorder, it is difficult to fix a precise incidence because essential tremor may be mild enough to go unnoticed in 50% or more of affected people.[4,5] In many instances, the disease is familial and can be inherited in an autosomal dominant fashion; the remainder of cases appear to be sporadic.[1,4-6] Absence of a family history of tremor does not preclude a diagnosis of essential tremor.

The diagnosis of essential tremor, like that of most movement disorders, is clinical—that is, there are no pathognomonic laboratory or radiological abnormalities. The most characteristic feature of the disease is tremor, which is further described below. The tremor begins insidiously and progresses at a variable rate,[7] although generally slowly. Most commonly, the tremor begins in the upper extremities, and it is usually mildly asymmetric.[8] Tremors are classified according to the circumstances in which they occur. Broadly, these can be divided into rest and action tremors. Tremor at rest occurs when the affected body part is at repose and completely supported against gravity, and is typical of Parkinson's disease (PD). Action tremors are further subdivided into posture-holding tremors, which occur when a limb is held outstretched against gravity; kinetic tremors, which occur with voluntary movement (eg, writing, pouring); and task-specific tremors, which occur only during a specific activity. For instance, enhanced physiologic tremor (ie, the tremor that occurs in most normal individuals) occurs with voluntary movement and posture holding, whereas dystonic tremor may be task-specific. Essential tremor is an action tremor that occurs during voluntary movement and posture-holding, without task-specific characteristics.[9] Much has been written about tremor frequencies. In general, essential tremor occurs at a rate of 4 to 10 Hz (Figure 13–1), whereas enhanced physiologic tremor occurs at a rate of 8 to 12 Hz.

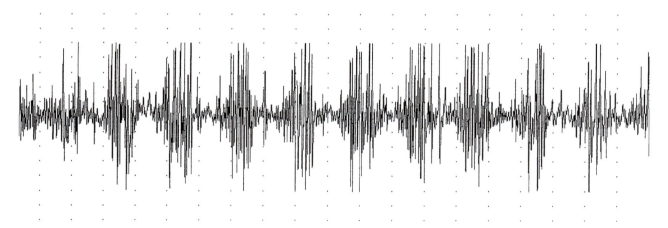

FIGURE 13–1. This EMG recording of the thyroarytenoid muscle of a patient with essential voice tremor during sustained /i/ phonation clearly reveals the rhythmic waxing and waning activation of the muscle typical of tremor, in this case at a rate of 5 Hz. Normally, muscle activation should be continuous during this activity (each horizontal division = 100 msec; each vertical division = 100 μvolts).

Intention ("cerebellar") tremor is slower, occurring at a rate of 2 to 5 Hz.[4,9] As is evident, there is considerable overlap in the frequencies of different tremors and, as a result, clinical circumstance (resting versus action) is a more useful diagnostic feature than is tremor frequency.

ESSENTIAL VOICE TREMOR

Essential tremor, when it affects the voice, is usually not restricted to the intrinsic muscles of the larynx. Other muscles of the phonatory apparatus that are often variably involved include extrinsic laryngeal muscles, pharyngeal and palatal muscles, the muscles of articulatory structures, as well as muscles of the diaphragm, chest wall, and abdomen, which affect phonatory expiration.[10-12] The term "essential voice tremor" thus describes the clinical situation better and is more apt than "essential laryngeal tremor."

Because of this broad involvement of different muscle groups, a given patient with essential voice tremor may present with variability in frequency as well as (or in place of) intensity. Most often, though, patients complain of intensity fluctuations associated with a perception of increased phonatory effort. Muscular discomfort and fatigue may result from efforts to stabilize the vocal tract. Symptoms are usually present across all phonatory activity, although they may be difficult to perceive during whispering in which variable glottic aperture may have relatively little acoustic impact. For this reason, patients with severe vocal tremor may adopt whispering as their customary mode of phonation, rendering the diagnosis obscure until revealed by louder sustained vowel phonation or endoscopic examination. Usually there is no dysphagia or dyspnea. Occasional patients complain of dyspnea; however, this represents breathlessness during voicing from glottic insufficiency, similar to that experienced by patients with unilateral vocal fold paralysis, rather than true difficulty breathing. Precise questioning will usually reveal the difference.

Patients with essential glottic tremor generally report slowly worsening symptoms over months to years. Voicing worsens with anxiety or stress[13] and is especially troublesome under more demanding acoustic conditions, such as speaking against background noise, addressing a classroom or conference, or using the telephone. In common with other manifestations of essential tremor, alcohol may effect a voice improvement. That these features are also found in spasmodic dysphonia is a source of diagnostic confusion.

Brief reflection on the overall prevalence of essential tremor and of laryngeal involvement discussed above suggests that only a small proportion of patients with vocal tremor present for evaluation by the otolaryngologist. Were it otherwise, essential vocal tremor would certainly form a greater proportion of our caseload than, say, spasmodic dysphonia. This in turn suggests a relatively low prevalence of severe or incapacitating vocal symptoms, although effective pharmacologic treatment (prescribed by neurologists) or simply a lack of information about appropriate specialty care may also contribute to this phenomenon.

A brief neurologic examination encompassing the upper extremities and gait in addition to the head and neck will serve to identify and distinguish among associated action and rest tremors and reveal signs of PD such as bradykinesia and cogwheel rigidity in the limbs. Laryngeal examination is best performed with a flexible transnasal endoscope, as the lingual traction necessary for transoral examination prevents connected speech, and the required posture may suppress characteristic signs. Rhythmic, oscillatory motion of the palate, pharynx, and/or vocal folds is diagnostic. Vocal fold tremor is bilateral and grossly symmetric. Tremor may be present across all laryngeal tasks, including quiet respiration as well as phonation; the traditional distinction between rest and activity appears unhelpful in the larynx. In fact, neither during breathing nor during phonation is the larynx truly at rest. Its activity is probably better defined as posture-holding during both of these tasks, which renders the clinical finding of tremor during "rest" more intelligible. Instrumental measures of voice have revealed (1) elevated jitter and shimmer and (2) decreased harmonic-to-noise ratio, s/z ratio, and maximum phonation time, which are abnormalities shared with other conditions of glottic insufficiency.[14]

If both history and examination are characteristic, further investigation is unnecessary. If findings are atypical or ambiguous, and especially if onset of symptoms is rapid, it is prudent to consult a neurologist. Ruling out thyrotoxicosis and drug-induced tremor—in the otolaryngologic pharmacopeia, adrenergic decongestants are the most common source—will prevent an unnecessary referral.

DIFFERENTIAL DIAGNOSIS

Asymptomatic Tremor

Occasionally, the examiner will incidentally note several cycles of vocal fold tremor during respiration or as the larynx assumes phonatory posture during laryngeal exam. In the absence of associated findings or complaints, the nature of this is an academic question. There is no evidence that this is a reflection of underlying neural dysfunction.

Parkinsonian Tremor

Tremor, most commonly involving the strap muscles and producing vertical laryngeal movement, is present in 55% of patients with idiopathic PD.[15] However, both associated physical findings and speech characteristics differ. Examination may reveal lack of facial affect and upper extremity rigidity with cogwheeling, shuffling gait, and other manifestations of bradykinesia. Any tremor present will tend to be more evident at rest rather than during activity. Most important, the speech of PD, although often breathy and of low intensity, does not demonstrate these characteristics in a rhythmic fashion. Rather, the characteristic hypophonia of PD is relatively constant, a

manifestation of incomplete glottic closure and poor breath support resulting from chest wall rigidity, often exacerbated by articulatory difficulties and sometimes by cognitive problems associated with the disease. These issues are discussed in detail in the previous chapter.

Myoclonus and Tics

The vocal characteristics of myoclonus and tics will occasionally resemble the cyclic phonatory changes of tremor. However, the rhythmic and oscillatory nature of the motion of essential tremor usually serves to distinguish it from these entities. Myoclonus, which can affect the same variety of muscles as tremor, resembles a sudden jerk, usually followed by a slower return to the null position. Hiccough is a common form of myoclonus, and serves to illustrate the essential quality of myoclonic movement. Tic disorders, including Gilles de la Tourette syndrome, are heterogeneous and may involve the larynx. In general, tics are suppressible for a time. Patients usually describe associated sensory phenomena as well as an urge to perform the tic motion, features absent from essential tremor. It is not often that tic or myoclonic activity is truly rhythmic.

Spasmodic Dysphonia and Tremor

Sometimes, the involuntary vocal fold adduction or abduction of spasmodic dysphonia will occur with rhythmic or near-rhythmic regularity, creating a pattern of phonatory breaks nearly indistinguishable from that of severe essential tremor.[16,17] Dystonic tremor has been noted in up to one-third of spasmodic dysphonia patients,[18] a feature spasmodic dysphonia shares with other focal or segmental dystonias, such as torticollis and writer's cramp.[1,9] Like dystonic activity as a whole and unlike essential tremor, dystonic tremor is often task-specific and may decrease with a sensory trick (a method of touching an affected body part to reduce the severity of the involuntary motion).[9] In the larynx, a dystonic tremor may be more evident during connected speech than during singing or sustained-vowel phonation and may be suppressed by insertion of a flexible fiberoptic laryngoscope. Dystonic tremor is usually somewhat aperiodic, although this may be extremely hard to appreciate. Ultimately, a therapeutic trial may be required to distinguish essential voice tremor from laryngeal dystonia. In the author's experience, botulinum toxin treatment of spasmodic dysphonia that is consistently followed by prolonged (greater than 10 days) and severe breathiness should raise the possibility of essential tremor. See chapter 14 for further details regarding spasmodic dysphonia.

TREATMENT

First-line treatment of essential tremor is pharmacologic. Propranolol and primidone are mainstays of treatment, with proven efficacy in controlled clinical trials. Their utility in treating voice tremor is less well documented. Propranolol is a beta-adrenergic blocker that reduces tremor amplitude by means of peripheral modulation of beta-adrenergic receptors in skeletal muscle, resulting in symptomatic relief in up to 50% of patients.[19] Primidone is an anticonvulsant that is effective in the control of tremor symptoms in about 50% of patients; the mechanism is not fully understood but it may involve enhancement of gamma-aminobutyric acid neurotransmission in the central nervous system.[19] Neither primidone[20] nor propranolol[21] has been shown to improve voice tremor in studies of small numbers of patients. Methazolamide, a carbonic-anhydrase inhibitor, appeared to improve vocal symptoms in more than half of patients (16 of 28) treated in an open trial,[22] results not supported by a subsequent blinded investigation.[23] A case of effective treatment with gabapentin has been reported.[24] These few reports notwithstanding, pharmacologic treatment of voice tremor has been sparsely studied; further investigation is called for.

Botulinum toxin treatment of essential voice tremor is predicated on the assumption that vocal fold tremor and resulting inappropriate glottal aperture account for the greater part of the symptoms of essential tremor of the phonatory tract. Generally, botulinum toxin is injected into one[27] or both thyroarytenoid muscles[19,25-28] in the manner of treatment of adductor spasmodic dysphonia and in comparable doses. According to patient self-perception of vocal quality, botulinum toxin injections were useful to 67 to 80% of cases. Acoustic measures documented benefit less often, leading investigators to hypothesize that much of the perceived improvement resulted from decreased phonatory effort. The reader is referred to the primary reports for details of treatment and results (Table 13-1).

Botulinum Toxin Treatment: Essential Voice Tremor Versus Spasmodic Dysphonia

Botulinum toxin treatment of essential voice tremor yields qualitatively different results than the treatment of spasmodic dysphonia, and personal experience with such treatment has not been entirely consistent with the sanguine reports in the literature. Botulinum toxin does not eliminate the tremor, but rather decreases tremor amplitude. However, this does not always translate reliably into acoustic improvement or greater voice functionality. Not infrequently, treatment of adductor muscles yields prolonged and troublesome breathy dysphonia. Neither injecting abductor muscles nor limiting treatment to one side has yielded reliably better results. Such results are also typical of botulinum toxin treatment of hand and head tremor, in which muscle chemodenervation has not offered consistent and predictable functional benefit.[5,34] Many patients with essential voice tremor do not elect to continue long-term botulinum toxin treatment for essential voice tremor, in sharp contrast to those with spasmodic dysphonia.

This striking difference may be due to distinctions in the pathophysiology of essential tremor and dystonia. There is some evidence to suggest that an afferent signal plays some role in dystonia, and that botulinum toxin may achieve part of its therapeutic effect by altering feedback to the central nervous system.[29,30] On the other hand, essential tremor is likely the result of abnormalities in cerebellar-thalamic outflow pathways without an afferent component, potentially compromising an important part of the effect of botulinum toxin.

TABLE 13–1. Botulinum Toxin Treatment of Essential Voice Tremor: Summary of Studies

Study	Type of Study	Number of Subjects	Muscles Injected	Dose Used	Patient Subjective Evaluation	Blinded Perceptual Evaluation	Acoustic Analysis
Hertegard et al[25]	Open trial	15	Bilateral TA, occasionally thyrohyoid & cricothyroid	0.6 to 5U per side (TA)	10 of 15 (67%) reported benefit	Significant mean improvement on VAS	Significant decrease of F_0 & F_0 variation
Warrick et al[27]	Open trial with crossover (unilateral vs. bilateral injection)	10	Bilateral TA / Unilateral TA	2.5U per side / 15U	8 of 10 (80%) wished to be treated again	No statistically significant improvement	No statistically significant change
Koller et al[19]	Open trial	?	Bilateral TA	1.0 to 2.5U per side	Significant mean improvement on 0–100 scale of function	Not reported	Not reported
Adler et al[28]	Dose-randomized open trial	13	Bilateral TA	1.25U, 2.5U or 3.75U per side	Significant mean improvement on 5-point tremor severity scale	Significant mean improvement on 5-point tremor severity scale	Significant mean improvement in F_0 variation

U = Units of botulinum toxin type A; TA = Thyroarytenoid; VAS = 100 mm visual analog scale; F_0 = fundamental frequency

Extralaryngeal muscles are commonly involved in essential voice tremor, and extending botulinum toxin treatment to these may offer improved results,[25] although swallowing difficulties are likely to impose limits on such treatment. Because essential voice tremor is a clinically heterogeneous disorder, it may also be possible to select patients who are more likely to benefit from botulinum toxin treatment based on differences in muscle involvement seen in the clinical examination; these studies remain to be performed.

Thalamic deep brain stimulation (DBS) by means of implanted electrodes is an evolving method of treating disabling, medication-resistant essential tremor and PD. This method is increasingly taking the place of thalamotomy. Initial reports of postoperative dysarthria, particularly after bilateral procedures, created reservations regarding the utility of DBS in the treatment of essential voice tremor, as both speech and voice are tightly time-gated activities requiring a high degree of coordination. However, mounting evidence suggests that DBS may be efficacious in the treatment of voice tremor.[31-36]

Essential voice tremor is a clinically heterogeneous disorder that may involve a variety of muscles of the phonatory apparatus, both laryngeal and extralaryngeal. It is probably more common than is generally suspected. Diagnosis as well as differentiation from similar disorders affecting the larynx depends on thorough clinical examination. Its salient feature is kinetic (action-induced) tremor, which produces rhythmic fluctuation in voice intensity and/or pitch, and an absence of rigidity, bradykinesia, and spasms typical of other disorders of involuntary motion.

Despite limited evidence of efficacy, it seems reasonable to begin with pharmacologic treatment, particularly when patients with essential voice tremor have other troublesome manifestations of the disease (eg, tremor of the upper extremities) that may benefit from such treatment (Figure 13–2). Patients whose only complaint is voice tremor, on the other hand, may choose between pharmacologic treatment and botulinum toxin injections as initial treatment. Benefit is by no means universal, and functional

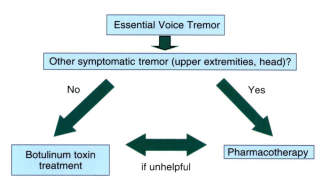

FIGURE 13–2. Management algorithm for essential voice tremor.

voice improvement often remains. The effect of combined chemodenervation and medical treatment remains to be determined. Voice tremor alone has yet to become an indication for deep brain stimulation, although the possibility exists in truly crippling cases. As in most voice disorders due to benign pathology, a well-informed and well-advised patient is usually the person best suited to weigh treatment options.

Review Questions

1. Which features are typical of essential tremor?
   a. More common with age
   b. Autosomal recessive inheritance
   c. Slow progression
   d. The voice is affected in half of patients
   e. The tremor improved with alcohol intake

2. Which clinical characteristics are typical of essential tremor?
   a. Asymmetric.
   b. Resting tremor
   c. Cogwheeling
   d. Bradykinesia
   e. Action-induced

3. What features of connected speech suggest essential voice tremor?
   a. Weak, breathy voice with poor articulation
   b. Strangled voice breaks
   c. Rhythmic fluctuation in intensity and/or pitch.
   d. Irregular breathy voice breaks
   e. "Scanning speech"

4. Which method of examining the larynx is least likely to obscure the typical signs of essential tremor?

5. Which medications have a documented benefit in essential voice tremor?
   a. Propranolol
   b. Primidone
   c. Methazolamide
   d. None of the above

REFERENCES

1. Factor SA, Weiner WJ. Hyperkinetic movement disorders. In: Weiner WJ, Goetz CG, eds. *Neurology for the Non-Neurologist*. Philadelphia, Pa: Lippincott, Williams & Wilkins; 1999:143–177.

2. Koller WC, Busenbark K, Miner K. The relationship of essential tremor to other movement disorders: report on 678 patients. *Ann Neurol.* 1994; 35:717–723.

3. Findley LJ, Gresty M. Head, facial and voice tremor. *Adv Neurol.* 1988;49:239–253.

4. Elble RJ. Diagnostic criteria for essential tremor and differential diagnosis. *Neurology.* 2000;54 (suppl 4):S2–S6.

5. Louis ED. Essential tremor. *Lancet Neurol.* 2005;4: 100–110.

6. Louis ED, Ottman R. How familial is familial tremor? The genetic epidemiology of essential tremor. *Neurology.* 1996;46:1200–1205.

7. Louis ED, Ford B, Barnes LF. Clinical subtypes of essential tremor. *Arch Neurol.* 2000;57:1194–1198.

8. Jankovic J. Essential tremor: Clinical characteristics. *Neurology.* 2000;54 (suppl 4):S21–S25.

9. Fahn S, Greene PE, Ford B, Bressman SB. *Handbook of Movement Disorders*. Philadelphia, Pa: Current Medicine, Inc; 1998.

10. Tomoda H, Shibasaki H, Kuroda Y, Shin T. Voice tremor: dysregulation of voluntary expiratory muscles. *Neurology.* 1987;37:117–122.

11. Koda J, Ludlow CL. An evaluation of laryngeal muscle activation in patients with voice tremor. *Otolaryngol Head Neck Surg.* 1992;107:684–696.

12. Finnegan EM, Luschei ES, Barkmeier JM, Hoffman HT. Synchrony of laryngeal muscle activity in persons with vocal tremor. *Arch Otolaryngol Head Neck Surg.* 2003;129:313–318.

13. Mendoza E, Carballo G. Vocal tremor and psychological stress. *J Voice.* 1999;13:105–112.

14. Gamboa J, Jimenez-Jimenez FJ, Nieto A, et al. Acoustic voice analysis in patients with essential tremor. *J Voice.* 1998;12:444–452.

15. Perez KS, Ramig LO, Smith ME, Dromey C. The Parkinson larynx: tremor and videostroboscopic findings. *J Voice.* 1996;10:354–361.

16. Aronson AE, Hartman DE. Adductor spastic dysphonia as a sign of essential voice tremor. *J Speech Hear Disord.* 1981;46:52–58.

17. Barkmeier JM, Case JL, Ludlow CL. Identification of symptoms for spasmodic dysphonia and vocal tremor: a comparison of expert and nonexpert judges. *J Commun Disord.* 2001;34:21–37.

18. Blitzer A, Brin MF, Stewart CF. Botulinum toxin management of spasmodic dysphonia (laryngeal dystonia): a 12-year experience in more than 900 patients. *Laryngoscope.* 1998;108:1435–1441.

19. Koller WC, Hristova A, Brin M. Pharmacologic treatment of essential tremor. *Neurology.* 2000;54 (suppl 4):S30–S38.

20. Hartman DE, Vishwanat B. Spastic dysphonia and essential (voice) tremor treated with primidone. *Arch Otolaryngol.* 1984;110:394–397.

21. Koller WC, Graner D, Micoch A. Essential voice tremor: treatment with propranolol. *Neurology.* 1985;35:106–108.

22. Muenter MD, Daube JR, Caviness JN, Miller PM. Treatment of essential tremor with methazolamide. *Mayo Clin Proc.* 1991;66:991–997.

23. Busenbark K, Ramig L, Dromey C, Koller WC. Methazolamide for essential voice tremor. *Neurology.* 1996;47:1331–1332.

24. Padilla F, Berthier ML, Campos-Arillo VM. Temblor essencial de la voz y tratamiento con gabapentina. *Rev Neurol.* 2000;31:798.

25. Hertegard S, Granqvist S, Lindestad PA. Botulinum toxin injections for essential voice tremor. *Ann Otol Rhinol Laryngol.* 2000;109:204-209.

26. Warrick P, Dromey C, Irish J, Durkin. The treatment of essential voice tremor with botulinum toxin A: a longitudinal case report. *J Voice.* 2000; 14:410-412.

27. Warrick P, Dromey C, Irish JC, Durkin L, Pakiam A, Lang A. Botulinum toxin for essential tremor of the voice with multiple anatomical sites of tremor: a crossover design study of unilateral versus bilateral injection. *Laryngoscope.* 2000a;110: 1366-1374.

28. Adler CH, Bansberg SF, Hentz JG, et al. Botulinum toxin type A for treating voice tremor. *Arch Neurol.* 2004;61:1416-1420.

29. Hallett M. How does botulinum toxin work? *Ann Neurol.* 2000;48:7-8.

30. Sulica L. Contemporary management of spasmodic dysphonia. *Curr Opin Otolaryngol Head Neck Surg.* 2004;12:543-548.

31. Carpenter MA, Pahwa R, Miyawaki KL, Wilkinson SB, Send JP, Koller WC. Reduction in voice tremor under thalamic stimulation. *Neurology.* 1998;50: 796-798.

32. Yoon MS, Munz M, Sataloff RT, Spiegel JR, Heuer RJ. Vocal tremor reduction with deep brain stimulation. *Stereotact Funct Neurosurg.* 1999;72: 241-244.

33. Taha JM, Janszen MA, Favre J. Thalamic deep brain stimulation for the treatment of head, voice and bilateral limb tremor. *J Neurosurg.* 1999;91: 68-72.

34. Pahwa R, Lyons K, Koller WC. Surgical treatment of essential tremor. *Neurology.* 2000;54(suppl 4): S39-S44.

35. Lyons KE, Pahwa R. Deep brain stimulation and essential tremor. *J Clin Neurophysiol.* 2004;21:2-5.

36. Lyons KE, Pahwa R, Comella CL, et al. Benefits and risks of pharmacologic treatment for essential tremor. *Drug Safety.* 2003;26:461-481.

14

Spasmodic Dysphonia

Joel H. Blumin, MD, FACS
Gerald S. Berke, MD, FACS

KEY POINTS

■ Spasmodic dysphonia is a neurologic voice disorder that
affects the fluency of connected speech.

■ The majority of patients with adductor spasmodic dysphonia
have a stereotypical staccato, strangled speech quality.

■ The diagnosis of muscle tension dysphonia should be
considered in the differential diagnosis and ruled out before
entering the patient into treatment.

■ Botulinum toxin remains the mainstay of treatment,
although many patients have been successfully treated by a
surgical approach.

Spasmodic dysphonia is an idiopathic focal dystonia of the larynx. A *dystonia* is a neuromuscular disorder characterized by involuntary, sporadic, and irregularly occurring muscle contractions. Dystonias can be generalized or focal, affecting the entire body or only a specific muscle group. Certain dystonias, like spasmodic dysphonia, tend to be task-specific and do not affect the muscle group during vegetative function or at rest. Dystonias are chronic conditions and, like other movement disorders, are not typically associated with dementia or other cognitive deficits.

HISTORY, ETIOLOGY, AND DEMOGRAPHICS

Traube is credited with first writing about the condition we know today as spasmodic dysphonia.[1] In 1871, he coined the term "spastic dysphonia" to describe a patient with a nervous hoarseness. Others have noted the stereotypical speech patterns and described them as a "vocal fold stutter" or talking "while being choked."[2,3] For almost a century, it was assumed that the disorder was of a psychiatric etiology[4] and only recently was it identified as a neurologic disorder similar to other dystonias. The terms "spasmodic dysphonia" and "laryngeal dystonia" were recommended by Brin and Blitzer to specifically associate the disorder with other dystonias.[5] Many patients with spasmodic dysphonia have a high incidence of other neurological disorders including other dystonias.[6,7] Abnormalities have been shown in the brainstem reflexes and other aspects of central processing in those with spasmodic dysphonia.[8] A subset of patients with dystonia demonstrate a familial and genetic origin for their disorder.[5,9-11] Diagnostically, spasmodic dysphonia and muscle tension dysphonia should be considered in patients with a characteristic strained-strangled voice quality.[12] Muscle tension dysphonia is a term that describes a voice disorder that stems from behavioral misuse of laryngeal tension during voicing.[13] Estimates from the National Spasmodic Dysphonia Association suggest that spasmodic dysphonia affects approximately 35,000 to 50,000 Americans. These estimates are rough and were derived from extrapolations of populations with dystonia in general. No formal population study on the incidence of spasmodic dysphonia has been performed, but, in general, this is a rare disease.

The etiology of spasmodic dysphonia is considered to be idiopathic. Several studies have looked for commonalities in those patients with spasmodic dysphonia.[5,14] This disease affects women two to three times as often as men. The mean age of onset is in the 5th to 6th decade with a wide range of onset, from teenager to octogenarian. Ten to 20% of patients associate a blunt trauma (such as motor vehicle accident) or an upper respiratory infection with the time of onset. Whether this is causative or happenstance is unknown. Childhood measles or mumps infections have been noted in 45 to 65% of patients and, although this incidence may reflect a bias of the studied cohorts, the numbers are greater than the general population and may suggest a viral association.[14] Other neurologic diseases, such as herpes zoster, have been associated with latent viral infections.

PATHOPHYSIOLOGY, SYMPTOMOLOGY, AND DIAGNOSIS

Spasmodic dysphonia affects a patient's ability to produce fluent connected speech. It is a task-specific dystonia: the affected task is voice production, and the specific muscles affected are those that control movement of the vocal folds. In general, spasmodic dysphonia does not affect the muscles associated with resonance (pharynx, palate) or articulation (tongue, lips). However, some patients have dystonias in other muscle groups. It is not uncommon to have multiple focal dystonias clustered in a given patient. Meige's syndrome, for example, is a dystonia of the face, tongue, jaw, and lips as well as larynx and can affect a patient's ability to articulate.[15]

A specific pathologic finding that leads to the development of spasmodic dysphonia has not been demonstrated. Spasmodic dysphonia is thought to be a disorder of central nervous system processing, although the exact mechanism has not been elucidated. Research has suggested an abnormality of motor responses to sensory input and feedback from the larynx, possibly by disinhibition of laryngeal motor responses.[8,16] Changes in laryngeal muscle and nerve histology have been demonstrated but likely suggest an end result of central remodeling rather than a peripheral injury or myositis.[17]

Spasmodic dysphonia is subcategorized into multiple subtypes depending on a patient's predominate symptomatology and clinical findings.[7] Approximately 80 to 90% of patients with spasmodic dysphonia have the adductor type. These patients have involuntary spasms of the laryngeal adductors, namely, the thyroarytenoid and the lateral cricoarytenoid. Some patients also have spasms of the intra-arytenoid muscles.[18] Patients with adductor spasmodic dysphonia tend to have a stereotypical strained-strangled quality of speech. More specifically, these patients exhibit vocal breaks or stops when attempting to produce a speech task loaded with voiced consonants (b, d, g, z, v, j, m, n). The symptoms are less pronounced when the task is loaded with voiceless consonants (p, t, k, s, f, ch) or when phonating a less complicated utterance, such as the production of a continuous vowel sound.[6,19,20]

Abductor spasmodic dysphonia affects up to 17% of patients who have spasmodic dysphonia.[4] In this disorder, the spasms are primarily noted in the laryngeal abductor, the large posterior cricoarytenoid muscles. Patients with this disorder have spasms that produce inappropriate loss of laryngeal resistance resulting in a perceptual quality of intermittent breathiness. They also have difficulty during connected speech tasks, but their problem is more noted when the task is loaded with voiceless consonants and utterances with softer attacks (eg, "how hard did he hit him?").

Although the majority of patients have a spasmodic dysphonia that falls into one of the major subcategories, some may have a mixed disorder characterized by both abductor and adductor phonatory breaks. Some authors believe that all spasmodic dysphonia patients have both types of disorder but are more dominant for a certain subtype at a given point in time, and the dominant symptoms can change over the course of a patient's life.[21,22] Many patients also consciously and unconsciously alter laryngeal resistance as a strategy for coping with these disorders. This can result in perceptual voice qualities that deviate significantly from the stereotypical disorder where they lose some of the task specificity, and sound strained or breathy all the time, or change their fundamental frequency.[23,24]

Many patients with spasmodic dysphonia also have vocal tremor.[25,26] Vocal tremor typically affects muscle groups outside the larynx including strap and pharyngeal musculature. The auditory perception of this disorder is characterized by a tremulous, shaky, or quavering voice quality that occurs with all speech tasks. This tremor tends to be more resistant to treatment then the dystonia. Treatment of the spasmodic dysphonia can make a coexisting underlying tremor more noticeable.

The task specificity of spasmodic dysphonia goes beyond the consonant and vowel sounds within a given speech task. Many patients experience differences in voice difficulty depending on environment. For instance, almost all patients have more difficulty with telephone conversations then face-to-face conversations. They will also note that their voice is worse when reading a new passage aloud over reciting a memorized passage. Singing may be normal, as well as spontaneous emotional speech such as laughing or crying. The reason for these phenomena is unknown, but thought to be associated with differences in central nervous system processing of the different speech tasks. These features were noted by practitioners long ago and resulted in the incorrect consideration of spasmodic dysphonia as a psychiatric or psychological disorder.[21]

The diagnosis of spasmodic dysphonia can be difficult as there is no pathognomonic sign or specific test that will provide the diagnosis. In the past, the diagnosis was often delayed for years after the patient developed symptoms and sought medical care. Other more common voice and laryngeal disorders are often attributed to the patient before he or she finds an experienced practitioner who correctly recognizes their disorder.

The experienced clinician spends most of the interview *listening* to the patient's voice quality, especially during specific tasks, and the majority of the physical exam is spent ruling out other voice disorders. Although specific diagnostic tests and procedures can be helpful in supporting or discounting the disorder, the final diagnosis is usually associated with a clinical history and auditory perceptual findings that support the diagnosis. Imaging and laboratory testing are not routinely recommended; however, they can be helpful in ruling out other neurologic diagnoses, if suspected. Laryngeal electromyography is of limited diagnostic benefit[27]; however, in some patients with treatment-resistant spasmodic dysphonia, fine-wire electromyography of all intrinsic muscles has shown spasm in the intra-arytenoid muscle, an uncommon finding which may otherwise be overlooked.[18,25,28] Measurement of acoustic and aerodynamic perturbations may support the diagnosis, but are not diagnostic.

TREATMENT

All treatment for spasmodic dysphonia is aimed at reducing symptomatology and the impact of the voice disorder on a patient's daily function. No treatment is aimed at the source of disease and therefore cannot be considered truly curative. Four basic approaches exist and can be used singularly or in combination: speech therapy, pharmacologic agents, intramuscular injections of botulinum toxin, and surgical treatment (Figure 14–1).

Speech Therapy

Although some have reported speech therapy as a successful adjunct to botulinum toxin injection,[29] speech therapy as a sole treatment has a very limited role and often serves only to frustrate the patient with spasmodic dysphonia. Most

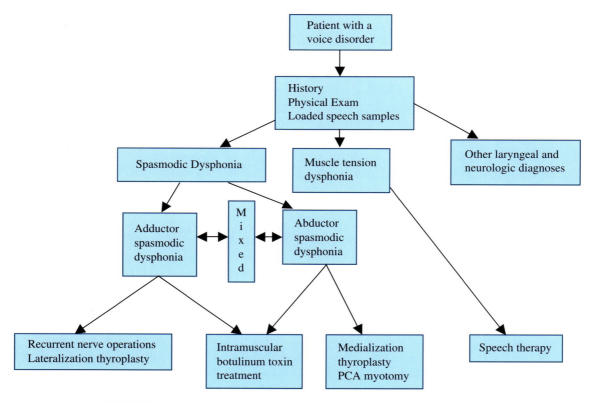

FIGURE 14–1. Management algorithm for spasmodic dysphonia.

believe that speech therapy with a goal for cure is an unreasonable expectation. Speech therapy is often used to distinguish patients with diagnostic difficulties, as those with spasmodic dysphonia, from patients with muscle tension dysphonia.[12,30]

Medical Therapy

Oral medical therapy has no proven benefit for patients with spasmodic dysphonia. There is no specific antidystonia agent, and although benzodiazepines, anticholinergics, dopamine depleters, and gabapentin are dosed empirically, they are often limited by central nervous system side effects including sedation.[31] Interestingly, many patients with spasmodic dysphonia note a diminution of symptoms with alcohol intake.

Botulinum Toxin Therapy

Fermentation of *Clostridium botulinum* produces a group of seven antigenically distinct exotoxin compounds that block neurotransmitter transmission at the mammalian neuromuscular junction.[32] Subtypes A, B, C, D, E, F, and G have been identified, but only A, B, E, F, and G have been known to cause the disease botulism. Botulinum toxin subtypes A and B are commercially available for clinical use, although they are not specifically the U.S. Food and Drug Administration approved for use in spasmodic dysphonia. Nonetheless, a large body of literature supports the use of intramuscular injections of botulinum toxin for treatment of spasmodic dysphonia[33] and its use is considered to be at the standard of care for this group of patients. Botulinum toxin type A has been used clinically to treat spasmodic dysphonia since 1984.[34] Type B has only become clinically available since 2000.[35] Type A is manufactured and distributed by a number of companies worldwide with Botox (Allergan, Inc, Irvine, Calif) dominating the commercial market. Type B is manufactured and distributed by Solstice Neurosciences, Inc. (South San Francisco, Calif) as Myobloc.

After being injected intramuscularly, botulinum toxin causes a flaccid paralysis by blocking presynaptic release of acetylcholine at the neuromuscular junction.[34] A dose-dependent effect and side-effect period are seen in patients with spasmodic dysphonia. Initially, patients will develop a breathy voice quality followed by a more fluent, less spastic voice quality. As the neuromuscular junctions recover, the patient gradually redevelops spastic voice.[36, 37] With toxin type A, the effect lasts about 3 months and once stable dosing is achieved, a given patient's response to injection is often quite reproducible. Toxin type B lasts a shorter period of time (approximately 6 weeks) and the conversion factor for type B is 50 to 80 times the dose of toxin A for similar effect.[35]

A variety of injection methods and dosing strategies are utilized by practitioners. No strategy has been shown to be superior to another. Most preferentially inject the thyroarytenoid muscle as the target for patients with adductor spasmodic dysphonia, although some recommend the lateral cricoarytenoid (the strongest laryngeal adductor) or the intra-arytenoid (when spastic activity has been identified on fine-wire electromyography).[7,24,28,38] The posterior cricoarytenoid muscle is the target for patients with abductor spasmodic dysphonia.[39] Injection technique is also highly variable from physician to physician and none has been demonstrated superior to another.[31] The toxin can be delivered to the muscle via a percutaneous[5] or permucosal approach,[40] with or without optical guidance, with[27] or without[41] electromyographic guidance. The posterior cricoarytenoid muscles can be approached from either a posteriolateral or a transcricothyroid membrane, transtracheal approach.[42] Dosages of toxin to muscle are typically low-dose with the majority of patients receiving about 3 units of type A toxin per muscle.[7] Others have recommended larger doses, even entering double digits per muscle, for longer effect. Unilateral or bilateral injections can be done.[43,44] Dosing strategies aim at maximizing the fluent voice, while minimizing the breathiness at the onset of toxin activity. These strategies vary from patient to patient depending on an individual's desires and level of voice use. As an example, a speaking professional performing radio voiceovers may come in for unilateral ½-unit doses every month, trading the frequency of dosing for minimal breathy side effect, whereas an elderly homemaker may come in every 6 months for a 5-unit bilateral dose, trading a few weeks of breathy voice for the inconvenience of the physician visit.

Although widely used as primary therapy for spasmodic dysphonia, botulinum toxin therapy does have its limitations. Many patients do not like the relative "roller-coaster effect" of the medicine, which produces a poor breathy voice shortly after injection, followed by a fluent voice, followed again by a dysphonic voice. Even though the toxin effect lasts a few months, a patient may state that his or her best voice only existed for several weeks in the middle of dosing. Other patients find traveling to a treating physician inconvenient, as treating patients with spasmodic dysphonia is not commonly practiced by the majority of otolaryngologists or neurologists. Some patients find erratic responses after each injection, thus never achieving a stable dose.

Botulinum toxin treatment of abductor spasmodic dysphonia seems to be less effective then treatment of adductor spasmodic dysphonia.[7,39] This may be related to the dual role of the abductor muscles as the most important laryngeal muscle of breathing. The belly of the muscle is larger than the other intrinsic laryngeal muscles and probably requires a larger dose for ultimate efficacy; however, the practitioner must treat at a lower dose to avoid total paralysis and airway obstruction.

Surgery

Adductor Spasmodic Dysphonia

An operative approach to spasmodic dysphonia predates the use of botulinum toxin. Dedo, in 1976, is credited for recognizing spasmodic dysphonia as a neurologic dysphonia with abnormal feedback between the end organ (larynx) and the central nervous system.[45,46] He proposed a procedure in which one recurrent laryngeal nerve is severed, thus interrupting the aberrant central-peripheral nervous system interaction.[45,47] The initial reports of the recurrent laryngeal

nerve section were exciting; however, several manuscripts over the ensuing decade suggested that cure of spasticity was evident in about one-third.[48-50] The majority of patients traded the dysphonia of spasmodic dysphonia for that of a vocal fold paralysis with a breathy harsh sound. Electromyographic data showed that spontaneous reinnervation of the treated hemilarynx occurred despite nerve transaction.[51] Modifications of the original procedure were suggested; however, the patients developed either a breathy dysphonia or recurrence of spasm.[52-54]

Selective laryngeal adductor denervation and reinnervation represents a more extensive modification of the original nerve severing procedure.[55-57] Four significant modifications of the original recurrent laryngeal nerve section were instituted. First, a bilateral recurrent laryngeal nerve operation should be more effective than a unilateral procedure; however, severing both recurrent nerves would put the patient at significant risk for dyspnea or airway obstruction. Second, the denervation should be specific to the adductors while preserving the innervation to the abductors of the larynx. Third, a method to prevent muscle atrphy associated with recurrent nerve transection was proposed. Lastly, late reinnervation from the "diseased" recurrent laryngeal nerve should be avoided. In the selective laryngeal adductor denervation and reinnervation procedure large windows are made into the thyroid cartilage bilaterally to widely expose the paraglottic space, revealing the intrinsic adductor muscles and the terminal portion of the recurrent laryngeal nerve. The anterior branch of the recurrent laryngeal nerve is identified under magnification and branches to the thyroarytenoid and the lateral cricoarytenoid muscles are severed and physically transposed outside the laryngeal cartilage to prevent reinnervation. A microneurorrhaphy is made between the proximal cut end of the sternohyoid branch of the ansa cervicalis to the distal branch of the recurrent laryngeal nerve just before it terminates in the thyroarytenoid muscle (Figure 14-2). This final step reinnervates the muscle providing thyroarytenoid muscle tone and, most importantly, prevents reinnervation from the proximal transected end of the recurrent laryngeal nerve. As a

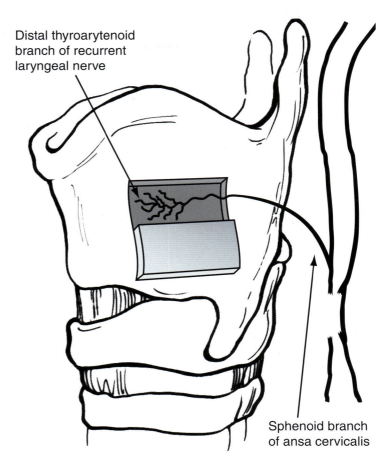

Distal thyroarytenoid
branch of recurrent
laryngeal nerve

Sphenoid branch
of ansa cervicalis

FIGURE 14–2. Microneurorrhapy between the proximal cut end of the ansa cervicalis to the distal branch of the recurrent laryngeal nerve.

part of the selective laryngeal adductor denervation and reinnervation procedure, the lateral cricoarytenoid is partially transected to weaken it because the terminal branch to the lateral cricoarytenoid is too small to be amenable to reliable reinnervation.[17,56]

Initial reports of this procedure are very promising with only a handful of treated patients failing therapy.[56] Although a degree of breathiness is noted from blinded observers, patients self-report a very high satisfaction rate in both voice quality and loss of spasticity.[58] This procedure has been repeated and further reported in the literature.[57] Long-term results on additional patients are quite enthusiastic.[58]

Another approach to spasmodic dysphonia is aimed at altering laryngeal biomechanics through framework surgery rather then by altering neuromuscular tensions. Isshiki and others have performed and modified this type II thyroplasty in which the vocal folds are lateralized away from each other.[59-62] The procedure is per-

formed under local anesthesia and the patient is allowed to talk, as in other phonosurgical procedures. A midline thyrotomy is made with care not to enter the mucosa. The cartilage halves of the thyroid ala are separated and then secured in position with a shim when the desired voice effect is heard. In this approach, the spasms of spasmodic dysphonia may still occur, but because the vocal folds are held apart, the audible quality of these spasms are lessened. Long-term results have been poor,[63] but this technique seems to have little morbidity and is a reasonable alternative for some patients.

Myotomy or myectomy alone of the thyroarytenoid has been proposed experimentally but has had limited success in clinical treatment of patients.[17,63] This can be performed through an open approach, or alternatively, via an endoscopic approach where a laser can be used to selectively vaporize and coagulate thyroarytenoid fibers. A cited advantage of the open approach is that it can be performed in the

Alternative Therapies

As a rare disease with an unknown etiology, discussions of diagnosis and treatment of spasmodic dysphonia often spark debate in both medical and lay communities. Although therapies offered by traditional allopathic medicine such as botulinum toxin and the different operations have defined track records with reasonable science behind them, other nontraditional treatments for spasmodic dysphonia are constantly being offered to patients. Herbal supplements, hypnotherapy, psychotherapy, and voice therapy for cure are offered to this vulnerable population of patients, often in exchange for significant cash outlays. Although some patients have been helped by such treatments, the data are anecdotal at best. It is likely hat many of the patients successfully treated did not actually have spasmodic dysphonia (a dystonia) but in reality had a nonorganic dysphonia such as muscle tension dysphonia. These nonorganic dysphonias often respond to psychological interventions including relaxation, motivation, and antidepressive techniques.

Other alternative therapies have been looked at by more credible sources. Some patients have seen improvements with acupuncture and a group of medical acupuncturists have reported on their data. Unfortunately, in their 2003 manuscript, Lee et al[64] were unable to show convincing evidence of success to blinded observers. Seven of ten patients reported improvements in voice symptoms, but only four of them continued with treatment. The National Institutes of Health is conducting an ongoing study on the effects of dextromethorphan, a commonly used over-the-counter cough suppressant, on voice disorders including spasmodic dysphonia. This medicine can inhibit laryngeal reflexes and decrease laryngeal tension.

With the expansion of the Internet, a person with a voice disorder is exposed to a veritable information overload before seeking professional medical care. Because voice disorders are not life-threatening, a patient may not even go to a physician or speech pathologist to seek an accurate diagnosis. Patients with nonorganic dysphonia can inaccurately diagnose themselves with spasmodic dysphonia and then report success after taking an herbal supplement, adding further confusion to a treatment decision made by those with the real diagnosis.

awake phonating patient, thus allowing the surgeon to titrate the extent of operation to voice quality.[65] Although the endoscopic approach avoids an apparent neck incision, one should weigh the negative effect of inducing mucosal scar and producing a harsh voice quality that is difficult to further remedy. Care should be made to keep the mucosal incisions lateral on the ventricular surface of the vocal folds. As a part of the selective laryngeal adductor denervation and reinnervation procedure, the lateral cricoarytenoid is partially transected to weaken it as the terminal branch of the recurrent laryngeal nerve is too small to be amenable to reliable reinnervation.[17,66]

Abductor Spasmodic Dysphonia

Because botulinum toxin treatment of abductor spasmodic dysphonia is less beneficial than in patients with adductor spasmodic dysphonia, alternative treatments have been developed. Some of the limitations to the treatment of abductor spasmodic dysphonia are related to difficulties associated with severe weakening of the posterior cricoarytenoid muscle, especially bilaterally. Both muscle-specific and framework procedures have been performed with limited success. Shaw and others reported on three cases treated by selective trimming (myoplasty) of the posterior cricoarytenoid muscle.[67] Others[68] have recommended permucosal selective electrocautery of the posterior cricoarytenoid muscle via the postcricoid area during a direct laryngoscopy approach. Some have reported limited success with medialization type I thyroplasty in these patients, using a concept similar to treating the adductor patients with a lateralization framework approach.[7,39] By moving the vocal folds together, the effect and auditory perception of the breathy voice break is lessened. This approach may be used as a supplement to botulinum toxin injection of the posterior cricoarytenoid muscle.

FUTURE DIRECTIONS

Although we continue to treat patients' symptomology, the true cure for spasmodic dysphonia and other dystonias probably lies in the central nervous system. In reality, we do not know if all patients with the symptoms of spasmodic dysphonia even have the same disease. Could there be multiple central disorders with a common end product of a spasmodic voice? The dystonia literature has pointed toward genetics as a possible source of disease. Familial segregation of dystonias has led toward identification of a number of dystonia genes and their protein products; however, none of these have been specifically implicated as the defect in spasmodic dysphonia. Further identification of the effects of gene mutation may yield better disease identification and, one hopes, a cure.

Our colleagues in neurosurgery are working with implantable devices capable of modifying in vivo neurologic communication in the basal ganglia.[68] Implantation of these deep brain stimulators has shown success in treating other movement disorders including Parkinson's disease, tremor, and generalized dystonia. As the electronics and programming of these products become more refined, a role in treating all centrally mediated motor disorders may develop.

Review Questions

1. You have diagnosed a patient with adductor spasmodic dysphonia and both you and she decide on treatment with botulinum toxin type A injections. Approximately how many units of toxin would you deliver to each thyroarytenoid muscle?
   a. 2 units
   b. 20 units
   c. 200 units
   d. 2000 units
   e. 20000 units

2. Spasmodic dysphonia is a psychiatric illness.
   a. True
   b. False

3. Abductor spasmodic dysphonia is characterized by:
   a. Vocal fold spasms most apparent while speaking passages weighted with voiced consonants
   b. Vocal fold spasms most apparent while speaking passages weighted with voiceless consonants

   c. Vocal fold tremor without spasm most apparent while speaking prolonged vowel sounds like "a" in ah

   d. Vocal fold spasms most apparent while speaking prolonged vowel sounds like "a" in ah

   e. b and d

4. Diagnosis of adductor spasmodic dysphonia is substantiated
   a. By findings of thalamic injury seen on magnetic resonance imaging
   b. By demonstration of a high titers of anti-cytomegalovirus IgG on plasma chemistry
   c. By listening for specific speech breaks during loaded sentences
   d. By demonstration of high vocal tract airflow during utterance of prolonged vowel sounds

5. Speech therapy with intent to cure is a reliable primary method of treating patients with spasmodic dysphonia.
   a. True
   b. False

REFERENCES

1. Traube L. *Gesammelte Beitrge Zur Pathologie Und Physiologie*. 2nd ed. Berlin: Verlag von August Hirschwald; 1871.
2. Critchley M. Spastic dysphonia ("inspiratory speech") *Brain*. 1939;62:96–103.
3. Bellussi G. Le disfonie impercinetiche. *Atti Labor Fonet Univ Padova*. 1952;3:1.
4. Bloch P. Neuro-psychiatric aspects of spastic dysphonia. *Folia Phoniatr (Basel)*. 1965;17:310–364.
5. Brin MF, Blitzer A, Stewart C. Laryngeal dystonia (spasmodic dysphonia): observations of 901 patients and treatment with botulinum toxin. *Adv Neurol*. 1998;78:237–252.
6. Aminoff MJ, Dedo HH, Izdebski K. Clinical aspects of spasmodic dysphonia. *J Neurol Neurosurg Psychiatry*. 1978;41:361–365.
7. Blitzer A, Brin MF, Stewart CF. Botulinum toxin management of spasmodic dysphonia (laryngeal dystonia): a 12-year experience in more than 900 patients. *Laryngoscope*. 1998;108:1435–1441.
8. Deleyiannis FW, Gillespie M, Bielamowicz S, Yamashita T, Ludlow CL. Laryngeal long latency re-sponse conditioning in abductor spasmodic dysphonia. *Ann Otol Rhinol Laryngol*. 1999;108: 612–619.
9. Bressman SB. Dystonia genotypes, phenotypes, and classification. *Adv Neurol*. 2004;94:101–107.
10. Saunders-Pullman R, Shriberg J, Shanker V, Bressman SB. Penetrance and expression of dystonia genes. *Adv Neurol*. 2004;94:121–125.
11. Bressman SB. Dystonia: phenotypes and genotypes. *Rev Neurol (Paris)*. 2003;159:849–856.
12. Roy N, Ford CN, Bless DM. Muscle tension dysphonia and spasmodic dysphonia: the role of manual laryngeal tension reduction in diagnosis and management. *Ann Otol Rhinol Laryngol*. 1996;105: 851–856.
13. Morrison M. Pattern recognition in muscle misuse voice disorders: How I do it. *J Voice*. 1997;11:108–114.
14. Schweinfurth JM, Billante M, Courey MS. Risk factors and demographics in patients with spasmodic dysphonia. *Laryngoscope*. 2002;112:220–223.
15. Tolosa E, Marti MJ. Blepharospasm–oromandibular dystonia syndrome (Meige's syndrome): clinical aspects. *Adv Neurol*. 1988;49:73–84.
16. Bielamowicz S, Ludlow CL. Effects of botulinum toxin on pathophysiology in spasmodic dysphonia. *Ann Otol Rhinol Laryngol*. 2000;109:194–203.
17. Chhetri DK, Blumin JH, Vinters HV, Berke GS. Histology of nerves and muscles in adductor spasmodic dysphonia. *Ann Otol Rhinol Laryngol*. 2003;112:334–341.
18. Hillel AD. The study of laryngeal muscle activity in normal human subjects and in patients with laryngeal dystonia using multiple fine-wire electromyography. *Laryngoscope*. 2001;111:1–47.
19. Sapienza CM, Walton S, Murry T. Adductor spasmodic dysphonia and muscular tension dysphonia: acoustic analysis of sustained phonation and reading. *J Voice*. 2000;14:502–520.
20. Roy N, Gouse M, Mauszycki SC, Merrill RM, Smith ME. Task specificity in adductor spasmodic dysphonia versus muscle tension dysphonia. *Laryngoscope*. 2005;115:311–316.

21. Cannito MP, Johnson JP. Spastic dysphonia: a continuum disorder. *J Commun Disord.* 1981;14:215–233.

22. Cyrus CB, Bielamowicz S, Evans FJ, Ludlow CL. Adductor muscle activity abnormalities in abductor spasmodic dysphonia. *Otolaryngol Head Neck Surg.* 2001;124:23–30.

23. Blitzer A, Brin MF, Fahn S, Lovelace RE. Clinical and laboratory characteristics of focal laryngeal dystonia: study of 110 cases. *Laryngoscope.* 1988; 98:636–640.

24. Blitzer A, Brin MF. Laryngeal dystonia: a series with botulinum toxin therapy. *Ann Otol Rhinol Laryngol.* 1991;100:85–89.

25. Klotz DA, Maronian NC, Waugh PF, Shahinfar A, Robinson L, Hillel AD. Findings of multiple muscle involvement in a study of 214 patients with laryngeal dystonia using fine-wire electromyography. *Ann Otol Rhinol Laryngol.* 2004;113:602–612.

26. Barkmeier JM, Case JL, Ludlow CL. Identification of symptoms for spasmodic dysphonia and vocal tremor: a comparison of expert and nonexpert judges. *J Commun Disord.* 2001;34:21–37.

27. Sataloff RT, Mandel S, Mann EA, Ludlow CL. Laryngeal electromyography: an evidence-based review. *Muscle Nerve.* 2003;28:767–772.

28. Hillel AD, Maronian NC, Waugh PF, Robinson L, Klotz DA. Treatment of the interarytenoid muscle with botulinum toxin for laryngeal dystonia. *Ann Otol Rhinol Laryngol.* 2004;113:341–348.

29. Murry T, Woodson GE. Combined-modality treatment of adductor spasmodic dysphonia with botulinum toxin and voice therapy. *J Voice.* 1995;9: 460–465.

30. Morrison MD, Rammage LA, Belisle GM, Pullan CB, Nichol H. Muscular tension dysphonia. *J Otolaryngol.* 1983;12:302–306.

31. Sulica L. Contemporary management of spasmodic dysphonia. *Curr Op Otolaryngol Head Neck Surg.* 2004;12:543–548.

32. Blitzer A, Sulica L. Botulinum toxin: basic science and clinical uses in otolaryngology. *Laryngoscope.* 2001;111:218–226.

33. American Academy of Otolaryngology–Head and Neck Surgery Foundation Policy Statements. Botulinum toxin treatment. Available at: http://www.entlink.net/practice/rules/botox_treatment.cfm. Accessed July 20, 1990.

34. Blitzer A, Brin MF, Fahn S, Lange D, Lovelace RE. Botulinum toxin (Botox) for the treatment of "spastic dysphonia" as part of a trial of toxin injections for the treatment of other cranial dystonias. *Laryngoscope.* 1986;96:1300–1301.

35. Adler CH, Bansberg SF, Krein-Jones K, Hentz JG. Safety and efficacy of botulinum toxin type B (myobloc) in adductor spasmodic dysphonia. *Mov Disord.* 2004;19:1075–1079.

36. Brin MF, Blitzer A, Fahn S, Gould W, Lovelace RE. Adductor laryngeal dystonia (spastic dysphonia): treatment with local injections of botulinum toxin (Botox). *Mov Disord.* 1989;4:287–296.

37. Ludlow CL, Naunton RF, Fujita M, Sedory SE. Spasmodic dysphonia: botulinum toxin injection after recurrent nerve surgery. *Otolaryngol Head Neck Surg.* 1990;102:122–131.

38. Grillone GA, Blitzer A, Brin MF, Annino DJ, Jr, Saint-Hilaire MH. Treatment of adductor laryngeal breathing dystonia with botulinum toxin type A. *Laryngoscope.* 1994;104:30–32.

39. Blitzer A, Brin MF, Stewart C, Aviv JE, Fahn S. Abductor laryngeal dystonia: a series treated with botulinum toxin. *Laryngoscope.* 1992;102: 163–167.

40. Ford CN, Bless DM, Lowery JD. Indirect laryngoscopic approach for injection of botulinum toxin in spasmodic dysphonia. *Otolaryngol Head Neck Surg.* 1990;103:752–758.

41. Green DC, Berke GS, Ward PH, Gerratt BR. Point-touch technique of botulinum toxin injection for the treatment of spasmodic dysphonia. *Ann Otol Rhinol Laryngol.* 1992;101:883–887.

42. Bielamowicz S, Squire S, Bidus K, Ludlow CL. Assessment of posterior cricoarytenoid botulinum toxin injections in patients with abductor spasmodic dysphonia. *Ann Otol Rhinol Laryngol.* 2001;110:406–412.

43. Zwirner P, Murry T, Woodson GE. A comparison of bilateral and unilateral botulinum toxin treatments for spasmodic dysphonia. *Eur Arch Otorhinolaryngol.* 1993;250:271–276.

44. Bielamowicz S, Stager SV, Badillo A, Godlewski A. Unilateral versus bilateral injections of botulinum toxin in patients with adductor spasmodic dysphonia. *J Voice.* 2002;16:117–123.

45. Dedo HH. Recurrent laryngeal nerve section for spastic dysphonia. *Ann Otol Rhinol Laryngol.* 1976;85:451–459.

46. Dedo HH, Townsend JJ, Izdebski K. Current evidence for the organic etiology of spastic dysphonia. *Otolaryngology.* 1978;86:875–880.

47. Dedo HH, Behlau MS. Recurrent laryngeal nerve section for spastic dysphonia: 5- to 14-year preliminary results in the first 300 patients. *Ann Otol Rhinol Laryngol.* 1991;100:274–279.

48. Aronson AE, DeSanto LW. Adductor spastic dysphonia: 1½ years after recurrent laryngeal nerve resection. *Ann Otol Rhinol Laryngol.*1981;90:2–6.

49. Aronson AE, De Santo LW. Adductor spastic dysphonia: three years after recurrent laryngeal nerve resection. *Laryngoscope.* 1983;93:1–8.

50. Dedo HH, Izdebski K. Problems with surgical (RLN section) treatment of spastic dysphonia. *Laryngoscope.* 1983;93:268–271.

51. Sulica L, Blitzer A, Brin MF, Stewart CF. Botulinum toxin management of adductor spasmodic dysphonia after failed recurrent laryngeal nerve section. *Ann Otol Rhinol Laryngol.* 2003;112:499–505.

52. Biller HF, Som ML, Lawson W. Laryngeal nerve crush for spastic dysphonia. *Ann Otol Rhinol Laryngol.* 1983;92:469.

53. Netterville JL, Stone RE, Rainey C, Zealear DL, Ossoff RH. Recurrent laryngeal nerve avulsion for treatment of spastic dysphonia. *Ann Otol Rhinol Laryngol.* 1991;100:10–14.

54. Weed DT, Jewett BS, Rainey C, et al. Long-term follow-up of recurrent laryngeal nerve avulsion for the treatment of spastic dysphonia. *Ann Otol Rhinol Laryngol.* 1996;105:592–601.

55. Sercarz JA, Berke GS, Ming Y, Rothschiller J, Graves MC. Bilateral thyroarytenoid denervation: a new treatment for laryngeal hyperadduction disorders studied in the canine. *Otolaryngol Head Neck Surg.* 1992;107:657–668.

56. Berke GS, Blackwell KE, Gerratt BR, Verneil A, Jackson KS, Sercarz JA. Selective laryngeal adductor denervation–reinnervation: a new surgical treatment for adductor spasmodic dysphonia. *Ann Otol Rhinol Laryngol.* 1999;108:227–231.

57. Allegretto M, Morrison M, Rammage L, Lau DP. Selective denervation: reinnervation for the control of adductor spasmodic dysphonia. *J Otolaryngol.* 2003;32:185–189.

58. Chhetri DK, Mendelsohn A, Blumin JH, Berke GS. Long-term follow-up results of the selective laryngeal adductor denervation-reinnervation surgery for adductor spasmodic dysphonia. *Laryngoscope.* 2006;116:635–642.

59. Isshiki N, Tsuji DH, Yamamoto Y, Iizuka Y. Midline lateralization thyroplasty for adductor spasmodic dysphonia. *Ann Otol Rhinol Laryngol.* 2000;109: 187–193.

60. Isshiki N, Haji T, Yamamoto Y, Mahieu HF. Thyroplasty for adductor spasmodic dysphonia: further experiences. *Laryngoscope.* 2001;111:615–621.

61. Tucker HM. Laryngeal framework surgery in the management of spasmodic dysphonia. Preliminary report. *Ann Otol Rhinol Laryngol.* 1989;98:52–54.

62. Tucker HM. Anterior commissure laryngoplasty for adjustment of vocal fold tension. *Ann Otol Rhinol Laryngol.* 1985;94:547–549.

63. Chan SW, Baxter M, Oates J, Yorston A. Long-term results of type II thyroplasty for adductor spasmodic dysphonia. Laryngoscope. 2004;114(9): 1604–1608.

64. Lee L, Daughton S, Scheer S, et al. Use of acupuncture for the treatment of adductor spasmodic dysphonia: a preliminary investigation. *J Voice.* 2003;17:411–424.

65. Genack SH, Woo P, Colton RH, Goyette D. Partial thyroarytenoid myectomy: an animal study investigating a proposed new treatment for adductor spasmodic dysphonia. *Otolaryngol Head Neck Surg.* 1993; 08:256–264.

66. Koufman JA, Rees CJ, Halum SL, Blalock D. Treatment of adductor-type spasmodic dysphonia by surgical myectomy: a preliminary report. Ann Otol Rhinol Laryngol. 2006;115(2):97–102.

67. Shaw GY, Sechtem PR, Rideout B. Posterior cricoarytenoid myoplasty with medialization thyroplasty in the management of refractory abductor spasmodic dysphonia. *Ann Otol Rhinol Laryngol.* 2003;112:303–306.

68. Koufman JA. Management of abductor spasmodic dysphonia by endoscopic partial posterior cricoarytenoid (partial) myectomy. *Phonoscope.* 1999;2:159–166.

69. Marks WJ. Deep brain stimulation for dystonia. *Curr Treat Options Neurol.* 2005;7:237–243.

B. Inflammatory and Structural Disorders

15

Localized Inflammatory Disorders of the Larynx

Natasha Mirza, MD, FACS

KEY POINTS

- Most acute laryngeal inflammation is self-limiting; whereas viral laryngitis may result in secondary bacterial infections, empiric antibiotic therapy has not been shown to be beneficial.

- Severe infections of the upper airway, such as *supraglottitis* and *bacterial tracheitis*, must be aggressively treated with antibiotics and supportive care; management of the airway is the paramount concern.

- Laryngeal *candidiasis* occurs in immune-compromised persons.

- A persistent lesion of the larynx must always be considered to be a possible malignancy; although rarely indicated in the acutely inflamed larynx at the first visit, biopsy should be considered for persistent lesions.

- Posterior laryngeal granuloma has a high rate of recurrence following excision. Treatment involves antireflux medication and possibly speech therapy.

Local laryngeal inflammatory conditions cover a spectrum of infectious and irritative lesions. They also include immune mediated conditions whereby the laryngeal tissues mount a response to an exogenous or endogenous insult. They are all characterized by a local reaction to an insult with changes in the laryngeal tissues that can either be localized to one site, involve several subsites, or involve the entire larynx.

The management of inflammatory conditions of the larynx depends to a great extent on the etiology of the condition. This is, however, not often easily apparent when the patient first presents. The clinical course can be variable and the symptoms and signs nonspecific. Several of these disorders, such as acute viral laryngitis, are among the most common conditions affecting the upper aerodigestive tract. Recognition and knowledge of the more elusive conditions is necessary so that the appropriate tests are ordered, cultures and biopsies are taken, and eventually the appropriate management instituted.

Most cases where there is laryngeal involvement present with dysphonia, odynophonia, and occasionally cough and dyspnea. Complaints related to swallowing problems and odynophagia are rarer and may represent advanced infection or inflammation.

Biopsy may be required in cases that are not self-limiting. For most patients, this means a trip to the operating room for direct laryngoscopy and an evaluation of the trachea and bronchi if possible. All suspicious lesions should be biopsied to help make a conclusive diagnosis and also to rule out malignancy, a constant concern. Cultures of the surface of the lesions and also of the biopsied material are also helpful in some situations.

In this chapter, we review some of the laryngeal lesions with an infectious, immune, or irritative etiology, their typical presentation, laryngeal findings, and management (Figures 15–1 and 15–2). These will be distinguished by whether or not they typically involve the entire larynx at the time of presentation.

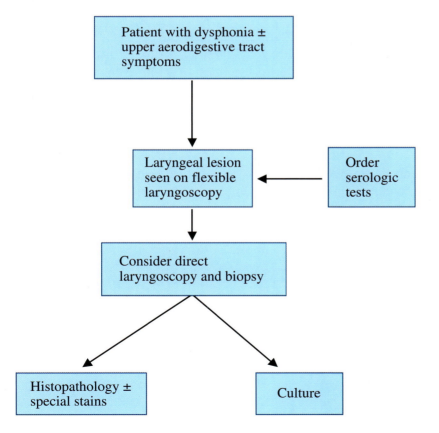

FIGURE 15–1. Clinical approach to a patient with a suspected inflammatory laryngeal lesion.

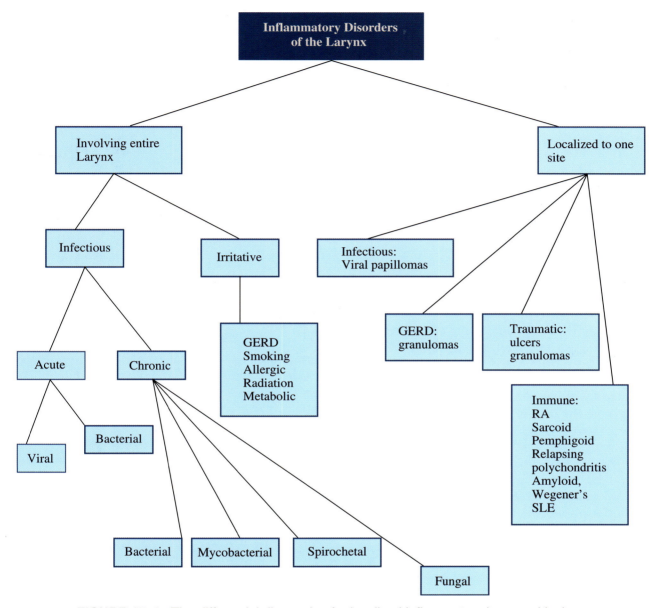

FIGURE 15–2. The differential diagnosis of a localized inflammatory laryngeal lesion.

LESIONS INVOLVING ENTIRE LARYNX

Acute Infections: Viral

The most common cause of laryngeal symptoms is acute viral laryngitis related to an upper respiratory tract infection. Presenting symptoms include dysphonia and even loss of voice, cough, fever, and often symptoms of rhinitis. Laryngoscopic findings include erythema and edema which involves the vocal folds and often the supraglottis as well. Treatment includes voice rest and hydration. Most conditions are self-limited and resolve in about 1 week.

In more advanced cases, *viral* laryngotracheitis can result in more profound illness with airway obstruction. In children and adults *parainfluenza* or *influenza*[1,2] viruses are leading causes of croup. In addition to general supportive measures, dexamethasone appears to be beneficial in reducing the overall severity of advanced cases of laryngotracheitis during the first 24 hours after infection.[3]

Acute Infections: Bacterial

Bacterial laryngitis is not common, although when it does occur, it can be quite severe. Two clinical entities, epiglottitis and bacterial laryngotracheitis, are discussed below. When the larynx appears to be infected and purulent debris is present on the laryngeal mucosa, it is tempting to treat the patient with antibiotics If the patient does not exhibit signs of toxicity, as in the more severe forms, this is not likely to be beneficial. Two studies, both from Sweden, compared penicillin and erythromycin, respectively, to placebo in patients with suspected bacterial superinfection involving the larynx.[4,5] The local symptoms and voice quality were felt to be equivalent between the two groups.

Bacterial tracheitis, a severe disorder, remains rare. The agent responsible is typically *Staphylococcus*, although *Hemophilus influenzae* and Group A *streptococcus* have also been implicated (among others). The characteristic patient will present with a high fever, dyspnea progressing to stridor, dysphonia, and cough. The diagnosis is made on the basis of thick purulence and crusts in the airway, erythema, and laryngeal edema. Blood cultures are often positive for the infectious agent. The mainstay of management is high vigilance; if the condition does not improve on antibiotics, hydration, and humidification, it is necessary to take the patient to the operating room and perform laryngotracheal toilet and suctioning. A tracheostomy is very rarely needed. The condition can be particularly dangerous in children due to the relatively small size of the central airways. One recent report has described an increase in the incidence of positive viral cultures (for influenza) and a lessening morbidity to the disease.[6]

Acute Supraglottitis/Epiglottitis

The infectious agent in adult supraglottitis (also known as *epiglottitis*, a less precise name) is usually *Hemophilus influenzae*. Although historically thought of as a children's disease, it has become relatively more common in adults. This is particularly true with the advent and widespread use of the *H. influenzae B* vaccine in children.[7] Presenting symptoms range from fever and odynophagia to stridor and drooling in the severe forms. Diagnosis in children is based on clinical suspicion and often a lateral neck film showing the "thumb sign" of epiglottic edema. In most adults, flexible laryngoscopy can be performed safely; this examination will reveal diffuse edema and erythema of the supraglottis. The diagnosis is based on clinical grounds and may be confirmed by blood cultures. Viral supraglottitis has also been described.[8] Surface cultures may be obtained if the patient has been taken to the operating room for airway management. The mainstay of management is to secure the airway. In children this involves an intubation in the OR whereas, in adults observation in the ICU, intubation, or even a tracheotomy may be necessary, though not common. A recent review of 23 adult cases from one institution in Ireland revealed that only three of the 23 required intubation or tracheotomy; indeed, all three had presented with rapidly progressing symptoms.[9] Although antibiotic therapy is critical, the concurrent use of antibiotics and steroids is a poorly defined but common practice.[10]

Chronic Infectious Conditions

1. Bacterial: Klebsiella (Rhinoscleroma)
2. Spirochetal: Syphilis, Lyme
3. Fungal: Candida
   Blastomycosis
   Histoplasmosis
   Coccidiomycosis
   Aspergillosis
4. Tuberculosis

Bacterial: Klebsiella

Respiratory scleroma is a rare, chronic progressive granulomatous disease that usually begins in

Symptomatic Relief of "Sore Throat"

Most patients do not present to the otolaryngologist for the evaluation and management of self-limiting benign inflammatory disorders of the upper aerodigestive tract. Nonetheless, the symptomatic treatment of patients with viral respiratory tract illness is a major over-the-counter industry and these problems represent a significant source of patient morbidity. Although many patients may receive temporary relief with alcohol/phenol based analgesia, prolonged use will exacerbate the problem. The term "pharyngitis medicamentosa" was coined for this clinical situation.[11]

Other than the sensible recommendations of hydration and the avoidance of irritants, what can reasonably be done for these patients once bacterial disease and its complications have been excluded? There has been significant interest in zinc preparations in the past decade, with mixed results.[12,13] Principal concerns with zinc studies include difficulties associated performing blinded studies with zinc products due their strong taste. In one double-blind placebo-controlled study, flurbiprofen, an anti-inflammatory, was given in lozenge form to patients complaining of sore throat. The treatment group had significant relief compared with placebo.[14]

the nose and then affects the upper and lower respiratory tract in approximately 40% of cases. The causative organism is *Klebsiella rhinoscleromatis* which is a gram-negative coccobacillus. The disease has three stages: catarrhal, granulomatous, and sclerotic. Patients initially present with dysphonia but airway obstruction generally occurs in the last stage of the disease. Patients rarely present with isolated laryngeal lesions, and there is usually a continuum of rhinologic and airway involvement. Laryngoscopic findings vary from isolated granulomas and nodules to stenosis at the glottic and subglottic levels. Management is based on first establishing a diagnosis with biopsies, which may show the specific Mikulicz cells which are large macrophages containing the bacilli and on cultures of the causative organism. Early cases may be successfully treated with oral tetracycline and the use of fluoroquinolones is being studied. In the more advanced cases it is important to secure the airway either with a tracheotomy or with endoscopic procedures such as dilatations and serial laser incisions and in some situations with a laryngofissure and open excision of the lesions. In a report of 22 patients, Shindo noted that 13 had laryngotracheal involvement, three of whom required emergency tracheotomy at some point for obstruction.[15]

Spirochetal

While laryngeal involvement can occur at any stage, Stage I and II syphilis may present with laryngeal ulcers and cervical lymphadenopathy. In the tertiary stage, the larynx may develop fibrosis and stenosis. Diagnosis can be made on the basis of serologic testing but, to prove that laryngeal lesions are associated with the syphilitic conditions, biopsies of lesions and identification of spirochetes are necessary. Treatment is with long-term antibiotics. This disorder is exceedingly rare today, but represented a significant source of chronic disease in the past.[16]

Fungal

Most of these infections occur in the endemic geographic areas in individuals who are also immunocompromised. Typical symptoms are vague and flulike with dysphonia and cough if there is laryngeal involvement. The diagnosis is made generally on the generalized symptoms but a biopsy of the laryngeal lesions is necessary to clinch the diagnosis.[17] Fungal stains are generally positive. Granulomas are found and the epithelium may show changes known as pseudoepitheliomatous hyperplasia, which can be mistaken for a malignancy. The main factor differentiating these conditions is the endemic region in which the individual resides. Treatment with long-term amphotericin-B is still the best modality; however, ketoconazole has also been tried for periods of 6 months or more.

Laryngeal candidiasis, in contrast to the disorders listed above, is a commonly seen fungal infection due to *Candida albicans*. This disease can occur in both immunocompromised patients and healthy patients with predisposing factors such as the use of corticosteroids, particularly inhaled steroids in asthmatics, broad-spectrum antibiotics, diabetes, burns, alcoholism, endotracheal intubation, and recent laryngitis. Sulica has published a recent review of this clinical entity.[18] Two forms of laryngeal candidiasis have been described. One is the benign, isolated laryngeal candidiasis commonly seen in asthmatics with chronic use of steroid inhalers (Figure 15–3). These otherwise healthy patients present with isolated hoarseness and typically no other symptoms. The clinical exam shows diffuse laryngeal erythema with an irregular, superficial white exudate usually involving the true vocal folds. The second form is invasive laryngeal candidiasis seen in the immunocompromised patient, which is typically more serious and can be life-threatening. In these patients, the infection is rarely limited to the larynx and may involve the esophagus, oropharynx, and lower airway. Invasive candidiasis presents with symptoms of hoarseness, odynophagia, and dysphagia. Laryngoscopy typically shows mucosal edema, ulceration, and possibly

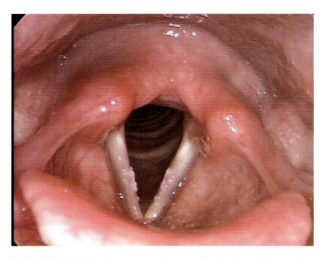

FIGURE 15–3. Laryngeal candiadasis. Note the bilateral white irregularities of the membranous vocal folds.

tissue necrosis. Significant airway obstruction can occur.

The diagnosis is confirmed with staining (fungal prep), culture, and/or biopsy. Further workup for immunosuppression is necessary in a patient with no known predisposing factors. This would include an HIV test as laryngeal candidiasis can be a presenting manifestation. For isolated laryngeal candidiasis, treatment usually consists of either topical antifungal gargles or troches versus systemic antifungals (ketoconazole or fluconazole) for 10 days to 2 weeks. Retreatment may be necessary due to the underlying predisposing factors. For invasive candidiasis, IV amphotericin-B is recommended and airway support as needed.

LOCALIZED INFLAMMATORY LESIONS OF THE LARYNX

Immune-Mediated

Many of the inflammatory disorders with local laryngeal manifestations are immune-mediated. They are discussed in detail in the following chapter, including rheumatoid arthritis and relapsing polychondritis. Other disorders are also presented, such as amyloidosis, sarcoidosis, and Wegener's granulomatosis. Loehrl and Smith have published an excellent review of these issues.[19]

Pemphigus Vulgaris and Pemphigoid

These two autoimmune disorders involve epithelial disease. Pemphigus vulgaris represents *intraepithelial* antibodies resulting in bleb for[20] Pemphigoid, on the other hand, is a *subepithelial* process, although many of the laryngeal presentations are similar. The patient may manifest local signs of inflammation with hoarseness or throat pain (Figure 15–4). In a recent review of *pemphigus* patients, 21/53 (40%) had laryngeal complaints, many of whom responded to an increase in systemic steroid therapy.[21] Cicatricial pemphigoid may affect the larynx; this subtype has a propensity for mucosa, most commonly affecting the oral cavity.[22] Advanced cases may result in laryngeal stenosis. The acute management of the patient, once the disorder is considered, is to rule out a superimposed fungal infection (see above) which may mimic the

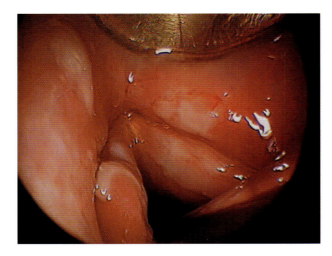

FIGURE 15–4. Direct laryngoscopy findings in a patient with active pemphigus vulgaris involving the larynx. A 70-degree telescope was used for this image.

local lesions in the larynx. With the cooperation of the patient's internist or dermatologist, the systemic immunosuppresion may be guided by the status of the laryngeal inflammation. Systemic therapy may also include more toxic agents such as dapsone, methotrexate, and cyclophosphamide.

Irritative and Inflammatory Lesions

Laryngeal Granuloma

These characteristic posterior laryngeal lesions are benign growths of hypertrophic granulation tissue; they most commonly occur at the vocal process of the arytenoid. They likely begin as ulcerations of the larynx (contact ulcers). Repeated trauma and inflammation then produce granulation tissue (Figures 13–5A and 13–5B). Although patients who develop these after intubation may be different, the typical patient with a spontaneous posterior granuloma suffers from laryngopharyngeal reflux. Ylitalo and others have demonstrated a high incidence of positive pH probe studies in these patients.[23] They have a high incidence of recurrence following surgical therapy and should only be excised for airway obstruction or concern over possible malignancy.

Patients present with odynophagia, odynophonia, and dysphonia. Whereas 24-hour pH probe monitoring may be helpful, empiric therapy with a proton-pump inhibitor is reasonable. Speech therapy, although controversial as a meaningful treatment for granuloma, may be beneficial.[24] Another option for patients is the use of botulinum toxin to create a chemical "voice rest."[25] The injection of botulinum toxin works by preventing the forceful adduction of the arytenoids which contributes to the local phonotrauma and high recurrence/persistence rates. In fact, Nasri et al have reported on the efficacious effect of Botox injections alone without excision of the granulomas by preventing mucosal damage caused by adduction of the arytenoids.[25] Studies are underway regarding the use of inhaled steroids for the treatment of posterior laryngeal granuloma.

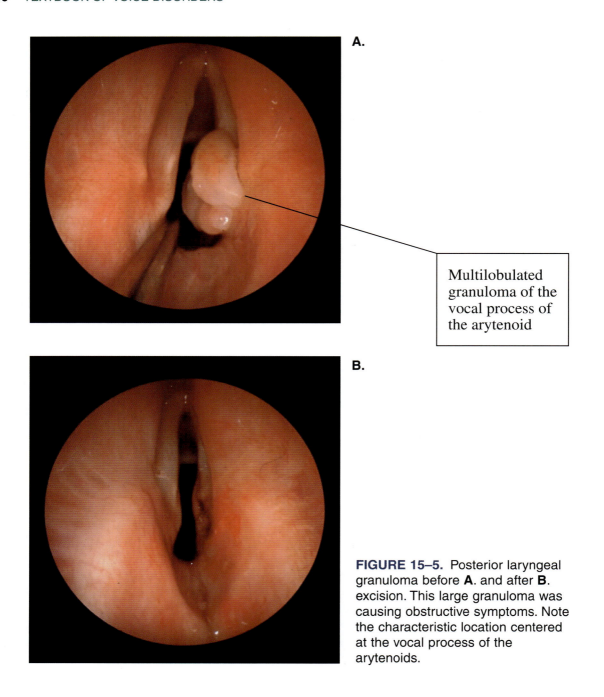

A.

Multilobulated granuloma of the vocal process of the arytenoid

B.

FIGURE 15–5. Posterior laryngeal granuloma before **A**. and after **B**. excision. This large granuloma was causing obstructive symptoms. Note the characteristic location centered at the vocal process of the arytenoids.

Teflon Granuloma

Teflon augmentation of the vocal folds was a popular and well-established technique for achieving medialization of a paralyzed vocal fold for most of the 1970s and 1980s. As laryngeal framework surgery became more popular, Teflon injection fell out of favor, particularly in light of the development of local reaction to the injected material over time. While the incidence of histo-

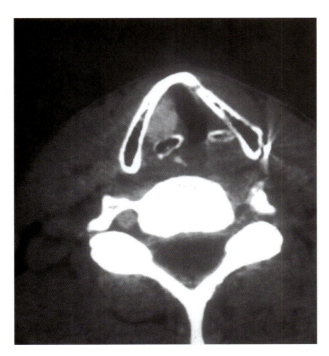

FIGURE 15–6. CT image of a right-sided Teflon granuloma.

logic reaction to Teflon is common, the clinical manifestations of this local inflammation are estimated to occur in 2 to 10% of patients; it is thought to be associated with over injection or misplaced Teflon.[26] The enlarging mass of Teflon/inflammation leads to dysphonia and airway compromise (Figure 15–6). Surgical removal may be required but must be considered carefully; advocates for endoscopic[27] and open[28] removal caution against the further disruption of normal tissue which may occur with surgical resection. A conservative endoscopic "contouring" of the involved vocal fold to create a straight edge for the working fold to vibrate against may be the best option in patients whose granuloma is intimately involved with the vocal ligament, as so many are.

This chapter has briefly outlined the clinical presentation and management of some of the inflammatory conditions of the larynx. While basic supportive treatment is appropriate for common self-limiting conditions such as acute viral laryngitis, serious disorders such as bacterial tracheitis and supraglottitis must be considered in the sick patient.

Biopsy may be considered for patients in whom malignancy is suspected or in the face of failure of medical management. Specific conditions, such as posterior granuloma and Teflon granuloma, must be handled with full knowledge of the natural history of these local processes.

Review Questions

1. An adult presents to your Emergency Room with progressive throat pain and dyspnea over a 24-hour period. His temperature is 102 degrees F. He has some stridor but is not in acute distress. You will most likely need to perform:
   a. Cricothyrotomy
   b. Elective endotracheal intubation
   c. Tracheotomy
   d. Transtracheal jet ventilation
   e. None of the above

2. A healthy, nondiabetic female has 2 weeks of sore throat following a sinus infection. Her rhinologic symptoms have resolved but she is hoarse and clearing her throat a great deal. Laryngeal examination reveals diffuse white specks on the vocal folds, which themselves are reddened. She:
   a. Has candidiasis; treat with antifungals
   b. Cannot have candidiasis without being diabetic or otherwise immunocompromised
   c. Should not be treated without cultures of the vocal folds
   d. This is a manifestation of reflux
   e. Should resume antibiotics for her sinusitis, now involving the larynx

3. A 45-year-old homeless man is admitted for shortness of breath. His chest x-ray is clear but the admitting medical service notes sinusitis and laryngotracheitis. He is coughing and appears ill. His sputum reveals gram-negative coccobacillary organisms. Biopsy of his respiratory mucosa reveals Mikulicz cells. He has:
   a. Wegener's
   b. Amyloidosis
   c. Sarcoidosis
   d. Rhinoscleroma
   e. Teflon granuloma

4. A 55-year-old female is now 25 years s/p left thyroid lobectomy. She was treated for a vocal paralysis shortly after her surgery. After years of getting by with modest hoarseness and no dysphagia, she is now complaining of a globus sensation and her voice is more tense. Examination reveals:
   a. A bilobed granuloma at her vocal process on the nonparalyzed side
   b. A bilobed granuloma at her vocal process on the paralyzed side
   c. A Teflon granuloma in the paraglottic space on the nonparalyzed side
   d. A Teflon granuloma in the paraglottic space on the paralyzed side
   e. Gelfoam extruding from an old injection laryngoplasty site

5. A 65-year-old banker has chronic throat clearing. Examination reveals a smooth 5 mm bilobed granuloma at the vocal process on the left side. He is a nonsmoker. You:
   a. Reassure him that this is not cancer
   b. Recommend immediate biopsy
   c. Recommend antireflux treatment
   d. Inject botulinum toxin into the right vocal fold
   e. Inject botulinum toxin into the left vocal fold

REFERENCES

1. Cherry JD. State of the evidence for standard-of-care treatments for croup: are we where we need to be? *Pediatr Infect Dis J.* 2005;24(11 suppl): S198–S202.
2. Woo PC, Young K, Tsang KW, Ooi CG, Peiris M, Yuen K. Adult croup: a rare but more severe condition. *Respiration.* 2000;67(6):684–688.
3. Super DM, Cartelli NA, Brooks LJ, Lembo RM, Kumar ML. A prospective randomized double-blind study to evaluate the effect of dexamethasone in acute laryngotracheitis. *J Pediatr.* 1989; 115(2):323–329.
4. Schalen L, Eliasson I, Kamme C, Schalen C. Erythromycin in acute laryngitis in adults. *Ann Otol Rhinol Laryngol.* 1993;102(3 pt 1):209–214.
5. Schalen L, Christensen P, Eliasson I, Fex S, Kamme C, Schalen C. Inefficacy of penicillin V in acute laryngitis in adults. Evaluation from results of double-blind study. *Ann Otol Rhinol Laryngol.* 1985;94(1 pt 1):14–17.
6. Bernstein T, Brilli R, Jacobs B. Is bacterial tracheitis changing? A 14-month experience in a pediatric intensive care unit. *Clin Infect Dis.* 1998;27(3):458–462.
7. Gorelick MH, Baker MD. Epiglottitis in children, 1979 through 1992. Effects of *Haemophilus influenzae type b* immunization. *Arch Pediatr Adolesc Med.* 1994;148(1):47–50.
8. D'Angelo AJ Jr, Zwillenberg S, Olekszyk JP, Marlowe FI, Mobini J. Adult supraglottitis due to herpes simplex virus. *J Otolaryngol.* 1990;19(3): 179–181.
9. Madhotra D, Fenton JE, Makura ZG, Charters P, Roland NJ. Airway intervention in adult supraglottitis. *Ir J Med Sci.* 2004;173(4):197–199.
10. Shah RK, Roberson DW, Jones DT. Epiglottitis in the *Hemophilus influenzae type B* vaccine era: changing trends. *Laryngoscope.* 2004;114(3): 557–560.
11. Halwell R. Pharyngitis medicamentosa. *Arch Otolaryngol Head Neck Surg.* 1989;115(8):995.
12. Mossad SB, Macknin ML, Medendorp SV, Mason P. Zinc gluconate lozenges for treating the common cold.in children: a randomized double-blind, placebo-controlled study. *Ann Intern Med.* 1996; 125(2):81–88.
13. Macknin ML, Piedmonte M, Calendine C, Janosky J, Wald E. Zinc gluconate lozgenges for treating

the common cold in children: a randomized controlled trial. *JAMA.* 1998;279(24):1962–1967.

14 Blagden M, Christian J, Miller K, Charlesworth A. Multidose flurbiprofen 8.75 mg lozenges in the treatment of sore throat: a randomized, double-blind, placebo-controlled study in UK general practice centres. *Int J Clin Prac.* 2002;56(2): 95–100.15. Amoils CP, Shindo ML. Laryngotracheal manifestations of rhinoscleroma. *Ann Otol Rhinol Laryngol.* 1996;105(5): 336–340

15. Amoils CP, Shindo ML. Laryngotracheal manifestations of rhinoscleroma. *Ann Otol Rhinol Laryngol.* 1996;105(5):336–340.

16. Grunwald E. *Diseases of the Larynx.* Philadelphia, Pa: WB Saunders, 1900:64.

17. Makitie AA, Back L, Aaltonen LM, Leivo I, Valtonen M. fungal infection of the epiglottis simulating a clinical malignancy. *Arch Otolaryngol Head Neck Surg.* 2003;129(1):124–126.

18. Sulica L. Laryngeal thrush. *Ann Otol Rhinol Laryngol.* 2005;114(5):369–375

19. Loehrl TA, Smith TL. Inflammatory and granulomatous lesions of the larynx and pharynx. *Am J Med.* 2001;111(suppl 8A):113S–S117.

20. Pathak PN. Pemphigus of the larynx. *J Laryngol Otol.* 1971;85(1):81–82.

21. Hale EK, Bystryn JC. Laryngeal and nasal involvement in pemphigus vulgaris. *J Am Acad Dermatol.* 2001;44(4):609–611

22. Hanson RD, Olsen KD, Rogers RS 3rd. Upper aerodigestive tract manifestations of cicatricial pemphigoid. *Ann Otol Rhinol Laryngol.* 1988; 97(5 pt 1):493–499.

23. Ylitalo R, Ramel S. Extraesophageal reflux in patients with contact granuloma: a prospective controlled study. *Ann Otol Rhinol Laryngol.* 2002;111(5 pt 1):441–446.

24. Ylitalo R. Hammarberg B. Voice characteristics, effects of voice therapy, and long-term follow-up of contact granuloma patients. *J Voice.* 2000; 14(4):557–566.

25. Nasri S, Sercarz JA, McAlpin T, Berke GS. Treatment of vocal fold granuloma using Botulinum toxin type A. *Laryngoscope.* 1995;105:585–588.

26. Kasperbauer JL, Slavit DH, Maragos NE. Teflon granulomas and overinjection of Teflon: a therapeutic challenge for the otolaryngologist. *Ann Otol Rhinol Laryngol.* 1993;102(10):748–751.

27. Nakayama M, Ford CN, Bless DM. Teflon vocal fold augmentation: failures and management in 28 cases. *Otolaryngol Head Neck Surg.* 1993;109(3 pt 1): 493–498.

28. Netterville JL, Coleman JR Jr, Chang S, Rainey CL, Reinisch L, Ossoff RH. Lateral laryngotomy for the removal of Teflon granuloma. *Ann Otol Rhinol Laryngol.* 1998;107(9 pt 1):735–744.

16

Systemic Inflammatory Disorders Affecting the Larynx

Felicia L. Johnson, MD
James W. Ragland, MD

KEY POINTS

- Laryngeal inflammation is a nonspecific finding that has many etiologies; not all laryngeal inflammation is due to laryngopharyngeal reflux.

- The larynx may be the first area affected in many of these systemic inflammatory diseases with no other organ system involvement.

- Direct laryngoscopy with biopsy and histopathologic examination is warranted and may be necessary to make the diagnosis in many of these conditions.

- The incidence of laryngeal tuberculosis may be increasing; systemic mycobacterial disease is present in a minority of these patients.

- Directed surgical therapy in the larynx is beneficial in the management of some systemic inflammatory diseases in combination with medical therapy.

TUBERCULOSIS

Epidemiology/Pathogenesis

Laryngeal tuberculosis (TB) is a chronic often indolent bacterial infection caused by *Mycobacterium tuberculosis*. Previously, TB was one of the most common granulomatous diseases affecting the larynx. But with the development of antibiotics, laryngeal TB has become more uncommon, especially in developed countries. However, recently there has been a noted increase in the incidence of this disease in both developing and developed countries. This is thought to be due to the increasing number of patients with human immunodeficiency virus (HIV) infection and the emergence of multi-drug resistant mycobacterium. Also, in developed countries there has been a decrease in immunization for TB and an increasing immigration from countries with a high incidence of TB. A recent study by Shin et al[1] reported a changing trend in the patient population presenting with laryngeal TB. Their results show that the average age at the time of presentation is 42 years, older than that previously reported in the 1950s during which time the typical patient with laryngeal TB was 20 to 30 years old. They also reported a 2:1 male predominance in their patient population. The other significant finding in the Shin paper was the surprisingly low prevalence of active pulmonary TB in their patients with only 7 of 22 having active disease. This differs significantly with previous reports where laryngeal TB was almost always associated with advanced pulmonary disease.

The true pathogenesis of laryngeal TB is debated in the literature. There is a primary infection of the larynx in which the mycobacterial organisms directly infect the laryngeal mucosa in the absence of pulmonary disease. A secondary infection of the larynx may occur in several ways. The classically described pathway involves a patient with advanced pulmonary disease who subsequently inoculates the posterior larynx with infected sputum, resulting in laryngeal disease. Another mechanism is hematogenous or lymphatic drainage from affected tissues may seed the larynx. Most recent reports tend to favor the latter theory of pathogenesis in the current era of laryngeal TB, although primary cases of laryngeal disease have been reported. Shin et al[1] reported a 40% (9/22) incidence of primary laryngeal TB.

Clinical Presentation

Tuberculosis is often referred to as a masquerader as it can mimic carcinoma. The presenting symptoms can be identical to laryngeal carcinoma including hoarseness, odynophagia, dysphagia, cough, and weight loss. Indirect laryngoscopy can show a variety of lesions and can affect the supraglottis and glottis. The classically described posterior interarytenoid mucosal involvement seems to be less common as noted in the current literature. Instead, the most common sites of involvement include the true vocal folds, false vocal folds, and epiglottis. Shin et al[1] classified the types of lesions seen into four categories: nonspecific inflammatory, polypoid, white/ulcerative, and "ulcerofungative" lesions. Interestingly, they found that patients with active pulmonary disease tended to present with multiple lesions that were ulcerative in nature. Those patients without pulmonary disease typically presented with a single lesion that was nonspecific inflammatory in nature. This is a strong reminder to consider TB in the differential diagnosis of a patient presenting with what appears to be an early laryngeal carcinoma.

Evaluation and Testing

These cases rely on direct laryngoscopy and biopsy of affected tissues with appropriate staining for acid-fast bacilli. The specimen is also obtained to evaluate for the presence or absence of carcinoma. Other important tests needed when laryngeal TB is suspected include PPD testing, chest x-ray, and sputum cultures. Laryngeal histology is diagnostic showing caseating granulomas surrounded by pallisading epithelioid histocytes with lymphocytic infiltration and multinucleated giant cells. The differential diagnosis includes syphilis, sarcoidosis, Wegener's granulomatosis, cat-scratch disease, carcinoma, and fungal laryngitis. CT scans of the neck may also by helpful. The CT findings that are characteristic of laryngeal TB are bilateral involvement, thickening of the free margin of the epiglottis, and preservation of the pre-epiglottic/paraglottic spaces even in the presence of extensive mucosal involvement.[2,3]

Treatment

The standard treatment for laryngeal TB is long-term administration of multiple antituberculous medications with a general good prognosis. In Shin et al[1] the average time until resolution of laryngeal symptoms was 5.6 months, although several patients symptomatically improved within 1 to 2 months. The full scope of medical treatment for mycobacterial disease is beyond the scope of this chapter; the need for multiple drug therapy and the world-wide concern over emerging resistance should be noted.

BLASTOMYCOSIS

Epidemiology/Pathogenesis

Blastomycosis is a chronic pulmonary infection caused by the fungus *Blastomyces dermatitidis*. This organism is found in damp wooded areas and is endemic in the United States around the Great Lakes and the Mississippi and Ohio River valleys. Laryngeal involvement occurs in 2 to 5% of all cases.

Clinical Presentation

Patients may complain of severe hoarseness, cough, dysphagia, and dyspnea that has been present for many months. Typical laryngoscopy findings include erythematous granulomatous masses and/or exophytic bulky lesions with irregular borders involving the true vocal folds and occasionally the supraglottis. (see Figure 16–1). Advanced disease can present with vocal fold fixation. Like laryngeal TB, blastomycosis may also mimic carcinoma.

Evaluation and Testing

The diagnosis is made through direct laryngoscopy and biopsy of the tissue. Histopathologic examination will show caseating necrosis with an acute inflammatory infiltration and microabscesses. *Pseudoepitheliomatous hyperplasia* is characteristically seen in the laryngeal epithelium which can lead to a misdiagnosis of squamous cell carcinoma. Periodic acid-Schiff (PAS) and Gomori silver stains will show large broad-based budding yeast near the region of microabscesses. The chest x-ray is often normal and not helpful with the diagnosis.

Treatment

Blastomycosis is treated with either IV amphotericin-B or itraconazole for an average time of 6 months with good response. Surgical intervention is limited to biopsy or drainage of microabscesses as needed.

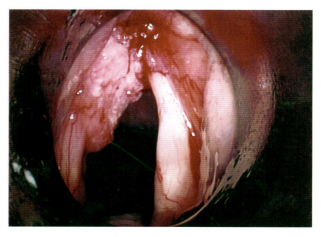

FIGURE 16–1. Blastomycosis affecting the larynx. The left membranous true vocal fold is the main site of involvement.

HISTOPLASMOSIS

Epidemiology/Pathogenesis

Histoplasmosis is caused by the dimorphic fungus *Histoplasma capsulatum* which is endemic to the Mississippi and Ohio River valleys. The mode of dissemination is via inhalation of spores from bird and bat feces. Symptoms at the time of the initial inoculation may be general and resemble a vague, flulike illness. Chronic pulmonary histoplasmosis can result in a disseminated form of the disease with hematogenous spread of the fungus which can ultimately involve the oral cavity, oropharynx, and larynx.

Clinical Presentation

The typical patient with laryngeal histoplasmosis is over 40 years of age and presents with symptoms of hoarseness, dysphagia, odynophagia, dyspnea, and hemoptysis. Patients may also present with painful oral cavity or oropharyngeal ulcerations. Indirect laryngoscopy may reveal a variety of lesions ranging from flat, white plaques to nodular granulomas that can eventually become ulcerative resulting in significant pain. The typical areas affected in the larynx with histoplasmosis include the true vocal folds, epiglottis, and false vocal folds.

Evaluation and Testing

Direct laryngoscopy with biopsy is necessary for diagnosis. Histopathology shows caseating granulomas with giant cells, lymphocytes, and large numbers of macrophages with intracellular yeast buds seen on PAS or Gomori methenamine silver stain. Chest x-ray may demonstrate pulmonary calcifications. Serology for *Histoplasma* antigen is generally not recommended for laryngeal histoplasmosis due to reported low sensitivities. The sensitivity varies with the severity and extent of the infection, with the greatest sensitivity seen in disseminated or acute diffuse pulmonary disease. Antigen detection is less useful in cases of subacute or chronic pulmonary disease and other manifestations of self-limited histoplasmosis, such as focal laryngeal histoplasmosis. The reported sensitivity in chronic pulmonary histoplasmosis ranges from 6 to14%.[4,5]

Treatment

The treatment for laryngeal histoplasmosis is oral itraconazole for 2 to 6 months with some protocols adding initial treatment with IV amphotericin-B. In general, the prognosis is good with complete resolution of the laryngeal disease.

SARCOIDOSIS

Epidemiology/Pathogenesis

Sarcoidosis is a chronic systemic granulomatous disease of unknown etiology. It is more prevalent in women and typically presents between the ages of 20 and 40. In the United States, it occurs more commonly in African-Americans and Hispanics. Various reports estimate the incidence of laryngeal involvement in sarcoidosis to be between 1 and 5%.[6-8] The pathogenesis of sarcoidosis is still unclear but it appears to be a host response to an unknown stimulus such as an infectious agent (*Mycobacteria* or *Propionibacteria* are two current putative causes) or in response to an environmental agent. Recently, several studies have shown a heightened T helper-1 immune response in patients with sarcoidosis.[9,10] It is unclear at this point whether this is a form of autoimmunity or rather an immunologic response to a previously described or undescribed stimulus.

Clinical Presentation

The most common presenting symptoms of laryngeal sarcoidosis are hoarseness, dysphagia, dyspnea, cough, and globus sensation. Typical laryngeal findings include pale, edematous mucosa with diffuse enlargement of the supraglottis particularly the epiglottis, aryepiglottic folds, arytenoids, and false vocal folds (see Figure 16–2). The true vocal folds are usually spared but the subglottis can be involved. Other head and neck signs of sarcoidosis may be present including parotid swelling and lymphoid hypertrophy. Vocal fold paralysis may be present, but always in association with mediastinal disease.

Evaluation and Testing

The diagnosis of laryngeal sarcoidosis is based on the typical supraglottic appearance and biopsy of the tissue. Histopathology demonstrates non-caseating granulomas and negative stains for fungus or acid-fast bacilli. The differential diagnosis includes tuberculosis, carcinoma, fungal laryngitis, amyloidosis, and radiation fibrosis. Other ancillary tests for systemic sarcoidosis include a chest x-ray, CBC, sedimentation rate, urine/serum calcium, protein electrophoresis, gallium-67 scan, and serum angiotensin-converting enzyme (ACE) levels. Abnormalities seen in systemic sarcoidosis include hilar lymphadenopathy on the chest x-ray, hypercalcemia, hypercalciuria, elevated gamma globulin, and inflammation in salivary and

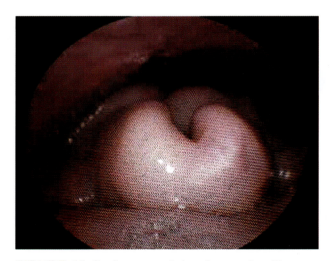

FIGURE 16–2. Laryngeal involvement with sarcoidosis; note the enlargement of the supraglottic structures.

lacrimal tissue on gallium scanning. Serum ACE levels are not useful for diagnostic purposes due to their low sensitivity; however, they can be useful to monitor the progression of the disease. Laryngeal sarcoidosis can occur in isolation with no systemic involvement and in one series occurred in 27% of the cases.[11]

Treatment

If the patient is currently asymptomatic or only mildly symptomatic, then close observation is reasonable. The mainstay of treatment for symptomatic laryngeal involvement is either systemic or intralesional steroids. In a review by Bower et al,[11] systemic steroids were very effective in the treatment of laryngeal sarcoidosis. In addition, intralesional steroid injections were found to be successful in selected patients with focal disease and no impending airway obstruction. A combination of both systemic and intralesional steroids were needed in a minority of patients. The precise indications for each of these treatments have yet to be defined. Other treatment options include tracheotomy for acute airway management, limited surgical resection, other cytotoxic medications, and low-dose external beam radiation. It is difficult to truly evaluate the efficacy of various treatments in laryngeal sarcoidosis because of the frequent spontaneous remissions that occur with this disease.

WEGENER'S GRANULOMATOSIS

Epidemiology/Pathogenesis

Wegener's granulomatosis (WG) is a systemic granulomatous disease of unknown etiology characterized by necrotizing granuloma and vasculitis involving the upper respiratory tract, lungs, and kidneys. Laryngeal involvement may occur in up to 23% of cases. Other areas of the head and neck, most notably the paranasal sinuses and the middle ear, are much more likely to be affected in WG.

Clinical Presentation

Patients with laryngeal involvement present with dyspnea and hoarseness. The main subsite of the larynx affected is the subglottis often resulting in severe subglottic stenosis. The clinical exam resembles that of idiopathic subglottic stenosis with no distinguishing characteristics. Other head and neck manifestations include recurrent sinusitis, septal perforation, saddle-nose deformity, and chronic serous otitis media.

Evaluation and Testing

Subglottic tissue biopsy is usually negative and not helpful in making the diagnosis. Patients should undergo direct microlaryngoscopy more for treatment than for diagnostic purposes. CT scans of the larynx and trachea may be helpful to determine the extent of the subglottic stenosis and the degree of cartilage involvement. Serology testing for antinuclear cytoplasmic antibodies (ANCA) is often helpful in making the diagnosis. There is a high specificity (more than 90%) with c-ANCA testing in Wegener's granulomatosis.[12] However, the sensitivity of c-ANCA depends on the extent of involvement and the current activity of the disease process. When a patient is in the granulomatous phase of this disease rather than the vasculitic phase, the sensitivity of this test is significantly lower. Also, p-ANCA testing can be positive in up to 20% of patients with WG.[13]

Treatment

If the patient is symptomatic from the subglottic stenosis, then treatment with surgical intervention is warranted. CO_2 laser incision with dilation and topical application of mitomycin-C and corticosteroids is the standard of care. It has been estimated that nearly 50% of all patients with WG will require a tracheotomy at some point in their disease process. Laryngotracheal reconstruction for those who fail endoscopic management is another option for treatment. Medical therapy is also warranted especially in patients with multi-organ involvement. Corticosteroids combined with cyclosporine or methotrexate are the only two regimens that have thus far been shown to induce remission of active WG affecting a major organ. Once remission has been induced, azathioprine and methotrexate have been used to maintain remission.

AMYLOIDOSIS

Epidemiology/Pathogenesis

Amyloidosis is an idiopathic dysproteinemia resulting in extracellular deposition of fibrillar proteins. It is not an inflammatory disorder in the traditional sense, but is included here as the clinical evaluation and decision-making are similar to

What if a Patient Doesn't Respond to Empiric Therapy?

Always consider other etiologies of laryngeal inflammation especially when a patient does not respond to empiric treatment. Many of these inflammatory diseases cannot be diagnosed without direct laryngeal examination and biopsy of the affected tissue. When something does not make sense, think of other less common etiologies in the differential diagnosis.

the other disorders presented in this chapter. This disease process may affect multiple organ systems; approximately 300 cases of laryngeal amyloidosis have been reported. Patients who present with laryngeal involvement often have no systemic signs of amyloidosis. There is equal distribution between males and females and the average age at the time of presentation is between the ages of 40 and 50.

Clinical Presentation

Patients with laryngeal amyloidosis present with symptoms of hoarseness, diplophonia, dyspnea, cough, hemoptysis, dysphagia, and globus sensation. Laryngoscopy reveals smooth although sometimes granular, pink/gray submucosal lesions. The lesions may even take on an orange hue. The site of laryngeal involvement varies with the most common site being the infraglottic aspect of the true vocal fold (Figure 16–3). Other sites of involvement include the ventricle, false vocal fold, aryepiglottic fold, and anterior subglottis.

Evaluation and Testing

Direct laryngoscopy with biopsy is necessary for diagnosis. The Congo red stain is diagnostic for

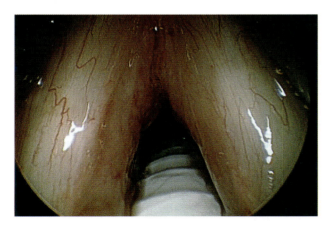

FIGURE 16–3. Laryngeal amyloidosis. The medial and infraglottic surfaces of the vocal folds are often involved.

amyloidosis showing apple-green birefringence with polarized light. Although the majority of patients with laryngeal amyloidosis do not have systemic disease, many authors still recommend a systemic workup to rule out other collagen vascular diseases, tuberculosis, and multiple myeloma. The differential diagnosis includes metastatic medullary thyroid cancer, laryngeal sarcoidosis, benign laryngeal polyps, carcinoma, benign minor salivary tumors, chondromas, neuroendocrine tumors, and lipoid proteinosis.

Treatment

Nondestructive surgical removal of amyloid deposits to restore laryngeal function is generally recommended in the literature. Dedo et al[14] showed that CO_2 laser excision of laryngeal amyloid deposits was effective in restoring vocal quality in a series of 10 patients with an average follow up of 6.5 years. There is no documented medical therapy which has been shown to be effective in isolated laryngeal amyloidosis.

OTHER SYSTEMIC INFLAMMATORY DISORDERS

Systemic lupus erythematosus (SLE) is an autoimmune collagen vascular disease that can present with laryngeal manifestations. The most commonly reported symptoms are hoarseness and dyspnea. Typical laryngoscopy findings include generalized vocal fold edema and/or ulcerations. Vocal fold paralysis and fixation have also been commonly reported. The histopathology is nonspecific. Urgent airway intervention such as a tracheotomy has been reported in some patients. Primary treatment of this disease is with medications such as steroids.

Rheumatoid arthritis (RA) is an autoimmune disorder resulting in polyarthropathy. Laryngeal involvement is not uncommon. The most common laryngeal finding is cricoarytenoid joint fixation, which may be present in as many as 25% of patients with generalized disease.[15] Other findings include rheumatoid nodules, which occur submucosally in the true vocal folds and result in decreased vibration of the vocal folds and dysphonia. Surgical removal of the nodules may be accomplished via a microflap approach, although this is controversial. One compelling recent publication has shed light on another clinical presentation in which the larynx is affected by RA, although not at the level of the larynx itself. Thompson reported on a series of patients with RA and vocal fold paralysis (some bilateral) due to cervicomedullary compression.[16] The site of compression was at the atlantoaxial joint and the skull base. All three patients in this paper had a long-standing history of RA and this did not represent a new diagnosis of the disease.

Relapsing polychondritis is a rare idiopathic autoimmune disease that causes cartilage inflammation. Laryngeal symptoms may include hoarseness, dyspnea, cough, stridor, pain, and sometimes hemoptysis. Laryngeal examination often reveals severe glottic and subglottic edema but no pathognomonic signs. Treatment is airway intervention as needed along with steroids and/or dapsone.

Review Questions

1. The following are true regarding patients with laryngeal amyloidosis:
   a. mean age at presentation is over 70 years of age
   b. predominantly female
   c. roughly 1 in 4 has systemic amyloidosis
   d. responds to medical therapy
   e. has a predilection for the subglottis

2. Laryngeal tuberculosis:
   a. occurs predominantly in young adults and the very old
   b. occurs predominantly in association with active pulmonary TB
   c. is becoming rarer
   d. is responsive to medication within several months
   e. none of the above

3. The most characteristic site of laryngotracheal involvement in sarcoidosis is:
   a. supraglottis
   b. anterior glottis
   c. posterior glottis
   d. subglottis
   e. trachea

4. A 45-year-old woman with a history of generalized rheumatoid arthritis presents with hoarseness of 4 months' duration. She is a nonsmoker. Her clinical examination reveals no stridor but she is moderately dysphonic. Videostroboscopy reveals a yellowish intracordal mass in the left vocal fold. It is transversely oriented. You also detect sluggish vocal fold motion on that side. Her skull base/neck/chest CT scan is unremarkable. You recommend:
   a. intralesional steroid injection
   b. microdirect laryngoscopy with excision of intracordal cyst and injection laryngoplasty at the same setting
   c. injection laryngoplasty
   d. laryngofissure with cyst excision
   e. trial of speech therapy followed by microdirect laryngoscopy with excision of intracordal cyst

5. A microbiological specimen taken from a larynx during direct laryngoscopy reveals several areas suspicious for cancer, though there is no definitive malignancy; special stains demonstrate broad-based budding yeast. The chest radiograph is negative. You suspect:
   a. carcinoma with bacterial superinfection
   b. carcinoma with fungal colonization
   c. disseminated Aspergillosis
   d. Blastomycosis of the larynx
   e. Sarcoidosis

REFERENCES

1. Shin JE, Nam SY, Yoo SY, et al. Changing trends in clinical manifestations of laryngeal tuberculosis. *Laryngoscope.* 2000;110:1950–1953.
2. Moon WK, Han MH, Chang KH, et al. Laryngeal tuberculosis: CT findings. *Am J Roentgenol.* 1996;166:445–449.
3. Kim MD, Kim DI, Yune HY, et al. CT findings of laryngeal TB: comparison to laryngeal carcinoma. *J Comput Assist Tomogr.* 1997;21:29–34.
4. Wheat LJ, Kohler RB, Tewari RP. Diagnosis of disseminated histoplasmosis by detection of *Histoplasma capsulatum* antigen in serum and urine specimens. *N Engl J Med.* 1986;314:83–88.
5. Williams B, Fojtasek M, Connolly–Stringfield P, et al. Diagnosis of histoplasmosis by antigen detection during an outbreak in Indianapolis, Ind. *Arch Path Lab Med.* 1994;118:1205–1208.
6. Devine KD. Sarcoidosis and sarcoidosis of the larynx. *Laryngoscope* 1965;75:533–569.
7. Krespi YP, Mitrani M, Husains S, et al. Treatment of laryngeal sarcoidosis with intralesional steroid injection. *Ann Otol Rhinol Laryngol.* 1987;96:713–715.
8. Ellison DE, Canalis RF. Sarcoidosis of head and neck. *Clin Dermatol.* 1986;44:136–141.
9. Robinson BW, McLemore TL, Crystal RG. Gamma interferon is spontaneously released by alveolar macrophages and lung T lymphocytes in patients with pulmonary sarcoidosis. *J Clin Invest.* 1985;75:1488–1495.
10. Moller DR, Forman JD, Liu MC, et al. Enhanced expression of IL-12 associated with Th1 cytokine profiles in active pulmonary sarcoidosis. *J Immunol.* 1996;156:4952–4960.
11. Bower JS, Belen JE, Weg JG, et al. Manifestations and treatment of laryngeal sarcoidosis. *Am Rev Respir Dis.* 1980;122:325–332.
12. Specks U, Wheatley CL, McDonald TJ. ANCA in the diagnosis and follow-up of Wegener's. *Mayo Clinic Proc.* 1989;64:28–39.
13. Gluth MB. Subglottic stenosis associated with Wegener's granulomatosis. *Laryngoscope.* 2003;113:1304–1307.
14. Dedo HH, Izdebski K. Laryngeal amyloidosis in 10 patients. *Laryngoscope.* 2004;114:1742–1746.
15. Montgomery WW. Cricoarytenoid arthritis. *Laryngoscope.* 1963;73:801–836.
16. Thompson-Link D, McCaffrey T V, Krauss WE, Link MJ, Ferguson MT. Cervicomedullary compression: an unrecognized cause of vocal cord paralysis in rheumatoid arthritis. *Ann Otol Rhinol Laryngol.* 1998;107(6):462–471.

17

Reflux and The Larynx

Riitta Ylitalo, MD, PhD

KEY POINTS

■ Detailed history and laryngoscopic examination constitute the basis for diagnosis of laryngeal and pharyngeal reflux (LPR). Fewer than 50% of patients with LPR will complain of heartburn.

■ Laryngoscopic examination will most commonly demonstrate findings in the posterior glottis and vocal folds.

■ Laboratory investigations include barium esophagography and ambulatory 24-hour pH probe; esophagoscopy is used to screen for complications related to GERD as well as for possible malignancy.

■ Acid suppression with proton pump inhibitors (PPI) on a long-term basis is the mainstay of treatment; a trial of PPIs may also be useful as a diagnostic maneuver.

Gastroesophageal reflux (GER) can be a normal physiologic phenomenon that occurs in most people, particularly after meals. Gastroesophageal reflux disease (GERD) develops when the reflux causes symptoms like heartburn and acid regurgitation, with or without esophagitis. Laryngopharyngeal reflux (LPR) happens when gastric contents pass the upper esophageal sphincter (UES) causing symptoms and tissue damage in the upper airway. All episodes of GER are not necessarily associated with LPR. Furthermore, the pattern of reflux is also different between LPR and GER patients. LPR occurs predominantly during the daytime in the upright position whereas GERD takes place more often in the, supine position. In fact, the patients may be quite different in terms of body habitus as well. Within the GI literature, reports have described the association[1,2] between obesity and GERD. In contrast, in a group of patients with laryngeal and pharyngeal symptoms, those with abnormal *pharyngeal* reflux events did not have a higher mean body-mass index (BMI) than those with normal studies.[3] A significantly higher percentage of *esophageal* reflux events was, however, seen in obese versus nonobese participants. The authors concluded that abnormal esophageal reflux (GERD) is associated with increasing BMI and obesity, although this was not true for patients with pharyngeal reflux.

It is estimated that up to 10% of patients visiting otolaryngology clinics have reflux-related disease, and up to 55% of patients with hoarseness have LPR.[4-6] Thus, LPR is considered one of the most important and common factors causing inflammation in the upper airways. The tissue damage—demonstrated in both animals and human beings—may be caused by direct exposure to acid, pepsin and bile, by vagally mediated reflexes,[7,8] or perhaps factors yet to be defined. The variance between esophageal symptoms/findings and upper aerodigestive tract disease may reflect the relative susceptibility of the laryngeal epithelium of the larynx and trachea/bronchi to reflux-related injury. LPR also occurs in healthy individuals without symptoms or laryngeal pathology but less frequently than in patients with reflux laryngitis.[9,10] Additionally, reflux-related laryngeal findings have been shown to have a slower resolution pattern and require higher medication levels than uncomplicated esophagitis. Reflux has been implicated in the pathogenesis of nearly all major categories of laryngeal disease, including stenosis, malignancy, benign lesions, dysphagia, and functional disorders.[4]

DIAGNOSIS

For the majority of otolaryngologists, the diagnosis of LPR begins with the history. It is then confirmed by laryngoscopy and subsequently validated by response to a trial of proton pump inhibitor therapy. Although some institutions do perform routine pH testing, for the majority of cases this testing is reserved for refractory or complicated cases.

Symptoms

In addition to hoarseness, the most common symptoms associated with LPR are cough, throat clearing, sore throat, globus, excess throat mucus, choking, and asthma. However, these entities have a multifactorial etiology and may be caused by recent sinusitis or other respiratory infections, smoking, voice abuse, and allergy, making the accurate diagnosis based on history a challenge. Belafsky et al developed the Reflux Symptom Index (RSI), a self-administered nine-item questionnaire to help categorize the severity of LPR (see Table 17–1). An RSI of greater than 13 is considered abnormal. Symptoms of GERD, which include heartburn, chest pain, indigestion or a regurgitation of acid, are important, but it should be noted that 50 to 80% of patients with LPR do not have these classic GERD symptoms.[11]

Laryngeal Examination

The most frequent laryngeal finding related to LPR is posterior laryngitis (PL) that occurs in up

TABLE 17–1. Reflux Symptom Index (RSI)[12] (A total score of 13 is thought to be clinically significant.)

Within the last month, how did the following problem affect you?	0—No Problem 5—Severe Problem					
1. Hoarseness or a problem with your voice	0	1	2	3	4	5
2. Clearing your throat	0	1	2	3	4	5
3. Excess throat mucus or postnasal drip	0	1	2	3	4	5
4. Difficulty swallowing food, liquid, or pills	0	1	2	3	4	5
5. Coughing after you eat or after lying down	0	1	2	3	4	5
6. Breathing difficulties or choking episodes	0	1	2	3	4	5
7. Troublesome or annoying cough	0	1	2	3	4	5
8. Sensations of something sticking in your throat or a lump in your throat	0	1	2	3	4	5
9. Heartburn, chest pain, indigestion, or stomach acid coming up	0	1	2	3	4	5

to 70% of LPR patients. It is characterized by edema or hypertrophy, and sometimes erythema and hyperemia on the posterior wall of the glottis. Occasionally the inflammation reaches up to the medial surface of the arytenoid cartilages and aryepiglottic folds. Most authors use the terms posterior laryngitis and reflux laryngitis synonymously, although this is not accurate. Furthermore, diffuse vocal fold edema, infraglottic edema reaching from the anterior commissure to the posterior wall, also referred to as *pseudosulcus*, and vocal fold granuloma are strongly associated with LPR (Figure 17-1). Of patients with pseudosulcus, 60 to 90% have LPR whereas 65% of granuloma patients are LPR positive. The nature of endolaryngeal mucus if it is thick and tenacious will also point to PL. Any or all of these findings can occur.[4] The difficulty in making a PL diagnosis is that the findings are sometimes quite subtle signs of inflammation and irritation and patients may display a quite normal looking larynx. Furthermore, it has been difficult to show any correlation between a sole laryngeal finding and the occurrence of hypopharyngeal reflux episodes.[10] As none of these findings alone is

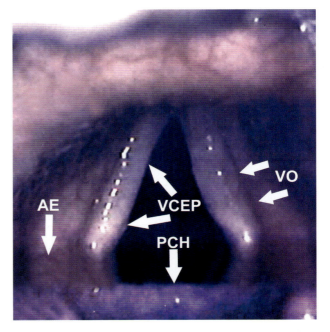

FIGURE 17–1. Magnified laryngoscopy showing some of the findings of reflux laryngitis with diffuse laryngeal edema, ventricular obliteration (*VO*), vocal fold edema and polypoid changes (*VCEP*), posterior wall hypertrophy (*PCH*), and arytenoid erythema (*AE*).

pathognomonic for LPR, a recently developed Reflux Finding Score (RFS) may be quite useful in categorizing the severity of the mucosal injury[13] (Table 17–2). Indeed, later work reported by Oelschlager described laryngoscopy as "complementary" to pH probe testing.[14] Patients both with significant scores on the RFS as well as positive pH probes were more likely to be responders to treatment than those with a low RFS.

In all suspected cases, endoscopic examination should include flexible or rigid laryngoscopy. As normal mucosa of the posterior glottis may look thickened during adduction, especially when the vocal folds are in the paramedian position, care should be taken to evaluate this part in full abduction. The evaluation of erythema is very dependent on the technical equipment, and should be limited to the estimation of color compared to that of the surrounding tissue.

On balance, findings on laryngoscopy are quite important and in fact predictive of clinical outcome in patients with the clinical diagnosis of LPR. A recent medical trial was published that reinforced the findings of Hanson et al years earlier[15]; in a prospective, double-blind-randomized, placebo-controlled study, two laryngeal findings—interarytenoid mucosal erythema and vocal fold abnormalities—were found to be predictive of symptomatic improvement following medical therapy.[16]

Empiric Trial of Acid Suppression as a Diagnostic Test

An empiric trial of PPI therapy over a prolonged period has been proposed as a valid diagnostic test for LPR. The typical regime is twice-a-day proton pump inhibitor (PPI) therapy for a duration of 1 to 4 months. This recommendation is based on the fact that we have not identified the specific symptom combination, or combination of symptoms and laryngeal signs, pathognomonic to LPR. Besides, ambulatory 24-hour double-probe pH measurement still has imperfect sensitivity and specificity, and is not available in all clinics. The prinicipal disadvantage of PPI therapy trial

TABLE 17–2. Reflux Finding Score (RFS)[13] (A total score of 7 is thought to be clinically significant.)

Subglottic Edema	2 = present 0 = absent
Ventricular Obliteration	2 = partial 4 = complete
Erythema/Hyperemia	2 = arytenoids only 4 = diffuse
Vocal Cord Edema	1 = mild 2 = moderate 3 = severe 4 = polypoid
Diffuse Laryngeal Edema	1 = mild 2 = moderate 3 = severe 4 = obstructing
Posterior Commissure Hypertrophy	1 = mild 2 = moderate 3 = severe 4 = obstructing
Granuloma/Granulation	2 = present 0 = absent
Thick Endolaryngeal Mucus	2 = present 0 = absent
	TOTAL

is its high cost, making some patients unwilling to engage in such a treatment trial, and possible placebo effect. However, the symptoms that do not improve after aggressive acid reduction therapy are unlikely to be caused by acid-related reflux.

DIAGNOSTIC STUDIES

pH Probe Testing

Although not perfect, at the present time pH probe testing is the best method of testing the presence of gastric refluxate in the area of the hypopharynx and larynx. The upper probe must be placed in a consistent zone at or above (2 cm) the functional upper esophageal sphincter (UES). This allows the lower probe to be placed

Controversy: Laryngoscopy in the Diagnosis of Reflux

Concerns have been raised by many authors regarding the significance of laryngoscopy and laryngeal findings in the support of the clinical diagnosis of reflux. Branski and colleagues[17] reported on a series of patients in whom reflux findings were scrutinized by five observers reviewing videotaped examinations. The conclusions of the paper were that significant variability exists in describing reflux-attributable findings. This paper has been cited while criticizing the assertion that physical examination of the larynx is an unpredictable diagnostic tool for the clinical evaluation of LPR. The study's limitations are important to note, however. First of all, the patients mostly complained of dysphonia—in fact, half of the subjects had vocal lesions on examination. It should not be surprising that a great deal of variability was found in assessment of reflux findings; this was not the primary source of laryngeal abnormality in most of these patients.

Perhaps the most cited paper in this arena came from Hicks and colleagues at the Cleveland Clinic.[30] In this important study, 100 "normal" subjects underwent laryngoscopy; their examinations were then reviewed by otolaryngologists and speech-language pathologists to estimate the presence of "reflux-attributable" lesions in these healthy volunteers. The key finding in this study, that nearly 80% of "normals" were found to have an interarytenoid bar or posterior commissure hypertrophy—helped to shed light on the possible insignificance of this one finding. Unfortunately, this revelation has been taken by many to be an indication that laryngoscopy in general is not useful in the clinical evaluation of reflux disease. Important findings, such as arytenoid erythema and vocal fold changes, continue to be valuable in the evaluation and treatment of LPR.

approximately 5 cm above the lower esophageal sphincter (LES). Normal pH values for the distal esophagus have been well established in the gastroenterology literature although there is still disagreement regarding pH values for the hypopharynx. A reflux *event* is currently defined as a fall in hypopharyngeal pH to less than 4.0 with a simultaneous drop to 4 or below in the distal esophagus. Acid exposure time (AET, percentage of time pH <4) is calculated as the frac-

tion of time below this level at a given probe site. At the upper probe, an AET greater than 0.01% total, 0.02% upright, or 0% supine has been reported to be pathologic. This limit may be reached during one reflux event in the 24-hour period[17] (Table 17–3). One area of controversy, however, stems from the activity of pepsin at different pH levels. Pepsin has been shown to retain activity at a pH of 5.0, suggesting that a threshold at pH 5.0 may be more valid[5] when assessing

TABLE 17–3. Ambulatory pH Measurements at Upper Probe in Patients with LPR Involved in Controlled Studies (n = 529)*

Authors	Year	Probe Level	No. of Patients and Sex	Reflux Events			Acid Exposure Time		
				No. Positive	Range	Mean	Range (s)	Range (min)	Mean %
Koufman[4]	1991	2 cm above UES	88 (NR)	44/88	NR	NR	NR	NR	NR
Shaker et al[9]	1995	2 cm above UES	14 (NR)	12/14	0–27	4.36	0–1,296	0–12.97	0.24
Toohill et al[19] and Ulualp et al[20]	1998 & 1999	2 cm above UES	12 (7M, 5F)	8/12	0–12	2.42	0–104	0–1.74	0.009
Kuhn et al[21]	1998	2 cm above UES	11 (2M, 9F)	7/11	0–9	2.30	0–216	0–3.6	0.07
Ulualp et al[22]	1999	2 cm above UES	20 (13M, 7F)	15/20	0–12	2.65	0–536	0–8.9	0.13
Ulualp et al[23]	1999	2 cm above UES	11 (NR)	7/11	0–12	2.64	0–605	0–10.1	0.01
Ylitalo et al[10]	2001	1 cm above UES	26 (14M, 12F)	18/26	0–26	1.50	0–1,050	0–17.5	0.034
Eubanks et al[24]	2001	1.5–2 cm above UES	222 (86M, 136F)	90/222	0–36	NR	NR	NR	NR
Oelschlager et al[25]	2002	1.5–2 cm above UES	76 (NR)	32/76	NR	3.4	NR	NR	NR
Loehrl et al[26]	2002	2 cm above UES	12 (NR)	9/12	NR	NR	NR	NR	NR
Powitzky et al[27]	2003	2 cm above UES	37 (NR)	29/37	0–47	6.9	NR	NR	NR

NR: sex not recorded by author, UES: upper esophageal sphincter
*Reprinted with permission from Merati et al.[18]

the clinical presence or absence of pathologic reflux. A patient with a pH above 4 at times during the study may have a "negative" or normal study, though the pepsin in that patient's refluxate maintains noxious and damaging activity in their pharynx, larynx, and esophagus. Indeed, up to 20 to 30% of patients with PL may have a negative pH study, but this also does not rule out reflux as the causative factor. Esophageal single-probe pH monitoring does not identify patients with pharyngeal reflux, but patients with abnormal esophageal acid exposure are three times more likely to have LPR than those with normal esophageal monitoring.

Esophageal Manometry

Esophageal manometry is particularly important for the accurate placement of pH probes. Another indication in reflux patients is preoperative assessment of those being considered for antireflux surgery if there is any question of alternative or confounding esophageal disease, especially achalasia or profound dysmotility. As a solitary test for the presence or absence of reflux, it is not accurate enough. It may be important in the postoperative assessment of lower esophageal function following antireflux surgery, particularly in combination with radiographic studies and endoscopy.

Esophagoscopy

Endoscopic examination of the esophagus, either by traditional sedated or nonsedated trans-nasal techniques (TNE), is generally used to screen complications related to GERD, or to exclude other diseases. Thus, it is performed to diagnose esophagitis or hiatal hernia, to screen for Barrett's esophagus, and to exclude other diseases or complications (esophageal cancer, peptic strictures) that may be detected on endoscopy. Indications for endoscopy may include dysphagia, bleeding, and weight loss, especially when patient history reveals smoking and alcohol abuse. Esophagoscopy alone, however, does not diagnose LPR. Esophagitis occurs in fewer than 20% of patients with LPR, whereas Barrett's esophagus is rare (<10%). It is the minority of patients with LPR, therefore, that have abnormal esophagoscopy.

Radiographic Imaging: Esophagography

The esophagram is an inexpensive and convenient technique used to detect significant deglutition or esophageal abnormalities that may otherwise be overlooked. It may be used to evaluate GERD patients with hiatal hernia, strictures, and esophageal rings. However, this examination is relatively insensitive in the evaluation of reflux. It is a short procedure that is noninvasive, requires no more than 30 minutes to perform and available in most clinical units.[28]

TREATMENT

The therapeutic approaches for LPR include lifestyle modifications, acid suppressive medications, and surgical therapy. Lifestyle modifications include elevation of the head of the bed, decreased intake of fat, citrus, tomato, chocolate, caffeine, and alcohol, cessation of smoking, and avoiding recumbancy and further eating 3 hours before bedtime. These measures are helpful if there is associated abnormal esophageal acid exposure. If only LPR is present these measures may be less meaningful because pharyngeal reflux occurs most often in upright position during the daytime. Although Hanson described a 50% response rate to these measures alone in patients with chronic laryngitis,[29] there is minimal supportive data on the efficacy of these measures in LPR.

Medical acid suppression is the most important and common method of treatment. Proton-pump inhibitors are the most widely used drugs for the treatment of reflux. They maintain a potent and consistent effect on gastric acid secretion with few adverse effects. Comparisons between the five available compounds (omeprazole, rabeprazole, lansoprazole, esomeprazole, and pantoprazole) show that they have a similar antisecretory potency on a milligram basis. Treatment recommendation at present is twice-daily dosing of PPIs for at least 3 to 4 months. Symptoms frequently improve before the laryngoscopic findings resolve. It should be kept in mind that, even if the pH is elevated with antireflux medication, reflux itself continues, meaning pharynx and larynx are still exposed to bile, pepsin, and other gastric contents. All available H2 receptor antagonists (H_2RA)—cimetidine, ranitidine, famotidine, and nizatidine—all inhibit acid secretion equally when taken in equipotent doses. They have a low incidence of side effects and are less expensive as compared to proton pump inhibitors (PPI). There has been some renewed interest in the H2 blockers as an adjunct to PPI treatment. A recent study by Park et al, however, failed to show any added benefit to the addition of H2 blockers to a regime of twice-daily PPIs in patients with laryngeal and pharyngeal complaints.[16]

Surgical Treatment

A complete description of the surgical management of reflux is beyond the scope of this chapter. The dominant procedure for the operative management of reflux disease continues to be the Nissen fundoplication. In this procedure, the fundus of the stomach is wrapped around the LES to provide a snug, mechanical antireflux barrier. It is most commonly performed laparascopically, and is referred to as a "laparoscopic Nissen fundoplication" (LNF). It should be considered in patients who obtain only partial relief from medications, or in those who prefer operative management to the possibility of long-term or even a lifetime of PPI treatment. Prior to embarking on a surgical intervention, the reasons for failure of medical acid suppression in some patients should be considered. In patients with good control of classic GER or LPR symptoms, fundoplication may be an option. In patients who do not respond to medication, their ongoing inflammation may be due to volume reflux of nonacidic entities, as noted above. These include pepsin and bile reflux. This group of patients may indeed respond to a laproscopic Nissen fundoplication, with reported success rates as high as 90%.[30] Operative management of LPR has not, however, been widely accepted.

The reflux of gastric and duodenal contents into the upper aerodigestive tract is common and is an important source of laryngeal disease. Fewer than 50% of patients present with heartburn; symptoms such as dysphonia, dysphagia, throat clearing, and even globus sensation are more typical. Laryngeal findings on examination are important and may be predictive of treatment outcome.

The variability of patient presentations and response to treatment may reflect the differences in cellular tissue response to injury as well as the presence of nonacidic injurious agents such as bile.

Empiric therapy with twice-daily proton-pump inhibitors is a reasonable initial step in the management of suspected laryngopharyngeal reflux. Long-term PPI treatment appears to be safe for the vast majority of patients. Nissen fundoplication has no role in the initial treatment of LPR although it may be highly beneficial in selected patients.

Review Questions

1. A 45-year-old male has been on PPI for 1 month with little clinical response; he stops taking his medication following a "negative" pH probe study. His LPR symptoms worsen. You ask the patient to resume the medical regime because:
   a. pH probe testing is not reliable
   b. the patient has not had an adequate length of treatment
   c. it will sterilize his oral flora
   d. surgery is not an option for a 45-year-old male.

2. The patient with a diagnosis of reflux laryngitis will:
   a. Not have an associated problem with gastroesophageal reflux disease (GERD)
   b. Have associated GERD in 20% of cases
   c. Have associated GERD in 50% of cases
   d. Have associated GERD in 95% of cases

3. When 24-hour ambulatory pH probe testing is preformed in patients with reflux laryngitis a positive result is:
   a. At least 10 hypopharyngeal events at pH 6 or below
   b. Acid exposure time of greater than 60 seconds per 24 hours
   c. A single drop in the pH below 5
   d. Acid exposure time (AET) of more than 0.01% at the upper probe.

4. Successful treatment for most LPR patients consists of:
   a. Proton-pump inhibitors
   b. Lifestyle modifications
   c. H2 blockers
   d. endoscopic cricopharyngeal myotomy
   e. a and b

REFERENCES

1. Smith KJ, O'Brien SM, Smithers BM, et al. Interactions among smoking, obesity, and symptoms of acid reflux in Barrett's esophagus. *Cancer Epidemiol Biomarkers Prev.* 2005;14(11 pt 1): 2481-2486.
2. Stein DJ, El-Serag HB, Kuczynski J, Kramer JR, Sampliner RE. The association of body mass index with Barrett's oesophagus. *Aliment Pharmacol Ther.* 2005;22(10):1005-1010.
3. Halum SL, Postma GN, Johnston C, Belafsky PC, Koufman JA. Patients with isolated laryngopharyngeal reflux are not obese. *Laryngoscope.* 2005; 115(6):1042-1045.
4. Koufman JA. The otolaryngologic manifestations of gastroesophageal reflux disease (GERD): a clinical investigation of 225 patients using ambulatory 24-hour pH monitoring and an experimental investigation of the role of acid and pepsin in the development of laryngeal injury. *Laryngoscope.* 1991;101:1-78.
5. Koufman JA. Aviv JE, Casiano RR, Shaw GY. Laryngopharyngeal reflux: position statement of the committee on speech, voice, and swallowing disorders of the American Academy of Otolaryngology-Head and Neck Surgery. *Otolaryngol Head Neck Surg.* 2002;127:32-35.
6. Ulualp SO, Toohill RJ. Laryngopharyngeal reflux, state of the art diagnosis and treatment. *Otolaryngol Clin North Am.* 2000;33(4):785-801.
7. Shaker R, Hogan WJ, Normal physiology of the aerodigestive tract and its effect on the upper gut. *Am J Med.* 2003;115(suppl 3A):2S-9S.
8. Shaker R, Dodds WJ, Ren J, Hogan WJ, Arndorfer RC. Esophagoglottal closure reflex: a mechanism of airway protection. *Gastroenterology.* 1992; 102(3):857-861.
9. Shaker R, Milbrath M, Ren J, et al. Esophagopharyngeal distribution of refluxed gastric acid in patients with reflux laryngitis. *Gastroenterology.* 1995;109:1575-1582.
10. Ylitalo R, Lindestad PA, Ramel S. Symptoms, laryngeal findings, and 24-hour pH monitoring in patients with suspected gastroesophago-pharyngeal reflux. *Laryngoscope.* 2001;111:1735-1741.
11. Belafsky PC, Postma GN, Koufman JA. Laryngopharyngeal reflux symptoms improve before changes in physical findings. *Laryngoscope.* 2001;111:979-981.
12. Belafsky PC, Postma GN, Koufman JA. Validity and reliability of the reflux symptom index (RSI). *J Voice.* 2002;16(2):274-277.
13. Belafsky PC, Postma GN, Koufman JA. The validity and reliability of the Reflux Finding Score (RFS). *Laryngoscope.* 2001;111:1313-1317.
14. Oelschlager BK, Eubanks TR, Maronian N, et al. Laryngoscopy and pharyngeal pH are complementary in the diagnosis of gastroesophageal-laryngeal reflux. *J Gastrointest Surg.* 2002;6(2): 189-194.
15. Hanson DG, Jiang J, Chi W. Quantitative color analysis of laryngeal erythema in chronic posterior laryngitis. *J Voice.* 1998;12(1):78-83.
16. Park W. Hicks DM, Khandwala F, et al. Laryngopharyngeal reflux: prospective cohort study evaluating optimal dose of proton-pump inhibitor therapy and pretherapy predictors of response. *Laryngoscope.* 2005;115(7):1230-1238.
17. Branski RC, Bhattacharyya N, Shapiro J. The reliability of the assessment of endoscopic laryngeal findings associated with laryngopharyngeal reflux disease. *Laryngoscope.* 2002;112(6):1019-1024.
18. Merati AL, Lim HJ, Ulualp SO, Toohill RJ. Meta-analysis of upper probe measurements in normal subjects and patients with laryngopharyngeal reflux. *Ann Otol Rhinol Laryngol.* 2005;114: 177-182.
19. Toohill RJ, Ulualp SO, Shaker R. Evaluation of gastroesophageal reflux in patients with laryngotracheal stenosis. *Ann Otol Rhinol Laryngol.* 1998; 107:1010-1014.
20. Ulualp SO, Toohill RJ, Shaker R. Pharyngeal acid reflux in patients with single and multiple otolaryngologic disorders. *Otolaryngol Head Neck Surg.* 1999;121:725-730.
21. Kuhn, J, Toohill, RJ, Ulualp SO, et al. Pharyngeal acid reflux events in patients with vocal cord nodules. *Laryngoscope.* 1998;108:1146-1149.
22. Ulualp SO, Toohill RJ, Hoffmann R, Shaker R. Pharyngeal pH monitoring in patients with posterior laryngitis. *Otolaryngol Head Neck Surg.* 1999; 120:672-677.
23. Ulualp SO, Toohill RJ, Hoffmann R, Shaker R. Possible relationship of gastroesophagopharyngeal acid reflux with pathogenesis of chronic sinusitis. *Am J Rhinol.* 1999;13:197-202.
24. Eubanks TR, Omelanczuk PE, Maronian N, Hillel A, Pope CE 2nd, Pellegrini CA. Pharyngeal pH monitoring in 222 patients with suspected laryngeal reflux. *J Gastrointest Surg.* 2001;5(2): 183-190.

25. Oelschlager BK, Eubanks TR, Maronian N, et al. Laryngoscopy and pharyngeal pH are complementary in the diagnosis of gastroesophageal-laryngeal reflux. *J Gastrointest Surg.* 2002;6(2):189–194.

26. Loehrl TA, Smith TL, Darling RJ, et al. Autonomic dysfunction, vasomotor rhinitis, and extraesophageal manifestations of gastroesophageal reflux. *Otolaryngol Head Neck Surg.* 2002;126(4):382–387.

27. Powitzky ES, Khaitan L, Garrett CG, Richards WO, Courey M. Symptoms, quality of life, videolaryngoscopy, and twenty-four-hour triple-probe pH monitoring in patients with typical and extraesophageal reflux. *Ann Otol Rhinol Laryngol.* 2003;112(10):859–865.

28. Kuhn JC, Massick D, Toohill RJ. *Role of the Esophagram in the Management of Dysphonia.* Presented at the Middle Section Triological Society; Kansas City, Missouri; January 24–26, 1997.

29. Hanson DG, Kamel PL, Kahrilas PJ. Outcomes of antireflux therapy for the treatment of chronic laryngitis. *Ann Otol Rhinol Laryngol.* 1995;104(7):550–555.

30. Lindstrom DR, Wallace J, Loehrl TA, Merati AL, Toohill RJ. Nissen fundoplication surgery for extraesophageal manifestations of gastroesophageal reflux (EER). *Laryngoscope.* 2002;112:1762–1765.

31. Hicks DM, Ours TM, Abelson TI, Vaezi MF, Richter JE. The prevalence of hypopharynx findings associated with gastroesophageal reflux in normal volunteers. *J Voice.* 2002;16(4):564–579.

18

Benign Lesions of the Larynx

Timothy D. Anderson, MD

KEY POINTS

■ As terminology of laryngeal lesions is inconsistent, a detailed description of the lesion is generally more informative than a diagnostic term with different meanings to various clinicians.

■ Diagnosis and management of benign laryngeal lesions require assessment of the underlying cause, the patients' vocal habits and needs, as well as laryngeal mechanics and structure.

■ Most patients with benign vocal fold lesions should undergo evaluation and treatment by a speech therapist prior to contemplation of surgical therapy.

■ Vocal fold scar currently has no reliability effective treatment. In patients who require microlaryngeal surgery, vocal fold scarring can be avoided by minimizing operative trauma and pursuing preoperative speech therapy to prevent abusive voice behaviors postoperatively.

■ Videostroboscopy can be extremely useful in the diagnosis and documentation of vocal fold lesions. Some diagnoses, most notably vocal fold scar, can only be made with the aid of stroboscopy. Documentation of the preoperative vibratory status of the vocal fold is important for guiding expectations of surgical results.

Benign laryngeal lesions are common problems. Most are evaluated due to voice changes; an accurate diagnosis and appropriate management are required to restore the voice. Many patients can be successfully managed without operative intervention. The most important step in successful management is to determine why the patient developed a voice problem in the first place. Without a clear understanding of the underlying factors contributing to the development of a benign laryngeal lesion, recurrence, poor surgical results, persistent voice problems are common. The general principles of evaluation and management of benign laryngeal growths are discussed first, followed by specific information regarding the most common lesions.

VOCAL TRAUMA

Vocal trauma is the most common cause of benign laryngeal lesions.[1] *Vocal fold nodules* are the most obvious example. Virtually all vocal nodules will resolve with changes in vocal use patterns. If the traumatic voice behaviors are not addressed prior to surgery, the patient will continue to abuse the voice in the postoperative period. At best, the nodules will recur. At worst, the patient will develop dense vocal fold scar and be permanently hoarse.

Given the high incidence of traumatic vocal behaviors in patients with benign vocal fold lesions, most patients with these problems should undergo evaluation and management by a speech-language therapist before surgery is contemplated.[2,3] Many patients will have adequate voice improvement with speech therapy alone and will not require surgery.[4,5] Patients who still require surgery will be better prepared for the postoperative recovery process and their surgical results will be better due to less trauma during the delicate early healing process.

DIAGNOSIS

Although visualization of the larynx is important in the diagnosis of laryngeal pathology, the history and complete otolaryngologic examination should be considered an essential part of the diagnostic process. Careful attention to voice use patterns, the sound of the voice, the history of the voice problem, and other symptoms or medical problems almost always reveals the diagnosis before examination of the larynx. Laryngeal examination then confirms the clinical suspicion. Laryngeal examination should not be confined to anatomy, but must also take into account voice use patterns and evaluate for the presence and severity of hyperfunctional voice disorders, reflux, and so forth. Video recording of the examination is helpful for patient counseling and medicolegal documentation and allows detailed review of the examination in challenging cases. Stroboscopy is the only widely available technique to evaluate the vibratory function of the vocal folds and is therefore extremely useful. Some diagnoses, such as diffuse vocal fold scar, can only be accurately diagnosed by stroboscopic examination. In many cases of benign vocal fold masses, determination of the degree of vocal fold stiffness can have important prognostic significance (see chapter 3, Videostroboscopy).

CLASSIFICATION

Diagnosis and treatment of benign laryngeal lesions depends on a detailed knowledge of vocal fold anatomy, as well as a clear understanding of the implications of the layered microstructure of the vocal folds. Hirano's description of the layered structure of the vocal fold is central to the surgical techniques of modern laryngology.[6] The relative paucity of fibroblasts in the superficial layer of the lamina propria (SLP) is thought to allow surgical disruption of this plane with relatively little postoperative scarring. Interwoven collagen fibrils and copious fibroblasts make the vocal ligament (deep layers of the lamina propria) a source of dense scar when surgically injured. Surgical results for lesions of the superficial layer of the lamina propria are generally excellent (polyps and nodules), as these do not result in a severe disruption or loss of SLP. Surgery for pathology that results in great disruption of the SLP (cysts and Reinke's edema) is less likely to produce perfect voices. Lesions involving the deep layer (sulcus vocalis) or all layers (vocal fold scar, invasive carcinoma) are surgical challenges and should be approached with trepidation given the risks of permanent vocal fold scar and impaired voice.

Several categorization schemes have been used to classify benign laryngeal lesions, all of which have some merit.[7-9] Anatomic descriptors have the advantage of clear pathologic correlations and knowledge of the location of lesions in the vocal fold microstructure has important surgical implications. Unfortunately, anatomic descriptions alone fail to consider causative factors that can be essential in proper management of benign laryngeal lesions. Anatomy also fails to consider the time course and differential expression of a single process—pathology of an acute hemorrhage, posthemorrhagic polyp, dilated ectatic vessel, and resolved hemorrhage with scar will all obviously be quite different, although they are all different aspects of a single pathophysiologic process. Categorization by cause of lesion is similarly flawed, as many "causes" are unproven or speculative and groupings are often arbitrary.

Nomenclature of Laryngeal Lesions

Unfortunately, a universally accepted terminology for benign laryngeal masses does not exist. Several attempts have been made to standardize the terminology by using videostroboscopic, pathologic, anatomic, or clinical behavior, but all have suffered from limitations that have prevented widespread acceptance.[7-9] When communicating with other otolaryngologists, adjectives describing the location and appearance of a lesion are generally preferred over arbitrary and frequently misunderstood labels. Similarly, published papers must be carefully read to determine what definitions are being used in order to properly evaluate techniques and results.

Terminology of Benign Laryngeal Lesions

Generally Accepted Terms	Terms with Varying Definitions
Sulcus vocalis	Nodule
Vocal fold scar	Polyp
Acute hemorrhage	Mass
Mucus retention cyst	Pseudocyst
Epithelial cyst	Granuloma
Papilloma	Varix
Reinke's edema	Edema
Polypoid degeneration	
Vascular ectasia	

Vascular Abnormalities

Acute Hemorrhage

Acute hemorrhage is an uncommon, but potentially devastating, problem that occurs due to trauma and rupture of a submucosal vessel. Bright red blood accumulates in the lamina propria, causing deformations of vocal fold shape, decreasing vibratory wave propagation, and leading to rapid hoarseness (Figure 18–1). Vocal trauma is frequently cited as the inciting cause, with singing, crying, screaming, and coughing most often reported.[10,11] Singers will often report that their voice becomes hoarse between notes. If the time to evaluation is delayed, the initial bright red color will often fade to shades of yellow and green as the hemoglobin is broken down, similar to bruising in other locations. At the time of acute hemorrhage, vocal fold vasculature is generally obscured by the submucosal blood and can only be seen after the hemorrhage begins to resolve.

Acute vocal fold hemorrhage seems to be more common in women than men and has been reported to be more common in the premenstrual period, although supporting data are weak. Use of blood thinners, including aspirin and ibuprofen, has also been implicated.[11,12] Some patients will suffer recurrent hemorrhage and may present with evidence of both acute and chronic

areas of hemorrhage. Many of these patients will have an abnormal appearance of the vocal fold vascularity. This can take the form of dilated capillaries (ectasia) or blebs in the vessels. Weak vessel walls may rupture more easily, while vessels that are not in the longitudinal axis of the vocal fold are exposed to massive shearing forces during vibration. Normal vessels in the vocal fold run predominately along the length of the vocal fold and are generally quite narrow.

Acute vocal fold hemorrhage is generally treated conservatively. Patients are generally kept on complete voice rest (no talking or singing for any reason) for at least a week. Cough should be treated aggressively with suppressants and use of anticoagulant medications minimized.[11,12] Many over-the-counter cold medications contain salicylates, and patients should be warned about these medications as well. Herbal remedies, including ginko and garlic, have blood-thinning properties and should be avoided.[13,14] The value of voice rest in subacute hemorrhage is unclear. High-level voice professionals should probably be advised to pursue a course of voice rest to maximize the chances of full recovery. Patients with less demanding voice requirements can frequently be observed, especially if they are already improving and have no evidence of incipient complications. Except in very unusual cases, there is no role for surgery in acute hemorrhage.

Posthemorrhagic Masses

Posthemorrhagic masses are red-brown masses that can occur anywhere on the vocal fold. They range from very small, sessile swellings (Figures 18–2 and 18–3) to huge, pedunculated masses. The pedunculated masses frequently ball-valve into the larynx during inspiration, causing intermittent periods of severe hoarseness when the mass is between the vocal folds alternating with periods of relatively normal voice when they move laterally above the vibratory edge of the vocal fold. There is almost always stiffness of the affected vocal fold, although preoperative stroboscopy is frequently difficult to interpret due to the damping effect of the masses and their interference with glottic closure and vocal fold

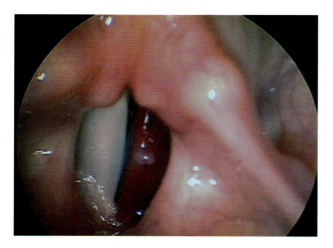

FIGURE 18–1. Acute left vocal fold hemorrhage.

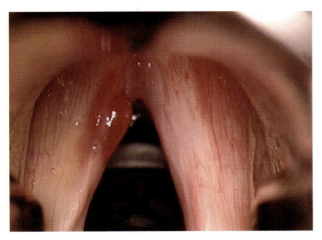

FIGURE 18–2. Small, broad-based, posthemorrhagic mass.

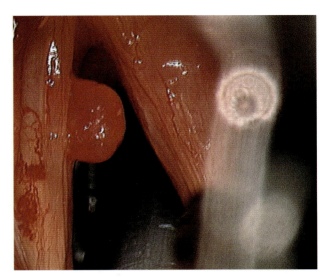

FIGURE 18–4. Posthemorrhagic mass with multiple vascular ectasias on superior surface of vocal fold.

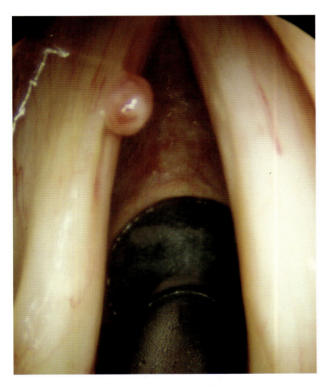

FIGURE 18–3. Small, broad-based, posthemorrhagic mass with underlying sulcus vocalis.

entrainment. With large masses, it is sometimes difficult to see any part of the vocal fold or even to determine which side is affected. Occasionally, posthemorrhagic masses can appear to be a

purplish submucosal cyst with surrounding edema. Abnormal vessels can frequently be seen in the region of the masses (Figure 18–4).

Posthemorrhagic masses likely form due to coalescence of clot from acute hemorrhage due to continued vocal fold use. Clot consolidation and contraction, damage of the gel-like lamina propria, inflammation from the clotting cascade, and macrophage activation all contribute to both scar formation and development of vocal fold masses. Once mature, these masses rarely involute, even with aggressive nonoperative therapy.

Treatment of posthemorrhagic masses is generally surgical. Preoperative speech therapy is helpful to minimize postoperative vocal trauma, but rarely results in significant voice improvement. Unfortunately, posthemorrhagic masses are generally associated with other vocal fold trauma, stiffness, and scarring, so surgery rarely results in perfect voice. However, as most patients have a severely disordered voice preoperatively, marked postoperative voice improvement is usually seen. Many surgeons advocate treating the abnormal vessels at the time of surgery to prevent recurrent hemorrhage.[15,16] Many techniques have been proposed, including CO_2 laser ablation, pulsed dye laser treatment, and resection of abnormal vessels. No randomized studies have evaluated any of these practices, but expert opinion supports their approaches.[15,16] Treatment of abnormal vascularity has also been recommended for patients with recurrent acute hemorrhages, with anecdotal supporting evidence.

Vascular Tumors

Occasional vascular tumors have been reported in the larynx, and generally have a very similar appearance to posthemorrhagic masses (Figure 18–5). Onset is generally chronic, although they can occasionally be associated with hemoptysis or airway obstruction. Erythematous masses involving the supraglottis or subglottis, or evidence of deep vocal fold involvement, should be approached cautiously, as the visible portion may be only a small portion of the entire mass. Workup for suspected vascular tumors should include a computed tomography (CT) and/or magnetic resonance imaging (MRI) to define the extent and vascularity of the lesion. Most vascular tumors are benign and can generally be cured if completely resected. Biopsy can result in massive hemorrhage and should be conducted under controlled circumstances.

Lesions Resulting from Overuse, Misuse, or Vocal Trauma

Transient, Mild Edema

Patients will frequently develop complaints of mild hoarseness that persists for several hours to days after vigorous voice use. Symptoms generally slowly abate with voice rest, but recur after the next performance, presentation, or conversation in a loud, smoky bar. When patients are examined while symptomatic, they generally give an impression of redundant contact of the vocal folds in the midportion during vibration. Rapid inspiration may result in subtle rounding of the vocal folds, suggesting mild increase in the volume of the lamina propria. Muscle tension dysphonia is almost always present, although singers will occasionally manifest mild postperformance edema despite excellent technique. Treatment generally includes reassurance and speech therapy to decrease hyperfunctional voice behaviors and improve vocal hygiene. In addition, reasonable voice use duration should be discussed with the patient. Some adults expect to sing for 1.5 hours for 2 sessions on a Friday, 3 sessions on a Saturday, followed by 3 sessions on a Sunday. Some patients cannot endure this grueling activity level and must learn reasonable voice expectations.

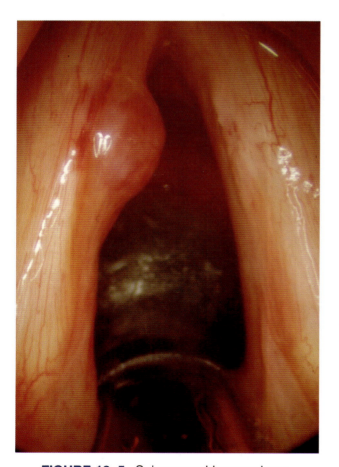

FIGURE 18–5. Submucosal hemangioma.

Vocal Nodules

Vocal nodules are symmetric masses that occur at the junction between the anterior and middle thirds of the vocal folds; this corresponds roughly to the midpoint of the musculomembranous vocal fold. They will frequently be the only area of contact between the vocal folds during soft phonation (Figure 18-6). There is generally little stiffness underlying these lesions, yet they do interfere with vibration. Nodules form at the region of maximal excursion of the vocal fold epithelium during vibration. These lesions generally involve the superficial lamina propria and epithelium, but do not involve the deeper layers. If aggressive vocal trauma persists, these lesions can evolve into relatively symmetric, firm large vocal fold nodules (Figure 18-7).

Patients with vocal fold nodules are characterized as outgoing, loud talkers with aggressive glottal attacks. The typical nodule patient is irrepressibly talkative with loud, pressed phonation.[17] The voice ranges from coarse and raspy to fuzzy. Singers with vocal fold nodules frequently complain of breaks in the passagio. Fibrotic masses, cysts, and other lesions are commonly misdiagnosed as nodules. Vocal fold nodules are bilateral; unilateral nodules, by definition, do not occur.

Vocal nodules almost always resolve with reduction in the underlying hyperkinetic voice behaviors.[18,19] In addition, vocal fold nodules are often associated with a clinical diagnosis of laryngopharyngeal reflux. Chronic throat clearing and the laryngeal inflammation may represent a secondary causative factor for the development of vocal fold nodules. Aggressive management with antireflux therapy is indicated in these patients. Chronic nodules occasionally require surgery after a prolonged trial of speech therapy fails to result in complete resolution. Although relative voice rest can be helpful early in the course of speech therapy, absolute voice rest is rarely necessary. Surgical intervention should be limited to the area of visible abnormality. Vocal fold stripping is never indicated for nodules due to the potential for widespread postoperative scarring and poor voice results. With modern phonomicrosurgical techniques, surgical success rates are generally excellent due to the superficial nature of these lesions.

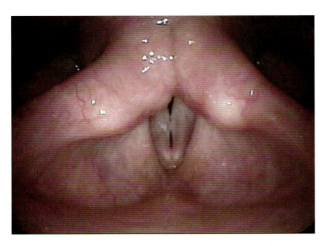

FIGURE 18–6. Subtle vocal nodules exhibiting premature contact during soft phonation.

Granulomas

Granulomas are exophytic lesions that occur most commonly on the medial surface of the vocal process of the arytenoid. Postintubation granulomas tend to be larger, pedunculated and more obvious (Figures 18-8 and 18-9) than granulomas resulting from hyperfunctional voice (Figure 18-10). Hyperfunctional granulomas are more sessile, frequently have an erythematous rim, and often present with pain on speaking or swallowing. In the earliest form, these hyperfunctional lesions are ulcerative (Figure 18-11). Because they are located on the posterior aspect of the cartilaginous vocal fold, granulomas cause few voice complaints. However, large granulomas can result in intermittent airway obstruction symptoms.

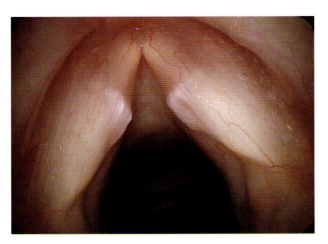

FIGURE 18–7. Firm vocal fold nodules.

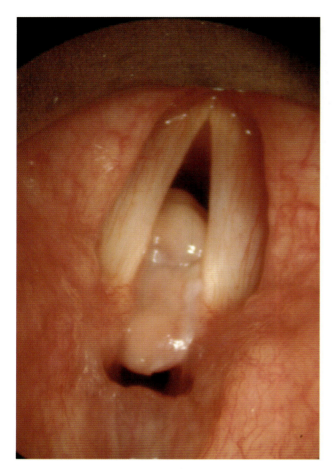

FIGURE 18–8. Intraoperative photo of a large post-intubation granuloma filling the interarytenoid region.

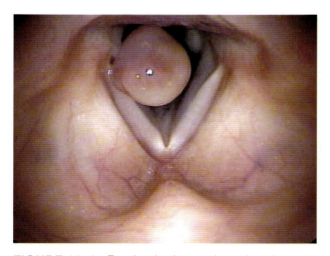

FIGURE 18–9. Postintubation pedunculated granuloma.

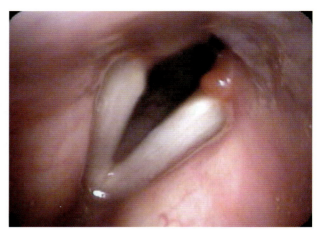

FIGURE 18–10. Granuloma secondary to hyperfunctional use.

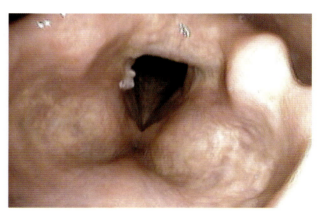

FIGURE 18–11. Small healing ulcer on the vocal process of the arytenoid due to trauma from hyperfunctional voice behaviors.

Granulomas are exuberant reparative processes that develop as the result of injury and inflammation. Ulceration is felt to form due to local trauma (throat clearing, coughing, hyperfunctional voice use, or intubation) as well as inflammation from laryngopharyngeal reflux. Granulomas can occasionally form at other sites on the vocal folds due to other sources of trauma and inflammation.

Granulomas are often quite frustrating to treat. Identification and elimination of underlying causes is paramount, with surgical resection reserved for refractory cases or large granulomas once the causative factors are controlled. As granulomas form in response to injury, surgical resection (with a resulting surgical injury) almost invariably leads to recurrence if any source of inflammation persists. Proton pump inhibitors are frequently helpful in the gradual control and elimination of granulomas, and antibiotics, inhaled steroids, and other medications may occasionally be useful.[20-23] Control of hyperfunctional voice behaviors is important to avoid further injury.[24] Botox injections are occasionally used to temporarily paralyze the affected vocal fold and thus reduce adductory forces.[25] Preliminary reports suggest that the pulsed dye laser may have a role in the treatment of granuloma.[26]

Vocal Fold Injury

Mucosal Tears

Violent vocal fold trauma can occasionally cause small mucosal tears rather than acute hemorrhage. These tears are generally quite subtle on examination and heal quickly, so a high index of suspicion is required to make an accurate diagnosis. Small linear areas of mucosal disruption with associated underlying stiffness are the most common finding. Patients most often report severe retching, persistent hard coughing, or similar trauma with abrupt change in voice. Hoarseness is frequently severe, especially when compared to the subtle findings on examination. The underlying cause of the trauma must be addressed to prevent further injury and voice rest is generally recommended.

Sulcus Vocalis

Sulcus vocalis is a narrow, linear depression in the surface of the vocal fold running longitudinally along the vocal fold (Figure 18–12). It must be distinguished from pseudosulcus vocalis, a wider furrow below the vocal fold that extends posterior to the vocal process of the arytenoid (Figure 18–13). Sulcus is a deficiency in the lamina propria of the vocal fold, and must therefore end at the tip of the vocal process of the arytenoid

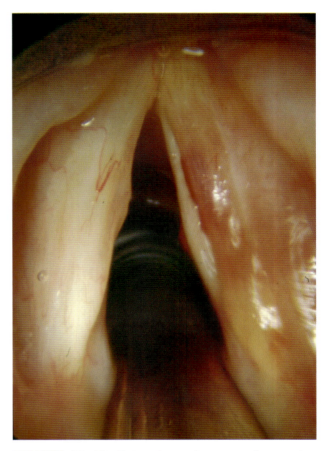

FIGURE 18–12. Extensive sulcus vocalis running the entire length of the right vocal fold.

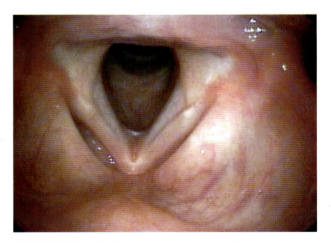

FIGURE 18–13. Pseudosulcus is defined as an apparent "groove" running the length of the vocal fold extending into the cartilaginous vocal fold. This "groove" represents subglottic edema.

as the layered structure of the vocal fold ends there as well. Pseudosulcus represents infraglottic edema. Sulcus vocalis frequently disrupts normal vibration of the vocal fold, especially if the sulcus extends to the vocal ligament. It may occur in the striking zone of the vocal fold and is not visible at all points of the vibratory cycle. Sulcus vocalis may occur in conjunction with unilateral vocal fold bowing or scar.

The pathogenesis of sulcus vocalis is debatable.[27] Theories include a response to injury with resultant loss of portions of the lamina propria with adherence of the epithelium to the vocal ligament. Some cases are clearly a congenital malformation of the vocal fold. Lastly, some speculate that some sulcus vocalis lesions develop due to rupture of a vocal fold cyst, with focal loss of SLP and adherence of the deep cyst epithelium to the vocal ligament.

Sulcus vocalis is extremely difficult to treat successfully. Multiple surgical options have been described, but the involvement of the vocal ligament and frequent associated scarring make surgical success a difficult proposition.[27-30] Occasionally, treatment of associated factors such as vocal fold bowing will result in marked voice improvements.[31]

Fibrotic Masses:

Fibrotic masses are dense, firm, white frequently unilateral masses. They often have dilated, ectatic vessels toward their base (Figure 18–14). They tend to be broad based and appear to be densely adherent to the vocal ligament. A contact lesion is often seen on the opposite vocal fold, centered at the point of contact with the fibrotic mass. The contact lesion is usually smaller than the primary lesion (Figure 18–15). Fibrotic masses with associated reactive swelling are frequently misdiagnosed as vocal nodules, but only the reactive mass will improve with speech therapy. Vocal fold vibration is generally severely disordered. The voice quality is variable, ranging from breathy to harsh depending on the dimensions of the mass and stiffness of the vocal fold.

Fibrotic masses may occur due to prior surgery, focal vocal fold trauma, or chronic vocal

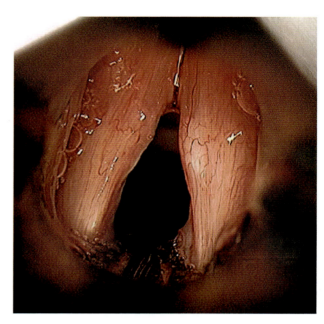

FIGURE 18–14. Bilateral fibrotic masses with abnormal vascularity.

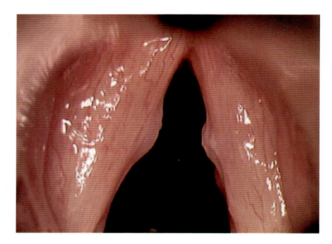

FIGURE 18–15. Irregular fibrotic mass of the right vocal fold with a smoother, softer left-sided reactive mass.

fold abuse. Often, the cause is unclear. These masses are associated with scar throughout the lamina propria, and clear demarcations between the fibrotic mass and scar is uncommon. Sulcus vocalis is occasionally noted at the time of surgery.

Speech therapy is worthwhile as an initial treatment as it will frequently reduce the size of a reactive mass. This occasionally results in marked voice improvement. Surgery is generally required, however. Surgery on fibrotic masses is difficult as the margins of the mass are generally unclear and frequently will extend to the vocal ligament and be densely adherent to the epithelium. If the contralateral vocal fold has good vibratory function, reasonable postoperative voice can be attained by simply resecting the mass and providing a smooth surface to allow good glottic closure.

Diffuse Vocal Fold Scar

Diffuse vocal fold scar is difficult to diagnose without stroboscopy. Scarred vocal folds will often look normal with conventional endoscopy, but stroboscopy will show absence of the mucosal wave or severely disordered and vibration. Some patients have dilated, abnormal vessels visible on the superior surface of the vocal fold. In severe scarring, marked compensatory hyperfunctional voice behaviors are frequently present and many

Parsing Hoarseness

Seth Dailey, MD

Patients with vocal problems will often use the term "hoarseness." Although indicative of an anatomic problem, this term does not aid the physician in detailing the specific nature of patients' concerns. The voice clinician may find it useful to distinguish if the voice issue is principally *aerodynamic* or *acoustic* in nature. It is important to note that a patient may have both types of complaints; they are not exclusive of one another.

Aerodynamic symptoms relate to the glottis as a valve—when the laryngeal valve mechanism is functioning properly, the valve is functioning efficiently. Any pathology (scar, polyp, nodules) that contributes to inefficient valving will produce effortful voicing, vocal fatigue, and difficulties with projection. These symptoms are generally speaking *aerodynamic* symptoms. Problems related to how the patient or other people perceive the sound of their voice can be termed *acoustic* symptoms.

Understanding which symptom category is of concern to the patient is important in evaluating potential treatment success. For example, a procedure for vocal fold scarring, if successful, is likely to significantly improve aerodynamic symptoms by improving the glottal gap; it is unlikely, however, to improve vocal quality (the acoustic symptoms). Conversely, a simple vocal polyp presents a case where acoustic and aerodynamic improvement is highly likely, and the patient can be counseled accordingly. As most patients who pursue medical attention for their vocal problems care a great deal about their phonatory function this mental tool for expectation management may aid in the counseling process and not set the patient and surgeon up for "failure" even if the operation is executed without error.

patients rely on false vocal fold vibration to produce a gravelly, low-pitched voice. Patients with dense scar will frequently complain more about the effort involved in producing voice, than the strained or breathy voice quality.

Vocal fold scar forms due to injury. The depth and severity of injury frequently correlates with the density of scarring. In addition to surgical injury, dense scar can result from infection, radiation therapy, chronic voice abuse, recurrent vocal fold hemorrhage, and other causes.

Treatment of vocal fold scar is generally unsatisfying. It is essential that the patient have reasonable expectations of any treatment that is contemplated. Treatments may improve voice stamina and ease of use, but improvements in voice quality are limited. Some authors feel that collagen injection into the scarred vocal folds may create some softening of scar due to collagenase activity.[32] Temporary closure of glottic gaps provides immediate benefit. However, in cases of severe scarring, closure of a glottic gap occasionally increases, rather than reduces, the effort required to produce voice. A variety of procedures have been described to reconstitute the lamina propria, including fat implantation, mucosal grafting, hyaluronic acid injection, and others.[33-36] Results have been mixed, with no procedure emerging as the cure for vocal fold scarring. Many patients will be best served by speech therapy to improve voice efficiency.

Structural Lesions

Cysts

Vocal fold cysts generally occur in the deeper layers of the SLP and may abut the vocal ligament. These lesions may represent either a mucus retention cyst or a squamous epithelial cyst. Epithelial cysts generally have a white color, are football shaped, and the edges of the cyst can be clearly distinguished from surrounding edematous lamina propria (Figure 18–16). Mucus retention cysts are often yellow in color. These lesions usually deform the surface of the affected vocal fold and may cause a contralateral reactive mass.

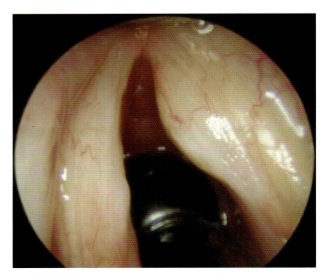

FIGURE 18–16. Large right epidermoid cyst.

Over time, cysts occasionally change in size, and may produce waxing and waning symptoms. Hoarse, pressed phonation is common, especially with larger cysts.

Epithelial-filled cysts may be congenital or traumatic in origin.[37] Mucus retention cysts are thought to be due to obstruction of a laryngeal mucous gland with gradual accumulation of material and do not have an epithelial lining (Figure 18–17). Ruptured cysts may generate vocal fold pits, sulcus vocalis, or mucosal bridges.[38]

Surgery is generally required for symptomatic cysts, although occasional patients will have adequate improvement with speech therapy alone.[38-39] As the cysts generally span the intermediate layer of the lamina propria, postoperative stiffness is common, even with meticulous surgical technique.

Polyps

Localized, soft masses on the medial surface of the vocal fold filled with clear fluid are common findings. When large and pedunculated, they are generally termed polyps; when sessile and smaller, they may be called polyps, nodules (if bilateral and symmetrical) or pseudocysts (Figure 18–18). If a polyp has recently hemorrhaged, it is usually referred to as a hemorrhagic polyp. For the

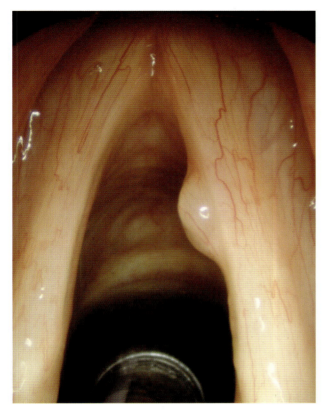

FIGURE 18–17. Small submucosal mucous retention cyst.

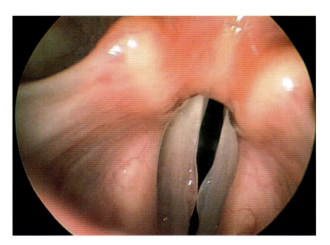

FIGURE 18–18. Bilateral pseudocysts.

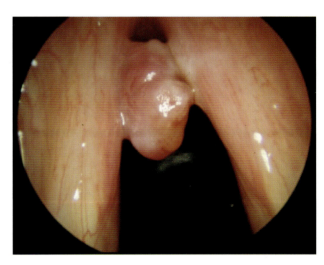

FIGURE 18–19. Polyp composed of granulation tissue and distended epithelium.

smaller lesions, a cyst wall is not identified during microsurgical exploration and a gel-like excess lamina propria is often found that is similar in consistency to that found in Reinke's edema. On examination, lucent areas are often seen just under the epithelium, suggesting the diagnosis. Larger superficial polyps can be located anywhere along the free edge or superior or inferior surface of the vocal fold and can cause intermittent voice complaints. Surgical exploration often reveals either granulation tissue or a myxomatous matrix with overlying distended epithelium. (Figure 18-19). Small polyps are soft and deformable on contact and generally exhibit normal or increased amplitude of the mucosal wave during voicing. Voices are generally lowered by the increased mass of the vocal fold.

Small and large polyps probably represent a final common pathway rather than being distinct pathologic entities.[40] Over time, some posthem-

orrhagic polyps may reabsorb all clot and hemoglobin and take on a softer, whitish appearance. Small polyps may form in response to injury or be localized areas of edema. Some cases may be focal areas of Reinke's edema. These lesions are often associated with a diagnosis of paresis. Generally, pathologic examination of the excised material will show a bland, virtually acellular matrix similar to normal lamina propria.

Treatment of small and large polyps must be individualized according to the patients' vocal demands and expectations, the size and location of the mass, and the severity of the voice changes. Larger masses, severely disordered voices, and high vocal demands all increase the likelihood that surgical resection will be required.

Lesions Associated with Smoking

Reinke's Edema

Reinke's edema (also called polypoid degeneration) occurs almost exclusively in heavy cigarette smokers and is much more noticeable in women, who complain of a masculinized voice. The increased mass of the vocal fold results in a lowered vibration frequency and a lower fundamental frequency. Physical examination reveals severely edematous, rounded vocal folds with increased mucosal wave amplitude and redundant contact. On inspiration, the vocal folds round out toward the posterior portion of the vocal fold (Figure 18–20). The vocal fold color becomes somewhat yellow or even yellow-green. Severe signs of laryngopharyngeal reflux are commonly present. Although voice quality is generally poor, the voice requires very little effort and hyperfunctional voice behaviors are rare.

Although polypoid degeneration of the vocal folds can be seen with severe hypothyroidism, most patients have normal thyroid function.[41] Formation of excess lamina propria probably occurs as a reaction and defense against chronic irritation from cigarette smoke and acid reflux.

Smoking cessation is an essential first step in the treatment of Reinke's edema. Many patients with mild Reinke's edema will have normalization of the voice within 6 to 12 months after stopping cigarettes. Surgical removal of excess lamina propria and mucosa is occasionally required.[42] Many surgeons prefer to only operate on one side at a time to reduce the risk of bilateral scarring, mucosal bridges, and other unusual complications.

Lesions Associated with Infections

Papilloma

In the adult, laryngeal papillomatosis can present as a solitary mass (Figure 18–21), diffuse vocal fold thickening and erythema (Figure 18–22), or as extensive glottic and supraglottic disease (Figure 18–23). Careful rigid stroboscopic examination will often reveal the typical punctate erythema with a grapelike surface typical of papilloma. Unfortunately, granuloma, squamous cell carcinoma, and other unusual tumors can have an identical appearance, so accurate diagnosis requires biopsy and pathologic examination.

Adult presentation of laryngeal papillomatosis is generally less severe than that seen in children, possibly due to maturity of the adult immune system. Human papilloma virus is the causative agent. Laryngeal papillomatosis is not thought to be easily transmittable and is associated with squamous cell cancer development.

Although adults generally have less severe disease, serial surgical excision is generally required. Many agents are used to modify the dis-

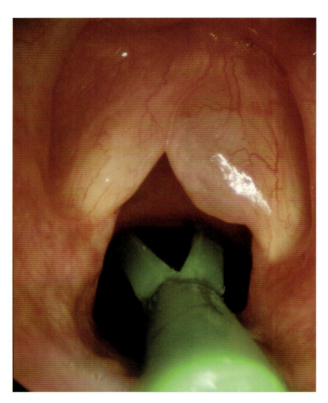

FIGURE 18–20. Reinke's edema.

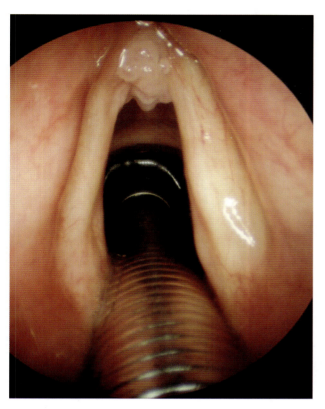

FIGURE 18–21. Isolated laryngeal papilloma.

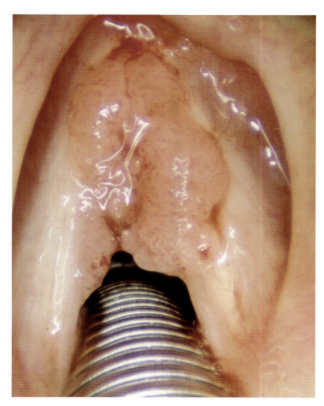

FIGURE 18–22. Diffuse laryngeal papilloma.

ease course, none of which results in complete control of disease while preserving laryngeal function. Currently, intralesional cidofovir injections seem to have promise, but not all patients seem to respond and optimal dosing and injection intervals are still unclear.[43] Because multiple procedures are generally required over time, each surgical procedure should cause minimal trauma to normal structures and minimize scarring and other complications. Powered instrumentation and the pulsed dye laser are currently being investigated as less traumatic methods for surgical papilloma control.[44-45]

Fungal Infections

Vocal fold fungal infections may present with hoarseness, coughing, or pain. Examination reveals glistening white lesions with rounded edges on the vocal folds with surrounding erythema and dilated vessels (Figure 18–24). Although originally

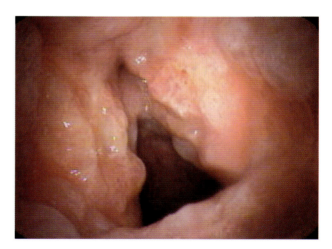

FIGURE 18–23. Extensive glottic and supraglottic papilloma.

described as a disease of immunocompromised patients, it is now known to occur in patients with local immunocompromise due to topical

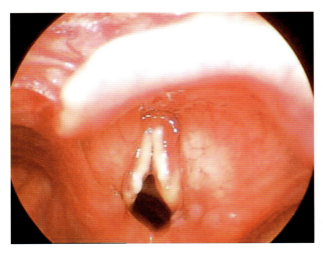

FIGURE 18–24. Fungal laryngitis. Note the rounded edges and the white lesions are not confluent at the anterior commissure.

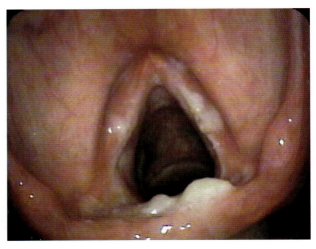

FIGURE 18–25. Ulcerative candida mimicking erythroleukoplakia.

steroid inhalers or after changes in the normal microbial environment.[46] In some cases, laryngeal *Candida* may appear as diffuse leukoplakia or mimic invasive carcinoma (Figure 18-25).[47-48]

In patients with risk factors for fungal overgrowth and a typical laryngeal appearance, it may be worthwhile to pursue empiric treatment with antifungal therapy prior to proceeding with an operative biopsy. Alternatively, in-office brush biopsy can be performed to confirm the diagnosis with minimal trauma. For further information, see chapter 15, Localized Inflammatory Disorders of the Larynx.

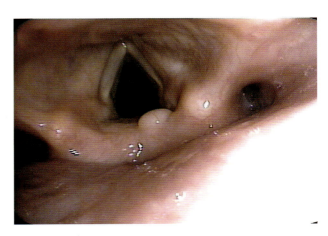

FIGURE 18–26. Neurofibroma.

Neoplasia

Benign laryngeal neoplasms are rare, require biopsy for diagnosis, and can generally be treated with complete surgical excision. Neurofibromas are the most common benign laryngeal tumors. They are generally small, rarely cause symptoms, and appear very similar to inclusion cysts (Figure 18-26). When grasped with forceps, they are much firmer than inclusion cysts, and obviously cannot be unroofed. Asymptomatic laryngeal masses with a benign appearance can be observed without biopsy in most cases.

Benign laryngeal lesions are commonly seen in general otolaryngology practice and usually are accurately diagnosed without a tissue biopsy. Stroboscopy is extremely helpful and necessary in some cases. Knowledge of the natural history and anatomic location of these lesions guides therapy and can have prognostic value. As terminology of many of these lesions changes over time, a precise description of the lesion aids communication between health care providers and avoids misunderstandings.

Review Questions

1. A 36-year-old woman complains of hoarseness for 6 months. She has been placed on voice rest and proton-pump inhibitors with little benefit. She is a nonsmoker and has no other symptoms. She eventually undergoes microdirect laryngoscopy, from which the following picture is obtained. Your clinical diagnosis is:

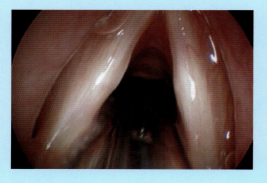

   a. Vocal nodule, unilateral
   b. Laryngeal papilloma
   c. Granuloma
   d. Hemorrhagic polyp
   e. Pseudopolyp

2. A 16-year-old aspiring singer has had 10 bouts of acute tonsillitis in the past 2 years. She is undergoing tonsillectomy and microdirect laryngoscopy. You note the findings seen below. Both vocal folds are soft on palpation. Your assessment and plan based on these findings is:

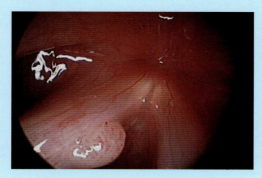

   a. Chronic laryngitis with normal vocal folds; no operative intervention on vocal folds at this time
   b. Bilateral intracordal cysts; bilateral microflap excision of vocal masses
   c. Bilateral intracordal cysts: no operative intervention on vocal folds at this time
   d. Vocal nodules: no operative intervention on vocal folds at this time
   e. Vocal nodules; staged micro-excision to avoid contamination from tonsillectomy

3. A 55-year-old banker has complained of vocal fatigue and hoarseness for 2 years. She has been on voice rest and speech therapy with no benefit. Her laryngeal hygiene is immaculate. At microlaryngoscopy, you note firmness in the left true vocal fold; the right is soft to palpation (see below). Your diagnosis is:

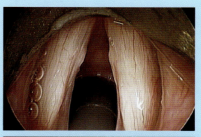
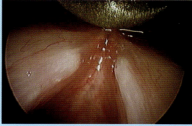

   a. T1 SCCA left true vocal fold (TVF)
   b. Intracordal cyst, left TVF
   c. Vocal nodules, bilateral
   d. Vocal nodule, left TVF with companion lesion on the right
   e. Sulcus vocalis

4. After deciding on a surgical plan, your surgical decision is to perform a microflap excision of the left true vocal fold mass. The mass is easily dissected at first, but eventually pops. You have removed the superficial aspect of the mass but you are not confident that the attachments to the vocal ligament are cleanly dissected (see below). At this point, you:

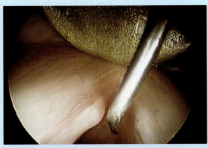

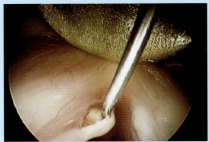

a. Open the vocal fold more widely, and attempt to regain the plane of dissection in previously uninvolved mucosa
b. Meticulously dissect the remnant from the ligament through the same incision
c. Use the laser to avoid any chance of scarring
d. Advance mucosa from nearby vocal fold to cover the defect
e. Abandon the procedure

5. Sulcus vocalis:
a. Requires surgical treatment
b. Represents a loss of the superficial layer of lamina propria
c. Represents a loss of middle layer of the lamina propria
d. Represents a loss of the deep layer of lamina propria
e. Responds to systemic steroid treatment

REFERENCES

1. Andrade DF, Heuer R, Hockstein NE, Castro E, Spiegel JR, Sataloff RT. The frequency of hard glottal attacks in patients with muscle tension dysphonia, unilateral benign masses and bilateral benign masses. *J Voice*. 2000;4(2):240–246.
2. Altman KW, Atkinson C, Lazarus C. Current and emerging concepts in muscle tension dysphonia: a 30-month review. *J Voice*. 2005;19(2):261–267.
3. Pedersen M, Beranova A, Moller S. Dysphonia: medical treatment and a medical voice hygiene advice approach. A prospective randomised pilot study. *Eur Arch Otorhinolaryngol*. 2004;261(6): 312–315.
4. MacKenzie K, Millar A, Wilson JA, Sellars C, Deary IJ. Is voice therapy an effective treatment for dysphonia? A randomised controlled trial. *Br Med J*. 200122;323(7314):658–661.
5. Carding PN, Horsley IA, Docherty GJ. A study of the effectiveness of voice therapy in the treatment of 45 patients with nonorganic dysphonia. *J Voice*. 1999;13(1):72–104
6. Hirano M. Morphological structure of the vocal cord as a vibrator and its variations. *Folia Phoniatr (Basel)*. 1974;26(2):89–94
7. Rosen CA, Murray T. Nomenclature of voice disorders and vocal pathology. *Otolaryngol Clin North Am*. 2000;33(5):1035–1046.
8. Milutinovic Z. Classification of voice pathology. *Folia Phoniatr Logop*. 1996;48(6):301–308.
9. Zeitels S, et al. Voice and Swallowing Committee, American Academy of Otolaryngology–Head and Neck Surgery. Management of common voice problems: Committee report. *Otolaryngol Head Neck Surg*. 2002;126(4):333–348.
10. Rosen CA, Murray T. Phonotrauma associated with crying. *J Voice*. 2000;14(4):575–580.

11. Kerr HD, Kwaselow A. Vocal cord hematomas complicating anticoagulant therapy. *Ann Emerg Med.* 1984:552-553.

12. Neely JL, Rosen C. Vocal fold hemorrhage associated with coumadin therapy in an opera singer. *J Voice.* 2000;14(2):272-277.

13. Koch E. Inhibition of platelet activating factor (PAF)-induced aggregation of human thrombocytes by ginkgolides: considerations on possible bleeding complications after oral intake of *Ginkgo biloba* extracts. *Phytomedicine.* 2005;12(1-2):10-16.

14. Hodges PJ, Kam PC. The peri-operative implications of herbal medicines. *Anaesthesia.* 2002;57(9):889-899.

15. Hochman I, Sataloff RT, Hillman RE, Zeitels SM. Ectasias and varices of the vocal fold: clearing the striking zone. *Ann Otol Rhinol Laryngol.* 1999;108(1):10-16.

16. Postma GN, Courey MS, Ossoff RH. Microvascular lesions of the true vocal fold. *Ann Otol Rhinol Laryngol.* 1998;107(6):472-426.

17. Hogikyan ND, Appel S, Guinn LW, Haxer MJ. Vocal fold nodules in adult singers: regional opinions about etiologic factors, career impact, and treatment. A survey of otolaryngologists, speech pathologists, and teachers of singing. *J Voice.* 1999;13(1):128-142.

18. McCrory E. Voice therapy outcomes in vocal fold nodules: a retrospective audit. *Int J Lang Commun Disord.* 2001;36(suppl):19-24.

19. Holmberg EB, Hillman RE, Hammarberg B, Sodersten M, Doyle P. Efficacy of a behaviorally based voice therapy protocol for vocal nodules. *J Voice.* 2001;15(3):395-412.

20. Hoffman HT, Overholt E, Karnell M, McCulloch TM. Vocal process granuloma. *Head Neck.* 2001;23(12):1061-1074.

21. Scheid SC, Anderson TD, Sataloff RT. Nonoperative treatment of laryngeal granuloma. *Ear Nose Throat J.* 2003;82(4):244-245.

22. Roh HJ, Goh EK, Chon KM, Wang SG. Topical inhalant steroid (budesonide, Pulmicort nasal) therapy in intubation granuloma. *J Laryngol Otol.* 1999;113(5):427-432.

23. Mitchell G, Pearson CR, Henk JM, Rhys-Evans P. Excision and low-dose radiotherapy for refractory laryngeal granuloma. *J Laryngol Otol.* 1998;112(5):491-493.

24. Leonard R, Kendall K. Effects of voice therapy on vocal process granuloma: a phonoscopic approach. *Am J Otolaryngol.* 2005;26(2):101-107.

25. Nasri S, Sercarz JA, McAlpin T, Berke GS. Treatment of vocal fold granuloma using botulinum toxin type A. *Laryngoscope.* 1995;105(6):585-588.

26. Clyne SB, Halum SL, Koufman JA, Postma GN. Pulsed dye laser treatment of laryngeal granulomas. *Ann Otol Rhinol Laryngol.* 2005;114(3):198-201

27. Ford CN, Inagi K, Khidr A, Bless DM, Gilchrist KW. Sulcus vocalis: a rational analytical approach to diagnosis and management. *Ann Otol Rhinol Laryngol.* 1996;105(3):189-200.

28. Welham NV, Rousseau B, Ford CN, Bless DM. Tracking outcomes after phonosurgery for sulcus vocalis: a case report. *J Voice.* 2003;17(4):571-578.

29. Hsiung MW, Kang BH, Pai L, Su WF, Lin YH. Combination of fascia transplantation and fat injection into the vocal fold for sulcus vocalis: long-term results. *Ann Otol Rhinol Laryngol.* 2004;113(5):359-366

30. Pontes P, Behlau M. Treatment of sulcus vocalis: auditory perceptual and acoustical analysis of the slicing mucosa surgical technique. *J Voice.* 1993;7(4):365-376.

31. Su CY, Tsai SS, Chiu JF, Cheng CA. Medialization laryngoplasty with strap muscle transposition for vocal fold atrophy with or without sulcus vocalis. *Laryngoscope.* 2004;114(6):1106-1112.

32. Bjorck G, D'Agata L, Hertegard S. Vibratory capacity and voice outcome in patients with scarred vocal folds treated with collagen injections—case studies. *Logoped Phoniatr Vocol.* 2002;27(1):4-11.

33. Benninger MS, Alessi D, Archer S, et al. Vocal fold scarring: current concepts and management. *Otolaryngol Head Neck Surg.* 1996;115(5):474-482.

34. Neuenschwander MC, Sataloff RT, Abaza MM, Hawkshaw MJ, Reiter D, Spiegel JR. Management of vocal fold scar with autologous fat implantation: perceptual results. *J Voice.* 2001;15(2):295-304.

35. Rosen CA. Vocal fold scar: evaluation and treatment. *Otolaryngol Clin North Am.* 2000;33(5):1081-1086.

36. Hirano S. Current treatment of vocal fold scarring. *Curr Opin Otolaryngol Head Neck Surg.* 2005;13(3):143-147.

37. Milutinovic Z, Vasiljevic J. Contribution to the understanding of the etiology of vocal fold cysts: a functional and histologic study. *Laryngoscope.* 1992;102(5):568-571.

38. Bouchayer M, Cornut G, Witzig E, Loire R, Roch JB, Bastian RW. Epidermoid cysts, sulci, and

mucosal bridges of the true vocal cord: a report of 157 cases. *Laryngoscope.* 1985;95(9 pt 1): 1087–1094.

39. Monday LA, Cornut G, Bouchayer M, Roch JB. Epidermoid cysts of the vocal cords. *Ann Otol Rhinol Laryngol.* 1983;92(2 pt 1):124–127.

40. Wallis L, Jackson-Menaldi C, Holland W, Giraldo A. Vocal fold nodule vs. vocal fold polyp: answer from surgical pathologist and voice pathologist point of view. *J Voice.* 2004;18(1):125–129.

41. White A, Sim DW, Maran AG. Reinke's oedema and thyroid function. *J Laryngol Otol.* 1991;105(4): 291–292.

42. Lumpkin SM, Bennett S, Bishop SG. Postsurgical follow-up study of patients with severe polypoid degeneration. *Laryngoscope.* 1990;100(4):399–402.

43. Shehab N, Sweet BV, Hogikyan ND. Cidofovir for the treatment of recurrent respiratory papillomatosis: a review of the literature. *Pharmacotherapy.* 2005;25(7):977–989.

44. Zeitels SM, Franco RA Jr, Dailey SH, Burns JA, Hillman RE, Anderson RR. Office-based treatment of glottal dysplasia and papillomatosis with the 585-nm pulsed dye laser and local anesthesia. *Ann Otol Rhinol Laryngol.* 2004;113(4):265–276.

45. El-Bitar MA, Zalzal GH. Powered instrumentation in the treatment of recurrent respiratory papillomatosis: an alternative to the carbon dioxide laser. *Arch Otolaryngol Head Neck Surg.* 2002;128(4): 425–428.

46. Mehanna HM, Kuo T, Chaplin J, Taylor G, Morton RP. Fungal laryngitis in immunocompetent patients. *J Laryngol Otol.* 2004;118(5):379–381.

47. Scheid SC, Anderson TD, Sataloff RT. Ulcerative fungal laryngitis. *Ear Nose Throat J.* 2003;82(3): 168–169.

48. Hanson JM, Spector G, El-Mofty SK. Laryngeal blastomycosis: a commonly missed diagnosis. Report of two cases and review of the literature. *Ann Otol Rhinol Laryngol.* 2000;109(3):281–286.

APPENDIX
Answer Keys for Chapter Review Tests

Chapter 1

1. a
2. d
3. e
4. e
5. b
6. b

Chapter 2

1. Laryngospasm and central apnea
2. Respiration and cough
3. Laryngopharyngeal reflux and stroke
4. Expiration and the laryngeal adductor response
5. Tracheobronchial cough and laryngeal cough

Chapter 3
1. True
2. False
3. True
4. False
5. False
6. False
7. False
8. False
9. True

Chapter 4

1. False
2. False
3. False
4. True
5. True
6. True

Chapter 5

1. No. The complexity of vocal function is not represented by a sample of simple sustained phonation. It is imperative that a variety of tasks be elicited, including connected speech samples.

2. Yes. Therapeutic probes can provide invaluable information regarding patients' ability to modify vocal behaviors, thereby confirming their candidacy for voice therapy, as well as providing insight into the specific techniques that would be effective.

3. No. These are complementary or supplementary tools, but not the primary basis for a differential diagnosis.

4. No. Consistent with any other sophisticated discipline, the advances of knowledge in voice science and treatment of voice disorders require continual education for both otolaryngologists and SLPs.

Chapter 6

1. a

2. e

3. c

4. a, b, and c

5. a

Chapter 7

1. Yes. Although the two behaviors are different in their demands, they involve the same organ. Vocal abuse can damage the tissues, thereby disrupting phonatory function for either or both activities.

2. No, not directly. Swallowing beverages bypasses the larynx so the liquid does not "bathe" the tissues. However, a "soothing" effect can be realized by secondary gain through increased secretions and/or muscle relaxation facilitated by enjoying liquids.

3. This is not well studied but the answer is probably no. Generally beverages that are cool or warm are preferable to those hot or cold—particularly if extreme. The chance

for tissue damage secondary to scalding or muscle contraction resulting from extreme cold should be avoided.

4. No. The physiology of whisper usually requires tight tissue contact and increased vocal fold tension, both conditions contraindicated for the inflamed tissues.

Chapter 8

1. The scope of practice for a speech-language pathologist when treating voice disorders does not include the diagnosis of organic changes that may have taken place on the vocal folds. It does include identifying the voice that presents with a current or potential problem, identifying and analyzing the problem, then providing the voice user with tools to modify vocal behaviors and use the vocal mechanism with optimal efficiency. In some cases, the larynx will be visualized and directly assessed by the SLP; in most cases, however, this is done initially by the otolaryngologist. The clinician may perceptually and acoustically identify dysphonia. It is then the clinician's responsibility to refer this patient to an otolaryngologist, ideally a laryngologist, to assess the anatomy and physiology of the larynx prior to continuing therapeutic intervention.

2. *Otolaryngologist:* The primary member of the team responsible for diagnosis and medical/surgical intervention.

   Speech-language pathologist: Conducts evaluation and treatment of the voice problem by promoting efficient use of the vocal mechanism.

   Singing voice specialist/teacher: Develops singing technique and singing voice production. This specialist may be beneficial to a nonsinger.

   Acting-voice specialist: Focuses on honing vocal skills such as projected speech and communication skills as they relate to vocally demanding professions.

The patient: The most important member of the team. This person's role is therapeutic and educational. The patient must be motivated, knowledgeable, and involved in therapy decision-making.

Voice researcher/scientist: Provides valuable insight and perspective with regard to the care of a voice patient because of specific knowledge and skills in acoustic measurement and voice production.

Singing voice coach: May provide valuable knowledge and perspective following rehabilitation work and will work on the development of artistic style and repertoire for the voice user.

Psychologist or psychiatrist: Provides the patient with counseling for the management of emotional reactions to the voice disorder, as well as psychological issues that may have contributed to its occurrence.

Physiatrist: Addresses areas of tension or injury throughout the body.

Each member of the team provides valuable knowledge of voice production and treatment and care of the voice. Based on the patient's history and voice disorder, each may require different team members. It is of value to cultivate these relationships within the community to develop a network of resources not only for the patient's benefit but as a professional sounding board. The different perspectives of each discipline can provide insight in our field and aid in providing the patient with well-rounded care.

3. History taking from a professional voice user and a nonprofessional are similar in that a complete medical history and history of the onset of the voice problems should be gathered, in addition to information on possible contributing factors, vocal hygiene, and voice use. The history taking is different for a professional voice user because there are special factors to consider. These may include, learning the vocal complaints as they relate to the "performance voice," inquiring about the history of professional voice user, and probing into the extent of the professional voice user's vocal training. A professional voice user's vocal demands and expectations are higher than the nonprofessional voice user and must be delved into thoroughly.

4. Breath support during phonation ideally involves abdominal expansion during inhalation and abdominal contraction during exhalation and phonation. "Abdominal breathing" also involves appropriate and coordinated activity of muscles of the chest, back, and elsewhere. Airflow during phonation refers to the release of air to produce phonation. Airflow sets the vocal folds into motion. However, abdominal breathing does not ensure efficient phonation. An abdominal breathing pattern may be present while airflow during phonation is decreased. This may be secondary to an inefficient abdominal movement pattern or hyperfunction in the vocal tract that inhibits appropriate airflow during voice production.

5. There are multiple factors to consider when choosing a therapeutic facilitator. These include the medical diagnosis, patient's primary vocal complaints, perceptual and acoustic evaluation, and physiology of the patient's current voice production versus the targeted efficient voice production. The facilitator should be chosen with these factors in mind and then modified based on the patient's response.

Chapter 9

1. d. The "sniffing" position provides the best view of the vocal folds. Anterior cricoid pressure may be needed in some cases and may be provided by 1-inch tape stretched across the neck of the patient from the operating table.

2. c. The presence of a mass on the vocal fold does not necessarily indicate surgery is needed. All other underlying problems should be treated first. Treatment of reflux and voice therapy might provide enough improvement to satisfy the patient's needs. Other underlying factors might be considered. One might wish to consider laryngeal EMG, given the preceding URI, to see if any subtle paresis is contributing. Allergy evaluation should be considered. The decision to recommend surgical excision should be reserved until all the potentially contributing factors have been considered and medical management has been exhausted.

3. e.

4. d. The use of the laser still requires deft ability with the nondominant hand. Excellent control of the micromanipulator is required to prevent inadvertent injury to healthy tissue. CO_2 laser does introduce some uncertainty in depth of thermal injury and introduces a small risk of airway fire which is easily avoided with appropriate preparation. CO_2 laser does provide better hemostasis; however, hemostasis is achievable with cold excision too using topical epinephrine. Ultimately, individual surgeon preference and experience are the determining factors as to which technique is best to use.

5. a. Overly aggressive excision of Reinke's edema can lead to severe scarring. One should consider operating on only one vocal fold initially. If scarring occurs, the contralateral side can usually compensate and yield an improved voice. If both sides are operated on and scar excessively, the patient may be left with a pressed, breathy voice that is difficult to correct.

Chapter 10

1. Myasthenia gravis. Characterized by fatigue with repetitive use and therefore an intermittent pattern, myasthenia gravis commonly presents in women between the second and fourth decades. Asking the patient to repeat syllables such as "ee-ee-ee" may elicit vocal fatigue.

2. c. glottal gap. Berke et al reported that 75% of patients who had a persistent glottal gap on stroboscopic examination were satisfied with vocal fold augmentation. Parkinson's patients usually demonstrate normal vocal cord mobility. The presence of significant laryngeal tremor and poor overall neurologic status indicate more advanced disease, which is less likely to benefit from augmentation.

3. b. Voice strain is seen in lesions involving the UMN or the basal ganglia.

4. Patients with Parkinson's disease usually demonstrate normal vocal cord mobility. Patients with multiple system atrophy, however, may have stridor during sleep. This is important to elicit during history taking. If the patient or family reports stridor, the diagnosis of MSA should be seriously considered.

5. d. Patients with essential tremor of the voice report subjective reduction in vocal effort after Botox injection, according to Warrick et al.

Chapter 11

1. This is nicely summarized in Table 17–3.

2. The precise answer is not known; each patient's co-morbid conditions, such as lung cancer or a history of head and neck radiation, may play a factor. The variability in laryngeal innervation may also play a role. There is no predictable pattern based on the "site of lesion."

3. a

4. Not necessarily; synkinesis is an example of reinnervation with poor voluntary motion.

5. This is outlined in the chapter. Briefly, these include tracheotomy, posterior cordotomy,

arytenoidectomy, medial arytenoidectomy, and lateralization (Lichtenberger technique).

6. c, although a may also occur depending on her degree of glottic insufficiency and likelihood of compensation

Chapter 12

1. d
2. b
3. b
4. c

Chapter 13

1. a, c, and e. When essential tremor is inherited, it is inherited in an autosomal dominant fashion. The voice appears to be affected in 25 to 30% of patients.

2. a and e. Tremor at rest, cogwheeling, and bradykinesia are signs of Parkinson's disease.

3. c. Patients with Parkinson's disease have hypophonia with articulatory difficulties. Strangled voice breaks are typical of adductor spasmodic dysphonia, and breathy breaks suggest abductor spasmodic dysphonia. "Scanning speech," which remains poorly defined, has been attributed to multiples sclerosis.

4. Flexible fiberoptic laryngoscopy.

5. d. No pharmacologic agent has a clearly documented benefit in essential voice tremor.

Chapter 14

1. a. In their review of over 900 patients with spasmodic dysphonia, Blitzer, et al[7] reported their mean dose of botulinum toxin A per

visit was ~3 units. This approximates clinical practice in the majority of those that treat patients with spasmodic dysphonia.

2. This dated concept has been debunked. Voice disorders are often made worse by psychiatric illness, but psychiatric illness is not the source of dysphonia. Sometimes, a nonorganic voice disorder can be misdiagnosed as spasmodic dysphonia, and vice versa.

3. b. Abductor spasmodic dysphonia is characterized by spasms that result in an intermittent breathy voice quality. This can be highlighted by asking the patient to speak a passage loaded with voiceless consonants. Patients with spasmodic dysphonia often have minimal spasm with less complex vocal tasks such as uttering prolonged vowel sounds.

4. c. The best examiner is an experienced listener. No laboratory or imaging study is specific for the diagnosis of spasmodic dysphonia.

5. b. Speech therapy can help make spasmodic dysphonia less symptomatic in a subset of patients; however, it cannot cure the dystonia. More times then not, sending a patient with spasmodic dysphonia for speech therapy serves more to frustrate him then cure him. Speech therapy may have a small role in having patients cope with some of the negative effects of botulinum toxin treatment.

Chapter 15

1. e. The patient described has supraglottitis, Intubation and surgical airway are options, most patients can be managed without this.

2. a. Either topical or systemic antifungals may be helpful.

3. d.

4. d

5. c. There is little role for surgery in a nonsmoker with a smooth, small lesion unless other concerns arise. Botulinum toxin would be quite uncommon as an initial treatment.

Chapter 16

1. c

2. d

3. a

4. e

5. d

Chapter 17

1. b. pH probe testing is fairly reliable although it may not be "positive" in cases of minimal pH change. Surgery is not an option at this point as he has not had adequate treatment —his age and sex do not exclude him from being a candidate,

however. It is generally felt that 3 to 6 months of treatment may be necessary to detect a clinical response to medical therapy.

2. b

3. d

4. d. PPIs are the mainstay of therapy along with lifestyle changes; the importance of these behavioral modifications is not well detailed, although it is reasonable to ask the patients to pursue healthy dietary choice and avoid laryngeal irritants such as tobacco, alcohol, and caffeine. H_2 blockers are widely used although their precise role in LPR patients is not clear.

Chapter 18

1. b

2. d

3. b

4. b

5. b

Index